DO NOT SPECIFIC   -24-02

REFERENCE USE ONLY

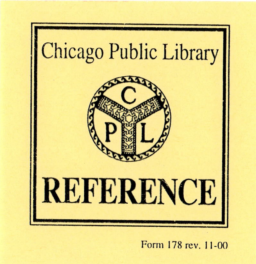

Poultry Meat Science

Poultry Science Symposium Series Volume Twenty-five

Poultry Science Symposium Series
Executive Editor (Volumes 1–18): B.M. Freeman

*Out of print
Volumes 1–24 were not published by CAB *International*. Those still in print may be ordered from:

Carfax Publishing Company
P.O. Box 25, Abingdon, Oxfordshire OX14 3UE, England

Poultry Meat Science

Poultry Science Symposium Series Volume Twenty-five

Edited by

R.I. Richardson

Division of Food Animal Science, University of Bristol, UK

and

G.C. Mead

Department of Farm Animal and Equine Medicine and Surgery,
The Royal Veterinary College, UK

CABI Publishing

CABI *Publishing* is a division of CAB *International*

CABI Publishing
CAB International
Wallingford
Oxon OX10 8DE
UK

CABI Publishing
10 E 40th Street
Suite 3203
New York, NY 10016
USA

Tel: +44 (0)1491 832111
Fax: +44 (0)1491 833508
E-mail: cabi@cabi.org

Tel: +1 212 481 7018
Fax: +1 212 686 7993
E-mail: cabi-nao@cabi.org

A catalogue record for this book is available from the British Library,
London, UK.

A catalogue record for this book is available from the Library of Congress,
Washington DC, USA.

ISBN 0 85199 237 4

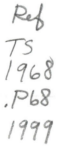

Typeset by Solidus (Bristol) Limited
Printed and bound in the UK at Biddles, Guildford and King's Lynn

CONTENTS

CONTRIBUTORS

R.J. Buhr, *Poultry Processing & Meat Quality Research Unit, United States Department of Agriculture, Agricultural Research Service, Russell Research Center, Athens, GA 30604, USA*

P.N. Church, *Food Technology Section, Leatherhead Food Research Association, Randalls Road, Leatherhead, Surrey KT22 7RY, UK*

J.E.L. Corry, *Division of Food Animal Science, School of Veterinary Science, University of Bristol, Langford, Bristol BS40 5DU, UK*

R.H. Davies, *Central Veterinary Laboratory, New Haw, Addlestone, Kent KT15 3NB, UK*

M. Enser, *Division of Food Animal Science, School of Veterinary Science, University of Bristol, Langford, Bristol BS40 5DU, UK*

S.J. Evans, *Central Veterinary Laboratory, New Haw, Addlestone, Kent KT15 3NB, UK*

L.J. Farmer, *Food Science Division, Department of Agriculture for Northern Ireland and The Queen's University of Belfast, Newforge Lane, Belfast BT9 5PX, UK*

D.L. Fletcher, *Department of Poultry Science, University of Georgia, Athens, GA 30602, USA*

G. Goldspink, *Department of Anatomy and Developmental Biology, The Royal Free Hospital School of Medicine, The University of London, Rowland Hill Street, London NW3 2PF, UK*

M.H. Hinton, *Division of Food Animal Science, School of Veterinary Science, University of Bristol, Langford, Bristol BS40 5DU, UK*

H. Hoogenkamp, *Protein Technologies International, Checkerboard Square, St Louis, MO 63164-00011, USA*

T.G. Knowles, *Division of Food Animal Science, School of Veterinary Science, University of Bristol, Langford, Bristol BS40 5DU, UK*

C.E. Lyon, *Poultry Processing & Meat Quality Research Unit, United States Department of Agriculture, Agricultural Research Service, Russell Research Center, Athens, GA 30604, USA*

M. Mahon, *School of Biological Sciences, 1.124 Stopford Building, University of Manchester, Oxford Road, Manchester M13 9PT, UK*

R. Mandava, *Nestle R&D Centre, P.O. Box 520, S-26725 Bjuv, Sweden*

G.C. Mead, *Department of Farm Animal and Equine Medicine and Surgery,*

The Royal Veterinary College, Boltons Park, Hawkshead Road, Potters Bar, Hertfordshire EN6 1NB, UK

M.A. Mitchell, *Roslin Institute (Edinburgh), Roslin, Midlothian EH25 9PS, UK*

E.T. Moran Jr, *Poultry Science Department, Auburn University, AL 36849–5416, USA*

R.W.A.W. Mulder, *DLO Institute for Animal Science and Health, P.O. Box 15, 8200 AB Lelystad, The Netherlands*

G.R. Nute, *Division of Food Animal Science, School of Veterinary Science, University of Bristol, Langford, Bristol BS40 5DU, UK*

E. O'Neill, *Department of Food Chemistry, University College, Cork, Eire*

A.B.M. Raj, *Division of Food Animal Science, School of Veterinary Science, University of Bristol, Langford, Bristol BS40 5DU, UK*

I. Richardson, *Division of Food Animal Science, School of Veterinary Science, University of Bristol, Langford, Bristol BS40 5DU, UK*

A. Sams, *Department of Poultry Science, Texas A&M University, College Station, TX 77843-2472, USA*

D.M. Smith, *Department of Food Science and Human Nutrition, Michigan State University, East Lansing, MI 48824-1224, USA*

A.B. Smyth, *Department of Food Chemistry, University College, Cork, Eire*

H.J. Swatland, *Department of Animal and Poultry Science, University of Guelph, Ontario N1G 2W1, Canada*

P.D. Warriss, *Division of Food Animal Science, School of Veterinary Science, University of Bristol, Langford, Bristol BS40 5DU, UK*

L.J. Wilkins, *Division of Food Animal Science, School of Veterinary Science, University of Bristol, Langford, Bristol BS40 5DU, UK*

L.F.J. Woods, *Food Technology Section, Leatherhead Food Research Association, Randalls Road, Leatherhead, Surrey KT22 7RY, UK*

C. Wray, *Central Veterinary Laboratory, New Haw, Addlestone, Kent KT15 3NB, UK*

S.Y. Yang, *Department of Anatomy and Developmental Biology, The Royal Free Hospital School of Medicine, The University of London, Rowland Hill Street, London NW3 2PF, UK*

PREFACE

This volume contains the papers presented at the 25th Poultry Science Symposium held at the University of Bristol, 17–19 September, 1997. The Poultry Science Symposia Series was begun in 1964 by the British Egg Marketing Board but has been organized since 1985 by the United Kingdom Branch of the World's Poultry Science Association and has become a bi-annual event. Each symposium is devoted to a specific topic within the field of poultry science. Lectures at the symposium are by invitation to those who are authorities in their own field. Although the symposium is organized by a national body the speakers and delegates are international. Meat science had a small section in Symposium 21, 'Recent Advances in Turkey Science', but has not been dealt with in any great detail since Symposium 15, 'Meat Quality in Poultry and Game Birds'. In a still expanding industry whose end product is quality meat, revisiting this field was timely.

A major objective was to produce an authoritative textbook reviewing a small area of poultry science in a style which is comprehensible to the non-specialist. Speakers were asked to write for an intelligent graduate student who has a good training in general biology or food science, but who has little specialized knowledge of meat science, or someone with a good knowledge of mammalian muscle biology who wishes to find out how birds differ from mammals as would technical managers from the poultry industry. This set the challenge of restating succinctly a good deal of general knowledge about avian meat science as a prelude to bringing their own topic up to the frontiers of present knowledge.

Divided into four sections, the first session dealt with the fundamental background to the study of meat quality, i.e. the latest knowledge on the structure and development of muscle tissue, followed by those topics which are essential to a good quality product, i.e. texture, colour and flavour. The second session dealt with more applied aspects, i.e. how production, nutrition, preslaughter handling and stunning and slaughter affected meat quality. Whenever we consider poultry meat we must ensure its micro-biological safety and this was the topic of session three which considered the production environment, hygiene during transport, stunning and slaughter, possible methods for decontaminating meat and for extending shelf-life. The final session dealt with harvested meat, how its quality could be assessed on-line, how harvesting itself affected quality, how you assessed quality with properly organized taste panels, and finishing with a look at the fundamentals of poultry meat functional properties which impacted on product development and quality, and a look at the technologies and range of products now available.

Although delegate numbers were down on other recent symposia, there was a happy blend of academia and industry to hear some excellent papers now presented in this volume. There was a happy atmosphere in the bar each evening and many acquaintances were made or re-made.

Ian Richardson

Geoff Mead

Organizing committee: R.I. Richardson (Chairman); K. McDonnell (Secretary); P. Bradnock; M. Enser; C. Fisher; P. Hocking; G.C. Mead; T.R. Morris; C. Nixey; M. Patterson; A.B.M. Raj.

ACKNOWLEDGEMENTS

The symposium Committee gratefully acknowledges generous financial support from the following organizations:

Roche Products Ltd
BOC Gases
BOCM PAULS Ltd

PART I
Biochemical basis of meat quality

CHAPTER 1
Muscle structure, development and growth

G. Goldspink and S.Y. Yang

Department of Anatomy and Developmental Biology, The Royal Free Hospital School of Medicine, The University of London, Rowland Hill Street, London NW3 2PF, UK

INTRODUCTION

Skeletal muscle provides the source of high-quality protein in most people's diet. Of the types of meat, poultry has become the least expensive because of strain selection for growth potential and improved feed conversion. However, it seems that the traditional selection for rapid live weight gain and food conversion may have been almost fully exploited. For example, in 1950 a 12-week period was required to reach the slaughter weight of 1.8–2.0 kg, whereas now it requires less than 6 weeks. The new molecular biology methods promise more specific ways of enhancing, not only muscle growth potential, but imparting disease resistance.

Poultry production represents one of the largest food industries worldwide. It is difficult to predict how this will develop in the future but no doubt attention will be aimed at improving meat quality as well as quantity and we can expect the introduction of more new types of poultry meat. As regards the latter it is difficult to see how muscle bulk can be further enhanced without increasing the incidence of pathological conditions such as skeletal deformities. However, the methods available for manipulating growth of farm animals now include a range of molecular biology methods which will allow us to alter the quality as well as the quantity of meat production on a much shorter time scale so that the balance of the musculoskeletal system (e.g. muscle : bone ratios) can be maintained. These methods include somatic gene transfer and the more controversial transgenic biology methods which involve introducing novel genes into the germ-line.

The purpose of this chapter is to review the available knowledge concerning the cellular and molecular regulation of muscle development. The intention is not to produce a fully comprehensive account of all the molecular biology data relating to muscle but to highlight those developments that have particular relevance to avian meat science and muscle developmental biology. The approach taken is an integrative one as the authors believe there is little point in discussing the molecular biology unless it is related to physiology and structural development of muscle.

MUSCLE STRUCTURE

Skeletal muscle is a syncytium that is formed by single nucleated mesodermal cells which undergo terminal differentiation to form myoblasts which then fuse to form multinucleated muscle fibres. These produce rod-like contractile structures, myofibrils, which are about 1 mm in diameter. The myofibrils are made up of protein filaments which in skeletal and cardiac muscle are arranged in units called sarcomeres (Fig. 1.1). Each sarcomere consists of one set of thick (myosin) filaments and two sets of thin (actin) filaments, and during the contraction of muscle the thin filaments are pulled in over the thick filaments so that each sarcomere shortens and generates force (Huxley, 1969). The force to produce contraction is generated by the myosin cross-bridge, the head of which (S1) is the molecular motor. This has a lever arm that is hinged, to which two smaller proteins, the myosin light chains (lcs), are attached. Each cross-bridge is an independent force generator, which interacts with a thin filament and pulls it towards the centre of the sarcomere. The cross-bridge then detaches from the thin filament and has to be reprised by adenosine triphosphate (ATP) before it can go through another cycle of force generation.

Barany (1967) was the first to relate the intrinsic velocity of contraction (V_{max}) of muscle fibres to the specific activity of their myosin ATPase by comparing the enzymatic activity of myosin isolated from different animals including the sloth. Earlier work in the authors' laboratory showed that the rate at which cross-bridges work and consume chemical energy varies considerably depending on the type of muscle fibre and the kind of activity for which it is adapted (Alexander and Goldspink, 1977). As discussed below, different types of muscle fibres, e.g. slow postural muscles, have different myosin cross-bridges to the fast phasic muscle fibres and this not only explains the differences in speed of contraction but also economy of force development and fatiguability (Goldspink, 1985). Both the myosin heavy chains (hcs) and myosin lc occur as several distinct isoforms, and different combinations of hcs and lcs may exist within the same muscle fibre, and within the same myosin filament. As described below these are coded for by different genes, the expression of these genes determines which type of molecular motor is produced. Experiments have indicated that the main determinant of the speed of contraction is the predominant type of myosin hc of the fibres. This has been shown by chemically skinning single isolated fast and slow fibres and exchanging the myosin lcs and measuring changes in the rate of shortening (Reiser *et al.*, 1985) and by the *in vitro* motility assay in which movement of actin filaments by isolated myosin S1 (myosin cross-bridge heads) coated on to microscope slides, can be demonstrated (Lowey *et al.*, 1993).

CELLULAR CHANGES ASSOCIATED WITH MUSCLE GROWTH

The postnatal increase in mass of muscles is due to hypertrophy rather than hyperplasia. After the myoblasts have fused to form myotubes and embryonic differentiation is complete there is no further increase in the number of muscle

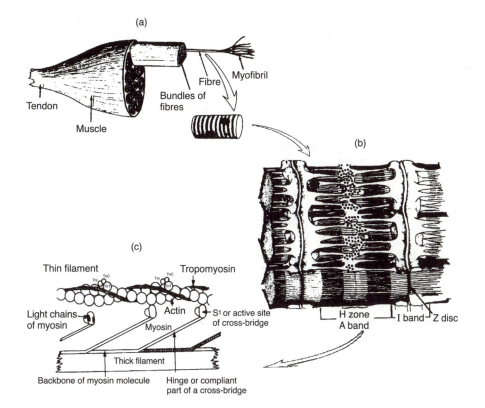

Fig. 1.1. Skeletal muscle structure. (a) Section through the belly of muscle showing bundles of striated muscle fibres. Within each fibre there are many myofibrils which are the contractile elements and which are also striated. Muscle fibres can just be seen with the naked eye and myofibrils can just be seen with the light microscope. (b) An electronmicrographic reconstruction showing the thick (myosin) and the thin (actin) filaments organized in units called sarcomeres. The generation of force takes place by the thin filaments being moved in over the thick filaments. The sarcoplasmic reticulum and transverse tubular systems involved in excitation–contraction coupling are visible surrounding the myofibril. The release of calcium from the sarcoplasmic reticulum activates the myosin cross-bridges which are the independent force generators that move the thin filaments. (c) Shows the molecular oganization of the thick and thin filaments. The thin filaments are decorated by the regulatory proteins, the tropomyosin/troponin complex. When activated by calcium the tropomyosin is pulled to one side exposing active sites on the filament to which the myosin cross-bridges attach. The cross-bridges are part of the double myosin heavy chain molecules. Part of the myosin heavy chain is the rod structure which is embedded in the thick filament. The cross-bridges project from the thick filament and have a hinge region which terminates in two heads with which the light chains are associated. The heads or S1 fragments are the business end of the molecule and contain the ATPase and actin binding sites. (Modified from Goldspink, 1996.)

fibres but the size of the fibres continues to increase throughout the growth period. This occurs because the myofibrillar content of the fibres increases markedly. Each myofibril reaches a certain size and splits into two or more daughter myofibrils due to a built in mismatch between the actin and myosin filament lattices. This causes the peripheral actin filaments to be pulled obliquely to the Z disc axis and this results in the Z discs ripping so that two or more daughter myofibrils are formed. In this way the myofibrillar mass is subdivided so that the SR and T systems can invade the mass which is particularly important in the case of fast fibres where rapid activation and relaxation from contraction are required. The work on this subject has been reviewed previously (Goldspink, 1984, 1996). However, the important question that now needs to be answered is, what causes the myofibrils to be built up in the first place so that, when they reach a critical size, they divide. This must involve the increased synthesis of actin, myosin and the other contractile proteins and therefore the problem has to be studied at the gene expression level.

Muscles also grow in length as well as girth and this has been shown to be associated with the increase in the length of the fibres by the serial addition of new sarcomeres on to the ends of the existing myofibril. The growth region for this is near the myotendon junction and beyond the point at which most of the myofibrils are attached to the basement membrane. It appears that as the bones lengthen during growth, the muscles are pulled out and the spaces at the ends of the fibres enable the new sarcomeres to be assembled on to the ends of the existing myofibril. In this way the length of the sarcomeres is constantly adjusted back to the optimum for force production during the growth process. Other morphological components of the fibres also increase including the nuclear content. This occurs because satellite cells fuse mainly at the ends and donate the nuclei that are required for longitudinal growth (Aziz-Ullah and Goldspink, 1974).

DIFFERENT TYPES OF MUSCLE FIBRES

Chicken skeletal muscle fibres, similarly to mammalian muscle fibres, can be divided into three different types of twitch muscle fibres. One of these is adapted for a high-power output over a short period (fast, glycolytic or type 2b) and another is adapted for a high-power output over a longer period of time (fast, oxidative, glycolytic or type 2a). Both of these type 2 fibres possess types of myosin and other contractile proteins that produce a fast cross-bridge cycle time and develop force rapidly. In larger mammals including humans the main fast type is the 2x and not the 2b as in the rat (Ennion *et al.,* 1995). The type 2a fibres have more mitochondria and a more oxidative metabolism than the 2b or the 2x fibres and are thus capable of sustaining high-power output over a reasonably long period of time. The other major type of fibre found in avian as well as in mammalian muscles is the slow oxidative or type 1 fibre that has a form of myosin which hydrolyses ATP slowly resulting in a slow cross-bridge cycle. This makes these fibres more efficient and more economical for producing slow repetitive movements and sustaining isometric force but not for generating power (work done per unit time). The type 1 fibres are particularly numerous in postural muscle such as the soleus, a muscle that is activated virtually all the time during standing, walking and running (Hnik *et al.*, 1985). In chickens there is another type of slow fibre, referred to as slow tonic, which is found in muscles such as the anterior latissimus dorsi. This muscle holds the wings back against the body and is therefore contracted most of the time. This it does with very little expenditure of ATP (Goldspink *et al.*, 1970). These very slow or tonic types of muscle fibres are not found in mammals.

Muscle fibre types differ phenotypically in that they not only express different subsets of myofibrillar isoform genes with different specific ATPase activities but also different types and levels of metabolic enzymes. The inherent ability of skeletal muscle to adapt to mechanical signals is related to its ability to induce or repress transcription of different isoform genes and to alter the general levels of expression of different subsets of genes. The fact that there are several myosin isoform genes means that muscle fibres possess the ability to alter their contractile properties during development and in response to levels of activity (Moore and Goldspink, 1985; Goldspink *et al.*, 1992). This involves both qualitative and quantitative changes in gene expression which result in alteration in the cross-sectional area of a given type of fibre.

It was found that fibre size and fibre type composition differed between meat-type and egg-type chickens. Growth coefficients obtained from early and late (before and after 15 weeks of age) stages indicated that muscle fibre growth differs among muscles, fibre types and developmental stages. The growth of type 1 fibres occurs mainly in the early stage (up to 15 weeks) and this correlates with bone growth which is completed in the chicken by 15 weeks. The late stage is characterized by a marked development of type 2a fibres and transformation from type 2b to 2a which results in remarkable growth of hind limb muscle. Iwamoto *et al.* (1993) suggested the transformation of small type 2a to large type 2b plays an important role in the further increase of muscle production.

MYOBLAST, SATELLITE CELL AND MUSCLE FIBRE NUMBER

Like mammalian species, avian skeletal muscle caudal to the branchial arches is derived from the myotome of the somites. One subset of myotomal cells commences to express muscle-specific genes within the somite, differentiating into epaxial trunk muscles, whereas another subset migrates to the somatopleure and becomes the progenitors of appendicular musculature including the limb muscles (Chevallier *et al.*, 1977; Christ *et al.*, 1977; Solursh *et al.*, 1987; Ordahl and Le Douarin, 1992). Precursor cells of limb muscle enter the limb bud and then undergo terminal differentiation (Stockdale, 1992). The myoblasts then fuse to form myotubes, which develop into muscle fibres with fibre number becoming fixed before hatching or shortly after hatching. During the postnatal growth of the animal, with the exception of fish, the growth of muscle occurs only due to hypertrophy and not hyperplasia. The muscle fibre increase in size happens in two ways: (i) by increase in length and (ii) by increase in circumference or girth. *In vitro* studies have shown that, once myoblasts have been incorporated into myotubes to become muscle fibres, the nuclei lose their ability to divide (Bintliff and Walker, 1960; Stockdale and Holtzer, 1961). *In vivo* studies, on the other hand, have demonstrated that there is a considerable increase in the number of nuclei during muscle growth in chicken (Moss, 1968). These apparently contrary findings are explained because the satellite cells in skeletal muscle provide a source of extra muscle nuclei during muscle growth (Moss and Leblond, 1971) and these fuse mainly with the ends of the muscle fibres (Aziz-Ullah and Goldspink, 1974) which are the growth regions for longitudinal growth (Griffin *et al.,* 1971).

The satellite cells, which are undifferentiated precursor muscle cells located between the membrane and basal lamina of the muscle fibre, are really residual myoblasts. A satellite cell is a mononucleated cell with a high nucleus-to-cytoplasm ratio and few organelles, such as mitochondria, Golgi apparatus, ribosomes and endoplasmic reticulum, all of which are necessary for protein synthesis (Bodine-Fowler, 1994). The number of satellite cells in muscle varies with age and the kind of muscle. Satellite cells account for about 30% of the nuclei in muscle fibres in the neonate and 2–4% in adult fibres (Snow, 1977; Schultz, 1989). In general, oxidative muscles have a much higher density of satellite cells than glycolytic muscles. The activity state of muscle is an important factor in the regulation of satellite cell proliferation. Increased functional demand that induces a hypertrophic response results in increased satellite cell mitotic activity, whereas decreased activity that results in atrophy results in decreased mitotic activity (Schultz, 1989).

Satellite cells have one surface in contact with the basal lamina of the myofibre. But despite this intimate contact, there is no evidence of electrical coupling between the cells (Bader *et al.,* 1988). They are mitotically quiescent in adult muscle but re-enter the cell cycle after muscle injury to generate a population of myoblasts, which may subsequently fuse to form new myofibres. In developing muscle, satellite cells are mitotically active and contribute virtually all of the nuclei in the secondary generation of myofibres. Identifying signals that govern satellite cell behaviour is of central importance in understanding muscle growth and regeneration as their abundance may determine the ultimate size to which a muscle can grow. However, the initial growth potential of a muscle is apparently determined by the number of myoblasts originally formed during embryonic development. Penney *et al.* (1983) showed that muscle mass in large and small strains of mice was related to the number of myoblast proliferations before fusion, and Stickland and Goldspink (1973, 1975) showed that pigs with a high fibre number had greater growth potential than those with a lower fibre complement. The use of the muscle fibre complement for growth potential was extended to poultry by Prentis *et al.* (1984). Therefore, it seems relevant to study the genes that determine cell number in muscle tissue.

MUSCLE GENES AND THE REGULATION OF THEIR EXPRESSION

Growth and phenotypic determination of muscle and any other tissue involves the coexpression of different subsets of genes. The myofibrillar protein genes have received the most attention as they exist as different isoforms and because of their functional significance. Muscle is the most abundant tissue in the body and myosin is the most abundant protein within muscle. Therefore, if we can understand how the myosin hc genes are regulated, we should be able to understand how muscle growth in general is controlled posthatching. Muscle is a versatile tissue as it can produce contractile proteins with different functional properties expressing different isoform genes. In the vertebrates different myosin hc isoforms are coded for by separate genes, some of which are preferentially expressed in fast skeletal muscle, slow skeletal muscle, cardiac muscle and smooth muscle. Also there are other types of myosin that constitute part of the cytoskeleton of both muscle and non-muscle cells. With regard to the latter, more than 10 different classes of myosin hcs have been described of which class II encompass the muscle myosin hc genes. The other classes are cytoskeletal myosins that have a molecular motor or S1 but no rod structure (Cheney and Mooseker, 1992; Howard, 1994). In human skeletal muscle there are at least seven separate skeletal myosin hc genes including the embryonic, neonatal and adult fast and slow myosin hc genes. *In toto* there are about 14 different members of the mammalian myosin hc genes in the mammalian myosin hc gene superfamily. In fish there are 28 unique myosin genomic sequences (Gerlach *et al.,* 1990) and in birds as many as 35 different myosin hc genes (Robbins *et al.,* 1986).

In contrast to the myosin hcs which are encoded by separate genes, myosin lcs 1 and 3 are coded for by split genes or transcriptional units. Animal genes contain both introns and exons. The latter are sequences coding for the amino acids which make up the specific protein whereas the introns are spacing sequences which are transcribed into RNA but not translated into protein. For the myosin lcs the different protein isoforms are obtained by alternative splicing. The process involves splicing together different exon RNA transcripts so that several permutations are possible from the same gene. Thus, a single gene can give rise to several mRNAs and, hence, to different myosin lc isoforms (Periasamy *et al.,* 1984). As far as the other myofibrillar proteins are concerned, actin is encoded by several genes, but only one, a skeletal actin isoform, is strongly expressed in adult skeletal muscle, although cardiac actin and cytoskeletal actin are expressed at low levels (Vandekerckhove and Weber, 1979). The troponins and tropomyosins exist in several different isoforms in cardiac muscle and in fast and slow skeletal muscle. These are also derived by alternative splicing of the primary transcript of the troponin and tropomyosin genes during RNA processing (Breitbart *et al.,* 1985; Wieczorek, 1988).

Most genes studied have a regulatory or promoter sequence upstream of the transcriptional start site, that is to say at their 5′ end . This is the sequence needed 'to drive' the gene. Experiments have shown that without this promoter sequence expression levels are very low. The promoter region contains certain regulatory elements including the so-called TATA box that has been described as the 'sign post' for RNA polymerase II which is usually just a few bases up from the start site for transcription. In addition to the TATA box there are often CCAAT boxes and E boxes (CAANTG) which are thought to be the binding site for transcriptional factors which 'up-regulate' or 'down-regulate' transcription. The E boxes represent binding regions for myogenic factors which determine whether a cell is going to be a muscle cell or not by specifically turning on the muscle genes (Buskin and Hauschka, 1989; Weintraub *et al.*, 1991).

In the 5′ regulatory sequence there are also positive and negative response elements for certain hormones. Thyroid hormone (T3) activates transcription of skeletal fast myosin hc gene as well as the cardiac α-myosin hc gene. The receptor for this steroid hormone is the cytosolic c-erb receptor, the second messenger of which binds with the thyroid response element within the myosin hc gene sequence of the particular gene (Izumo *et al.*, 1986). Other regulatory sequences, such as enhancers, may also be involved in facilitating the binding of the transcriptional factor proteins to DNA. These may be at the 5′ or 3′ end of the gene and many bases from the start sequence. Enhancer sequences are also sometimes found in untranslated introns as well as exons. In the myosin hc genes these are found in introns 1 and 2 which are untranslated (Chang *et al.*, 1993; Gauvry *et al.*, 1996). Enhancers are often quite remote in linear terms. However, they may be quite close to the start sequence when the three-dimensional structure of the chromosome DNA is considered. It is likely that enhancers facilitate the binding of *trans*-acting transcriptional factors to the promoter of the gene and thus increase the transcriptional rate of the gene in question. Enhancers also differ from promoters in that the orientation of the sequence does not seem to matter. That is to say, the sequence can be reversed yet the increase in the transcriptional level of the gene is still obtained. For further details the reader is referred to a general review of gene expression (Latchman, 1995). A knowledge of the function of these regulatory sequences for key muscle genes and subsets of muscle genes is, therefore, essential if growth is to be regulated in a scientific manner by the manipulation of gene expression including the introduction of engineered genes. These include the insulin-like growth factors I and II.

MOLECULAR EVENTS DURING DIFFERENTIATION OF MUSCLE

Muscle is a good tissue in which to study molecular mechanisms involved in cell differentiation as it is a tissue which produces large quantities of specialized proteins. The major problem in molecular biology is defining what turns on specific genes in certain cells during development and what determines whether a cell will become a nerve cell, fibroblast or muscle cell. Much research is now aimed at characterizing these transcriptional proteins which activate or repress gene expression. It appears that many genes have similar domains at the 5'-flanking region and therefore, it is likely that the same transcription factor proteins activate or repress several related genes, thus synchronizing their activity. The discovery of the first regulatory factors involved in terminal differentiation of pleuripotent embryonic cells into a given cell type was in skeletal muscle. A family of regulatory factor proteins has been identified including MyoD and myogenin (Weintraub *et al.*, 1989). These are believed to bind to response elements that are in the regulatory or 5'-flanking sequence of skeletal muscle genes which precedes the coding sequence. These proteins bind to the DNA at this point and initiate transcription of the muscle genes. These so-called myogenic factors are shown in Fig. 1.2.

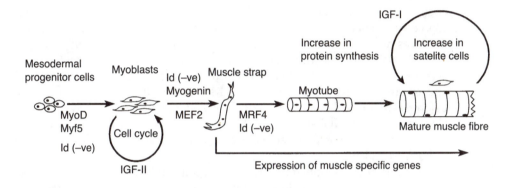

Fig. 1.2. Working model for the myogenic pathway in avian and mammalian muscle development. Muscle precursor cells migrate in a complex way to their place in the developing somites. Commitment to the myogenic lineage is first initiated by the expression of MyoD and Myf5. Muscle differentiation starts in the anterior somites and proceeds caudally. Early differentiation events are signified by the fusion of myoblasts into multinucleate myotubes; initiated in part by the expression of myogenin and MEF2. Later differentiation events and growth involve the expression of hormones including IGF-I which is produced systemically and locally, particularly by active muscle tissue.

In skeletal muscle there are two main phases during embryological differentiation of the tissue: a proliferative phase during which the number of myoblasts increases followed by the fusion of the myoblasts to form multinucleated muscle fibres. The growth factors that control the proliferative phase are different from those that trigger terminal differentiation and the formation of proper muscle fibres (Goldspink and Hansen, 1993). Increasing the number of myoblasts and the number of muscle fibres is an important strategy for increasing muscle mass (Stickland and Goldspink, 1973; Stickland *et al.*, 1975; Penney *et al.*, 1983). Therefore, attempts are being made to identify and isolate the genes which code for the growth factors that control the proliferative phase.

REGULATION OF MUSCLE MASS AND MUSCLE FIBRE TYPES BY GROWTH HORMONE AND INSULIN-LIKE GROWTH FACTORS

Growth hormone (GH) is a protein hormone produced by the pituitary which can stimulate the liver to produce two peptide growth factors termed insulin-like growth factor I and II (IGF-I and IGF-II). These have several physiological functions on different tissues which can be summarized into two main biological actions, i.e. an insulin-like metabolic action and a growth-promoting action including cell division. IGF-II is regarded as an embryonic form of IGF and its mitogenic activity is probably very important in determining cell number in muscle and other tissues. Both IGF-I and IGF-II are produced by the liver and their synthesis is to a large extent induced by circulating GH. In mammals, it has been shown that the liver is the main source of circulating IGF-I, except during intensive exercise when muscle produces and uses most of the circulating IGF-I (Brahm *et al.*, 1997). Under normal conditions the rates of hepatic secretion of IGF-I are sufficient to account for levels of IGF-I found in plasma as it is continuously synthesized and released by liver depending on GH status and it is synthesized rapidly before secretion (Schalch *et al.*, 1979; Schwander *et al.*, 1983). Interestingly, in chicken, the serum IGF-I concentration is not correlated with the serum GH level during embryonic development or during the posthatching period (Kikuchi *et al.*, 1991).

GH has been demonstrated to play an important role in promoting the growth of skeletal muscle in mammals. Administration of GH to pigs, for example, can increase their skeletal muscle growth (Chung *et al.*, 1985; Campbell *et al.*, 1989; Grant *et al.*, 1991; Goldspink and Hansen, 1993). In contrast to domestic mammals, exogenous chicken GH was shown not to increase lean body mass or improve production efficiency in chickens (Cogburn *et al.*, 1989). Halevy *et al.* (1996) showed that GH promotes more satellite cells to proliferate and leads to the addition of more nuclei to the growing muscle and suggested this effect was IGF-I independent. Using a breed of dwarf chicken that is unable to express the GH receptor, Tanaka *et al.* (1996) showed that IGF-I was still expressed in a range of tissues and thus it is concluded that the non-liver IGFs are GH and GH receptor independent. As these dwarf chickens show some growth it must be concluded that these extrahepatic IGFs do make an appreciable contribution to posthatching growth. By using chicken myotubes in primary culture derived from neonatal muscle satellite cells, Duclos *et al.* (1993) demonstrated that IGF-I exerts anabolic effects by stimulating protein synthesis and inhibiting protein degradation. The fact that IGF-I is more potent than insulin suggests that this effect was mediated by type I IGF receptor rather than by the insulin receptor. The stimulation of protein synthesis that is induced most likely results from several mechanisms, including increasing mRNA transcription and translation and stimulating amino acid transport.

So far, we know very little about the relationship between IGF-I and skeletal muscle gene expression. A study of effects of growth hormone treatments on the proportion of type 1 and type 2 fibres in skeletal muscle of hypophysectomized rats demonstrated that GH treatment, presumably acting through increased expression of IGF-I, elicited an increase in the relative proportion of type 1 fibres (Ayling *et al.,* 1989). *In situ* hybridization studies using the IGF-I probes, designed as described by Yang *et al.* (1996), on muscle sections from GH-deficient human patients demonstrated that 70% of IGF-I mRNA is distributed in type 1 fibres. Together, these observations indicate that GH and IGF-I may be related to the expression of specific myosin genes.

For many years it has been appreciated that there is local as well as systemic control of tissue growth, because if a muscle is exercised it is only that muscle which undergoes hypertrophy and not all the muscles of the limb. It has been shown that stretch is the major mechanical signal for the serial addition of new sarcomeres (Griffin *et al.,* 1971; Williams and Goldspink, 1971; Goldspink, 1984; Williams *et al.,* 1986), up-regulating protein synthesis (Goldspink and Goldspink, 1986; Loughna *et al.,* 1986) and changing gene transcription (Goldspink *et al.,* 1992; Yang *et al.,* 1997). Yang *et al.* (1996) have recently cloned the cDNA of a new growth factor that is expressed by skeletal and cardiac muscle when it is stretched and overloaded. Its sequence indicates that it is derived from the IGF-I gene by alternative splicing but has different exons, is not glycosylated and hence is smaller and has probably a shorter half-life than the liver IGF-Is. Thus, this isoform is likely designed for an autocrine/paracrine rather than the systemic type of action of the liver IGF-Is. The discovery of this growth factor provides a link between the mechanical stimulus and gene expression.

Although much of posthatching muscle growth is preprogrammed it is apparent that the quality and quantity of the proteins synthesized arises because different subsets of genes are activated to a greater or lesser extent by mechanical signals when muscles are actively used. The discovery of this local IGF-I expressed in active muscle provides a link between the mechanical stimulus and gene expression. The possibility of manipulating growth and phenotype by the introduction of these growth factors therefore exists as a way of modifying both muscle mass and phenotype. This would have to involve transferring engineered genes, as the proteins themselves would require repeated injections as they have a relatively short half-life and would be too expensive.

GENE TRANSFER

Emerging methods in molecular biology offer the prospect of introducing genes to enhance growth efficiency and food quality as well as disease resistance. Germ-line gene transfer in birds is technically somewhat more difficult than in mammals in which it can be achieved by injection of transgene into the nucleus of the ovum using embryological stem cells transfected with the transgene. At hatching the avian egg has 64,000 cells and it is necessary to transfer the gene into all cells. This is possible using a retroviral vector but this would generate consumer resistance to the use of an acquired immune deficiency syndrome (AIDS)-type virus. The other possibilities are to take the egg when it is still at the one-cell stage, before it is laid, and to introduce the transgene by injection (Love *et al.,* 1994). Another possibility is to intercept the primordial ovary cells in the developing chick as they travel through the bloodstream to the position where the ovary will develop (Vick *et al.,* 1993). These can be transfected and returned to the bloodstream so that the introduced gene will be present in the oocytes when they are formed.

There is also the more immediate possibility of somatic gene transfer by introducing engineered genes by injection of naked DNA. This can be done by using a gene gun and shooting minute metal particles coated with the DNA into skin or other tissues. Also an effective technique is to use direct intramuscular injection of the gene in a plasmid vector into muscle. Muscle has the somewhat unique ability to take up and express DNA following a simple intramuscular injection (Wolff *et al.,* 1990; Hansen *et al.,* 1991). As cell division in muscle fibres does not continue after myoblast fusion, the introduced gene which does not integrate into the chromosome is not lost and repeat injections are not necessary. We have shown that the expression is much higher when the DNA is introduced into young muscles (Wells and Goldspink, 1992) as presumably the factors involved in activating genes are present at higher levels. In recent experiments we introduced the cDNA of the new muscle growth factor which we have called mechanogrowth factor (MGF) into young mice by direct intramuscular injection and within 2 weeks there was a 20% increase in live weight gain above that of the age-matched control mice.

DNA vaccines delivered in the same manner offer a cheap and effective way of imparting disease resistance and the cDNA of growth factors could be introduced at the same time to provide cheap and effective improvements in poultry management.

ACKNOWLEDGEMENTS

The authors are grateful to Dr Paul Simons and Dr Steven Ennion for their helpful comments during the preparation of this review, and to the Wellcome Trust and Pfizer UK who supported different aspects of this work.

REFERENCES

Alexander, McN.R. and Goldspink, G. (1977) *Mechanics and Energetics of Animal Locomotion.* Chapman & Hall, London, pp. 1–20.

Ayling, C.M., Moreland, B.H., Zanelli, J.M. and Schulster, D. (1989) Human growth hormone treatment of hypophysectomized rats increases the proportion of type-1 fibres in skeletal muscle. *Journal of Endocrinology* 123, 429–435.

Aziz-Ullah and Goldspink, G. (1974) Distribution of mitotic nuclei in the biceps brachii of the mouse during post-natal growth. *Anatomical Record* 179, 115–118.

Bader, C.R., Bertrand, D., Cooper, E. and Mauro, A. (1988) Membrane currents of rat satellite cells attached to intact skeletal muscle fibers. *Neuron* 1, 237–240.

Barany, M. (1967) ATPase activity of myosin correlated with speed of muscle shortening. *Journal of General Physiology* 50, Suppl. 197–218.

Bintliff, S. and Walker, B.E. (1960) Radioautographic study of skeletal muscle regeneration. *American Journal of Anatomy* 106, 233–246.

Bodine-Fowler, S. (1994) Skeletal muscle regeneration after injury: an overview. [Review] *Journal of Voice* 8, 53–62.

Brahm, H., Piehl-Aulin, K., Saltin, B. and Ljunghall, S. (1997) Net fluxes over working thigh of hormones, growth factors and biomarkers of bone metabolism during short lasting dynamic exercise. *Calcified Tissue International* 60, 175–180.

Breitbart, R.E., Nguyen, H.T., Medford, R.M., Destree, A.T. and Mahdavi, V. (1985) Intricate combinatorial patterns of exon splicing generate multiple regulated troponin T isoforms from a single gene. *Cell* 41, 67–82.

Buskin, J.N. and Hauschka, S.D. (1989) Identification of a myocyte nuclear factor that binds to the muscle-specific enhancer of the mouse muscle creatine kinase gene. *Molecular and Cellular Biology* 9, 2627–2640.

Campbell, R.G., Steele, N.C., Caperna, T.J., Mcmurtry, J.P., Solomon, M.B. and Mitchell, A.D. (1989) Interrelationships between sex and exogenous growth hormone administration on performance, body composition and protein and fat accretion of growing pigs. *Journal of Animal Science* 67, 177–186.

Chang K.C, Fernandes, K and Goldspink G (1993) *In vivo* expression and molecular characterization of the porcine slow-myosin heavy chain beta gene. *Journal of Cell Science* 106, 331–341.

Cheney, R.E. and Mooseker, M.S. (1992) Unconventional myosins. [Review] *Current Opinion in Cell Biology* 4, 27–35.

Chevallier, A., Kieny, M. and Mauger, A. (1977) Limb-somite relationship: origin of the limb musculature. *Journal of Embryology and Experimental Morphology* 41, 245–258.

Christ, B., Jacob, H.J. and Jacob, M. (1977) Experimental analysis of the origin of the wing musculature in avian embryos. *Anatomy and Embryology* 150, 171–186.

Chung, C.S., Etherton, T.D. and Wiggins, J.P. (1985) Stimulation of swine growth by porcine growth hormone. *Journal of Animal Science* 60, 118–130.

Cogburn, L.A., Liou, S.S., Rand, A.L. and Mcmurtry, J.P. (1989) Growth, metabolic and endocrine responses of broiler cockerels given a daily subcutaneous injection of natural or biosynthetic chicken growth hormone. *Journal of Nutrition* 119, 1213–1222.

Duclos, M.J., Chevalier, B., Goddard, C. and Simon, J. (1993) Regulation of amino acid transport and protein metabolism in myotubes derived from chicken muscle satellite cells by insulin-like growth factor-I. *Journal of Cellular Physiology* 157, 650–657.

Ennion, S., Sant'ana Pereira, J., Sargeant, A.J., Young, A. and Goldspink, G. (1995) Characterization of human skeletal muscle fibres according to the myosin heavy chains they express. *Journal of Muscle Research and Cell Motility* 16, 35–43.

Gauvry, L., Ennion, S., Hansen, E., Butterworth, P. and Goldspink, G. (1996) The characterisation of the 5′ regulatory region of a temperature-induced myosin-heavy-chain gene associated with myotomal muscle growth in the carp. *European Journal of Biochemistry* 236, 887–894.

Gerlach, G.F., Turay, L., Malik, K.T., Lida, J., Scutt, A. and Goldspink, G. (1990) Mechanisms of temperature acclimation in the carp: a molecular biology approach. *American Journal of Physiology* 259, R237–R244.

Goldspink, D.F. and Goldspink, G. (1986)The role of passive stretch in retarding muscle atrophy. In: Nix, W.A. and Vrbova, G. (eds) *Electrical Stimulation and Neuromuscular Disorders.* Springer Verlag, Berlin, pp. 91–100.

Goldspink, G. (1984) Alterations in myofibril size and structure during growth, exercise and changes in enviromental temperature. In: Peachy, L.D., Adrian, R.H. and Geiger, S.R (eds) *Handbook of Physiology – Skeletal Muscle*. American Physiological Society, New York, pp. 593–554.

Goldspink, G. (1985) Malleability of the motor system: a comparative approach. *Journal of Experimental Biology* 115, 375–391.

Goldspink, G. (1991) Prospectives for the manipulation of muscle growth. In: Pearson, A.M. and Dutson, T.R. (eds) *Growth Regulation in Farm Animals. Advances in Meat Research, Volume 7*. Elsevier Applied Science, London, pp. 557–587.

Goldspink G. (1996) Muscle growth and muscle function: a molecular biological perspective. *Research in Veterinary Science* 60, 193–204.

Goldspink, G. and Hansen, E. (1993) Hormones involved in regulation of muscle differentiation and growth. In: Schreibman, M.P., Scanes, C.G. and Pang, K.T. (eds) *The Endocrinology of Growth, Development and Metabolism in Vertebrates*. Academic Press, San Diego, pp. 445–467.

Goldspink, G., Larson, R.E. and Davies, R.E. (1970) Thermodynamic efficiency and physiological characteristics of the chick anterior latissimus dorsi muscle. *Journal of Comparative Physiology* 66, 379–388

Goldspink, G., Scutt, A., Loughna, P.T., Wells, D.J., Jaenicke, T. and Gerlach, G.F. (1992) Gene expression in skeletal muscle in response to stretch and force generation. *American Journal of Physiology* 262, R356–R363.

Grant, A.L., Helferich, W.G., Kramer, S.A., Merkel, R.A. and Bergen, W.G. (1991) Administration of growth hormone to pigs alters the relative amount of insulin-like growth factor-I mRNA in liver and skeletal muscle. *Journal of Endocrinology* 130, 331–338.

Griffin, G.E., Williams, P.E. and Goldspink, G. (1971) Region of longitudinal growth in striated muscle fibres. *Nature – New Biology* 232, 28–29.

Halevy, O., Hodik, V. and Mett, A. (1996) The effects of growth hormone on avian skeletal muscle satellite cell proliferation and differentiation. *General and Comparative Endocrinology* 101, 43–52.

Hansen, E., Fernandes, K., Goldspink, G., Butterworth, P., Umeda, P.K. and Chang, K.C. (1991) Strong expression of foreign genes following direct injection into fish muscle. *FEBS Letters* 290, 73–76.

Hnik, P., Vejsada, R., Goldspink, D.F., Kasicki, S. and Krekule, I. (1985) Quantitative evaluation of electromyogram activity in rat extensor and flexor muscles immobilized at different lengths. *Experimental Neurology* 88, 515–528.

Howard, J. (1994) Molecular motors. Clamping down on myosin [news; comment]. *Nature* 368, 98–99.

Huxley, H.E. (1969) The mechanism of muscular contraction. [Review] *Science* 164, 1356–1365.

Iwamoto, H., Hara, Y., Ono, Y. and Takahara, H. (1993) Breed differences in the histochemical properties of the M. pubo-ischio-femoralis pars medialis myofibre of domestic cocks. *British Poultry Science* 34, 309–321.

Izumo, S., Nadal-Ginard, B. and Mahdavi, V. (1986) All members of the MHC multigene family respond to thyroid hormone in a highly tissue-specific manner. *Science* 231, 597–600.

Kikuchi, K., Buonomo, F.C., Kajimoto, Y. and Rotwein, P. (1991) Expression of insulin-like growth factor-I during chicken development. *Endocrinology* 128, 1323–1328.

Latchman, D. (1995) *Gene Regulation: a Eukaryotic Perspective*, Academic Press, London.

Loughna, P., Goldspink, G. and Goldspink, D.F. (1986) Effect of inactivity and passive stretch on protein turnover in phasic and postural rat muscles. *Journal of Applied Physiology* 61, 173–179.

Love, J., Gribbin, C., Mather, C. and Sang, H. (1994) Transgenic birds by DNA microinjection. *Bio/Technology* 12, 60–63.

Lowey, S., Waller, G.S. and Trybus, K.M. (1993) Skeletal muscle myosin light chains are essential for physiological speeds of shortening. *Nature* 365, 454–456.

Moore, G.E. and Goldspink, G. (1985) The effect of reduced activity on the enzymatic development of phasic and tonic muscles in the chicken. *Journal of Developmental Physiology* 7, 381–386.

Moss, F.P. (1968) The relationship between the dimensions of the fibres and the number of nuclei during normal growth of skeletal muscle in the domestic fowl. *American Journal of Anatomy* 122, 555–563.

Moss, F.P. and Leblond, C.P. (1971) Satellite cells as the source of nuclei in muscles of growing rats. *Anatomical Record* 170, 421–435.

Ordahl, C.P. and Le Douarin, N.M. (1992) Two myogenic lineages within the developing somite. *Development* 114, 339–353.

Penney, R.K., Prentis, P.F., Marshall, P.A. and Goldspink, G. (1983) Differentiation of muscle and the determination of ultimate tissue size. *Cell and Tissue Research* 228, 375–388.

Periasamy, M., Strehler, E.E., Garfinkel, L.I., Gubits, R.M. and Ruiz-Opazo, N. (1984) Fast skeletal muscle myosin light chains 1 and 3 are produced from a single gene by a combined process of differential RNA transcription and splicing. *Journal of Biological Chemistry* 259, 13595–13604.

Prentis P.F., Penney R.E.and Goldspink G (1984) Possible use of an indicator muscle in the future breeding experiments of the domestic fowl. *British Poultry Science* 25, 33–41.

Reiser, P.J., Moss, R.L., Giulian, G.G. and Greaser, M.L. (1985) Shortening velocity and myosin heavy chains of developing rabbit muscle fibers. *Journal of Biological Chemistry* 260, 14403–14405.

Robbins, J., Horan, T., Gulick, J. and Kropp, K. (1986) The chicken myosin heavy chain family. *Journal of Biological Chemistry* 261, 6606–6612.

Schalch, D.S., Heinrich, U.E., Draznin, B., Johnson, C.J. and Miller, L.L. (1979) Role of the liver in regulating somatomedin activity: hormonal effects on the synthesis and release of insulin-like growth factor and its carrier protein by the isolated perfused rat liver. *Endocrinology* 104, 1143–1151.

Schultz, E. (1989) Satellite cell behavior during skeletal muscle growth and regeneration. [Review] *Medicine and Science in Sports and Exercise* 21, S181–S186.

Schwander, J.C., Hauri, C., Zapf, J. and Froesch, E.R. (1983) Synthesis and secretion of insulin-like growth factor and its binding protein by the perfused rat liver: dependence on growth hormone status. *Endocrinology* 113, 297–305.

Snow, M.H. (1977) The effects of aging on satellite cells in skeletal muscles of mice and rats. *Cell and Tissue Research* 185, 399–408.

Solursh, M., Drake, C. and Meier, S. (1987) The migration of myogenic cells from the somites at the wing level in avian embryos. *Developmental Biology* 121, 389–396.

Stickland, N.C. and Goldspink, G. (1973) A possible indicator muscle for the fibre content and growth characteristics of porcine muscle. *Animal Production* 16, 136–146.

Stickland, N.C. and Goldspink, G. (1975) A note on porcine skeletal muscle parameters and their possible use in early progeny testing. *Animal Production* 21, 93–96.

Stickland, N.C., Widdowson, B.M. and Goldspink, G. (1975) Effects of severe energy and protein deficiencies on the fibres and nuclei in skeletal muscle of pigs. *British Journal of Nutrition* 34, 421–428.

Stockdale, F.E. and Holtzer, H. (1961) DNA synthesis and myogenesis. *Experimental Cell Research* 24, 508–520.

Stockdale, F.E. (1992) Myogenic cell lineages. [Review] *Developmental Biology* 154, 284–298.

Tanaka, M., Hayashida, Y., Sakaguchi, K., Ohkubo, T., Wakita, M. and Hoshino, S. (1996) Growth hormone-independent expression of insulin-like growth factor I messenger ribonucleic acid in extrahepatic tissues of the chicken. *Endocrinology* 137, 30–34.

Vandekerckhove, J. and Weber, K. (1979) The complete amino acid sequence of actins from bovine aorta, bovine heart, bovine fast skeletal muscle, and rabbit slow skeletal muscle. A protein-chemical analysis of muscle actin differentiation. *Differentiation* 14, 123–133.

Vick, L., Li, Y. and Simkiss, K. (1993) Transgenic birds from transformed primordial germ cells. *Proceedings of the Royal Society of London – Series B: Biological Sciences* 251, 179–182.

Weintraub, H., Davis, R., Tapscott, S., Thayer, M., Krause, M., Benezra, R., Turner, D., Rupp, R. and Hollenberg, S. (1991) The myoD gene family: nodal point during specification of the muscle cell lineage. [Review] *Science* 251, 761–766.

Weintraub, H., Tapscott, S.J., Davis, R.L., Thayer, M.J., Adam, M.A. and Lassar, A.B. (1989) Activation of muscle-specific genes in pigment, nerve, fat, liver, and fibroblast cell lines by forced expression of MyoD. *Proceedings of the National Academy of Sciences of the United States of America* 86, 5434–5438.

Wells, D.J. and Goldspink, G. (1992) Age and sex influence expression of plasmid DNA directly injected into mouse skeletal muscle. *FEBS Letters* 306, 203–205.

Wieczorek, D.F. (1988) Regulation of alternatively spliced alpha-tropomyosin gene expression by nerve extract. *Journal of Biological Chemistry* 263, 10456–10463.

Williams, P., Watt, P., Bicik, V. and Goldspink, G. (1986) Effect of stretch combined with electrical stimulation on the type of sarcomeres produced at the ends of muscle fibers. *Experimental Neurology* 93, 500–509.

Williams, P.E. and Goldspink, G. (1971) Longitudinal growth of striated muscle fibres. *Journal of Cell Science* 9, 751–767.

Wolff, J.A., Malone, R.W., Williams, P., Chong, W., Acsadi, G., Jani, A. and Felgner, P.L., (1990) Direct gene transfer into mouse muscle *in vivo*. *Science* 247, 1465–1468.

Yang, S.Y., Alnaqeeb, M., Simpson, H. and Goldspink, G. (1996) Cloning and characterization of an IGF-I isoform expressed in skeletal muscle subjected to stretch. *Journal of Muscle Research and Cell Motility* 17, 487–495.

Yang, S.Y., Alnaqeeb, M., Simpson, H. and Goldspink, G. (1997) Changes in muscle fibre type, muscle mass and IGF-I gene expression in rabbit skeletal muscle subjected to stretch. *Journal of Anatomy* 190, 613–622.

CHAPTER 2
Muscle abnormalities: morphological aspects

Mike Mahon
School of Biological Sciences,1.124 Stopford Building, University of Manchester, Manchester M13 9PT, UK

Recent overviews of the turkey industry have commented upon the greater production efficiency and increased weight of marketable birds but also on the health problems, stress susceptibility and downgrading of meat due to poor colour, texture and flavour (Ferket, 1995). This review and its sister review by Mitchell (Chapter 3) concerns both the morphological and physiological alterations which can occur in skeletal muscle due to disease or environmental factors and their effects on the poultry industry.

INTRODUCTION: MUSCLE PLASTICITY, ADAPTABILITY, VARIABILITY AND PATHOLOGY

Skeletal muscle is by nature a highly plastic tissue having a remarkable ability to adapt its morphology to suit functional demand. Hence, muscles located at different anatomical sites or found in different species or strains, or present at varying stages of growth or ageing often show great differences in their gross anatomical, microscopic and subcellular structure.[1] Even samples obtained from adjacent sites may show quantifiable differences (Mahon *et al.*, 1984). Therefore, without detailed knowledge of the normal structure of a specific muscle in each of these states it is difficult to detect any 'abnormalities' which may have occurred. Classic cases are the confusion between muscle 'anomalies' due to ageing (Froes *et al.*, 1987) or muscle sampled (Kristmundsdottir *et al.*, 1990) with those due to 'myopathy'. Pathology occurs when the muscle is unable to adapt to the demands placed upon it. This may be because the demand is too great, too acute or too continuous, or because a direct trauma or genetic defect (as in many neuromuscular diseases) has made the muscle incapable of showing the correct response. In many circumstances, however, given time, the muscle will recover from the insult or overload, regenerate or repair itself and adapt to the new circumstances. Thus, when

---

All figures in this chapter can be viewed in colour at http://www.biomed.man.ac.uk/mahon/muscle1999/
[1]See review by Schmalbruch (1985) and a recent account of avian muscle variations from Torrella *et al.* (1998).

studying samples of muscle tissue the observer must be acutely aware that only a 'snapshot in time' of a continuous process of adaptation and pathology is being seen. However, the importance of histological verification as the 'gold standard' in measuring muscle damage has been made clear (Bar _et al.,_ 1997).

Much of the available information on the processes involved in producing muscle abnormalities derives from a synthesis of data from experimental myology (mainly from work on rodents) and from clinical pathology (mainly from studies of human neuromuscular disorders, including single case histories). More recently, advances in molecular genetics over the last decade have helped elucidate the fundamental aetiology of most of the muscle diseases in man and other mammals and no doubt such knowledge will soon benefit the poultry industry.

In this part of the review, morphological changes and the key mechanisms involved in skeletal muscle adaptability and pathology in general will be covered followed by specific examples of muscle abnormalities in man, mammals and poultry. Only key references to the vast literature on human neuromuscular disorders are given and the reader is referred to our recent reviews, bibliographies and colour atlases, which also include accounts of the methodologies involved in such investigations (Cumming _et al.,_ 1994; Mahon, 1996; Weller _et al.,_ 1997) and the encyclopaedic coverage given by Carpenter and Karpati (1984); Mastaglia and Walton (1992); Vinken _et al._ (1992); Engel and Franzini-Armstrong (1994) and Walton _et al._ (1994). The emphasis here on poultry is on turkey muscle, particularly during growth in highly selected commercial breeds where muscle adaptability and abnormalities are rife. Much of the data on turkey muscle are from our own unpublished material and work in progress particularly from work done in conjunction with Sally Gilpin and Jo Mills and others cited in the acknowledgements.

Aspects of normal muscle structure relevant to this review are covered by Goldspink and Yang in Chapter 1 and the reader needs to be familiar with the terms muscle fascicle, muscle fibre, myofibril, myofilament and the concept of the motor unit and muscle fibre types. Reference will also be made to essential aspects of muscle development such as the myoblast, myotube and myosatellite cells (see Chapter 1).

BASIC RESPONSES OF THE MUSCLE FIBRE

Skeletal muscle is a highly differentiated and specialized tissue and its major component, the syncytial muscle fibres, have a limited response when challenged or damaged (Fig. 2.1). In most circumstances the changes are best viewed in thin stained sections cut transversely to the long axis of the muscle fibres (Fig. 2.2). Material for such investigations should be obtained fresh by simple excision after death or via a muscle biopsy needle (Fig. 2.3) under local anaesthetic. Samples are then rapidly frozen in liquid nitrogen to allow subsequent histological, histochemical, immunocytochemical and morphometric investigations without the loss of enzyme activity or the shrinkage which occurs when tissue is chemically fixed. Separate portions for ultrastructural

Fig. 2.1.

Fig. 2.2.

- **Hypotrophy or Atrophy**
- **Hypertrophy**
- **Degeneration**
- **Regeneration**
- **Cytochemical Alterations**

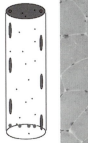
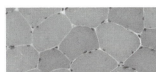

Fig. 2.3

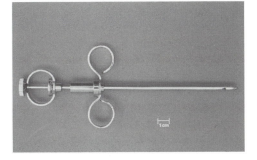

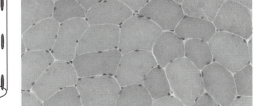

Fig. 2.1. Basic responses of the muscle fibre to internal or external factors.
Fig. 2.2. Transverse section of normal human quadriceps muscle fibres showing polygonal outlines, homogeneous cytoplasm, peripheral nuclei, and little interfibre connective tissue. Haematoxylin and eosin (H&E), × 200.
Fig. 2.3. Muscle biopsy needle used for obtaining samples of live individuals under local anaesthetic.

examination may be processed for electron microscopy (Loughlin, 1993; Cumming *et al.*, 1994). Other accompanying investigations often include biochemical, immunoblot, or molecular genetic analysis of biopsy samples; electromyography and nerve electrophysiology; and, in humans, a full clinical/ functional assessment of the individual from whom the biopsy was obtained. The latter is vital in interpreting and diagnosing neuromuscular diseases since the site of onset and time course of any disability is required to make full sense of the pathological observations as will become apparent from the following.

Hypotrophy and Atrophy

This is where the muscle fibre or fibres are smaller than they should be for a particular muscle at a particular age. *Hypotrophy* refers to situations where the muscle fibres have shown insufficient growth and never attained their normal calibre, which may be due to insufficient nutrition, endocrine, neural or mechanical stimulation or to an inherent genetic defect in their mechanisms of growth. In some cases this hypotrophy may be limited to a specific fibre type population (Fig. 2.4). *Atrophic* muscle fibres are those which have shrunk from their normal size and become small and rounded (often in clumps, Fig. 2.5) or thin and angular (often singular and squashed between normal-sized fibres,

Fig. 2.4.   **Fig. 2.5.**

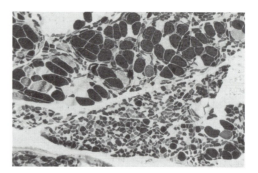

Fig. 2.6.   **Fig. 2.7**

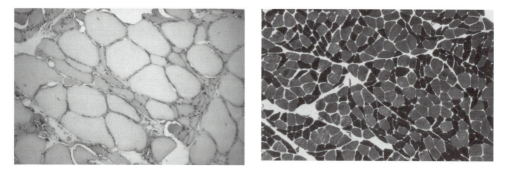

Fig. 2.4. Hypotrophic (small calibre) muscle fibres which have not achieved the normal size of their neighbours. H&E, × 200.
Fig. 2.5. Atrophic (small calibre) muscle fibres which have shrunk from their original size due to loss of innervation. ATPase, × 100.
Fig. 2.6. Scattered, ribbon-like, angulated muscle fibres squashed between normal-sized adjacent fibres. Acetylcholinesterase, × 200.
Fig. 2.7. Muscle biopsy from a 90-year-old human showing type 2 fibre atrophy and loss of type 1 fibres. ATPase, × 100.

Fig. 2.6). Again, the causes may be multiple and involve lack of nutrients, hormones, nervous stimulation or mechanical tension. As with hypotrophy, atrophic fibres may be restricted to a particular fibre type population, especially if the causes are hormonal or neural. Atrophic muscles associated with old age often feature type 2 fibre atrophy and type 1 fibre loss (*hypoplasia*) as shown in Fig. 2.7. Unfortunately, however, there is little quantitative data on the normal programmed loss (*apoptosis*) of muscle fibres throughout life to help interpret this data for most muscles.

Hypertrophy

This describes the abnormal enlargement of muscle fibres often due to increased workload, although it must be remembered that this is also the mechanism for normal muscle fibre growth (Chapter 1) since mature differentiated muscle fibres cannot normally divide and multiply (*hyperplasia*) except in rare rhabdosarcomas. Hypertrophic muscle fibres may be difficult to detect when all the muscle fibres in a given muscle are enlarged unless morphometric methods are employed (Fig. 2.8), but often stand out as large rounded profiles (sometimes with accompanying architectural defects such as splits, whorls or hyaline changes) when occurring singly (Fig. 2.9). In many circumstances hypertrophic fibres or hypertrophic portions of a muscle are the result of atrophy or damage in neighbouring regions causing some fibres to adapt in response to their new workloads, this is called *compensatory hypertrophy* (Fig. 2.10). The mechanisms involved in muscle fibre hypertrophy are complex and involve a combination of myofilament and sarcomere assembly, myofibril splitting and satellite cell activity which vary according to the exact stimulus and time course involved (Atherton *et al.*, 1981; Brotchie

Fig. 2.8.

Fig. 2.9.

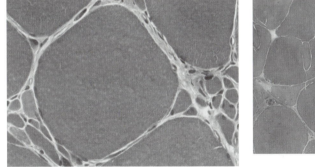

Fig. 2.10.

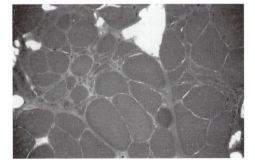

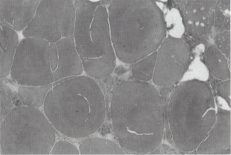

Fig. 2.8. Hypertrophic (enlarged) muscle fibres of normal appearance but attaining an average narrow fibre diameter of over 80 μm. Trichrome, × 400.

Fig. 2.9. Scattered hypertrophic fibres with abnormal internal architecture showing splits and whorls. Trichrome, × 200.

Fig. 2.10. Combination of atrophic fibres and fibres undergoing compensatory hypertrophy in the same fascicle. H&E, × 200.

et al., 1995; Rushton *et al.*, 1997) and are dealt with later under 'Control Factors in Growth and Regeneration, and Satellite Cells (see also Chapter 1).

Degeneration

Partly because muscle fibres have highly sensitive membranes and are extremely excitable and partly because they are so highly differentiated, when damaged they soon begin to degenerate. This process may ultimately lead to an irreversible cell death (*necrosis*) or a recovery involving repair and regeneration. In either case, attack by macrophages and removal of cell debris (*phagocytosis*) usually occurs as part of the acute inflammatory response. Furthermore, due to the elongated multinucleated structure of muscle fibres these processes may occur throughout the cell or in a restricted region (e.g. segmental necrosis) thus making interpretation of single section samples difficult. Typical features of damaged and degenerating muscle fibres are loss of membrane integrity, loss of myofibrillar material, and decreased histological staining in some areas and hypercontraction and hyalinization in other areas (Fig. 2.11). The activity of metabolic enzymes such as succinate dehydrogenase may also be reduced and numerous ultrastructural changes are observed. Many muscle enzymes, notably creatine kinase (CK; see Chapter 3), are leaked into the bloodstream and in extreme cases myoglobin may

Fig. 2.11.   **Fig. 2.12.**

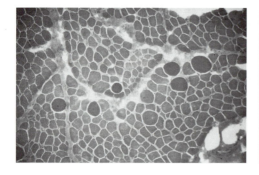   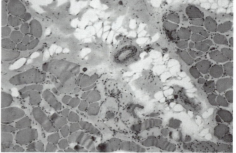

Fig. 2.13.

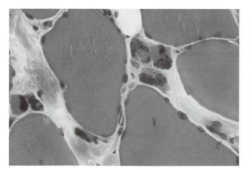

Fig. 2.11. Scattered hyaline (enlarged, rounded and darker staining) fibres in a biopsy from a child with Duchenne muscular dystrophy. H&E, × 100.

Fig. 2.12. Extensive connective tissue replacement and necrosis in a degenerating muscle. H&E, × 100.

Fig. 2.13. Late stages of muscle fibre degeneration in which some fibres remain as thin cells with pyknotic nuclear clumps. H&E, × 100.

appear in the urine. Later stages may show macrophage invasion (visible as excess granular internal nuclei or by intense localized hydrolase enzyme activity) and increased lysosomal activity (*autolysis*) and eventually complete loss of the muscle fibre and replacement by connective tissue (Fig. 2.12). In some cases atrophic pyknotic muscle fibres comprising little more than clumps of myonuclei may remain (Fig. 2.13). There is much experimental and clinical evidence to suggest that following the initial insult (whether physical, toxic, ischaemic, infective or immunological) or genetic defect, calcium influx plays a prime role in initiating and cascading the degenerative events (Salmons, 1997). The exact mechanisms of calcium-related degeneration and its potential importance to commercial poultry meat production is discussed later under 'Calcium Based Muscle Damage' and in Chapter 3.

Regeneration

Regeneration of whole fibres or segments of muscle fibres may occur as a response to and coincident with the degenerative process described above. Indeed, skeletal muscle has a tremendous ability to regenerate. If the initial insult or damage is not too great or continuous then the muscle fibre may repair itself or manufacture new muscle fibres which may fuse to the original one which was injured or defective (Fig. 2.14). This process usually involves the rapid activation, proliferation and migration of muscle precursor cells (or satellite cells, see Chapter 1) which then pass through the normal process of muscle fibre development (myoblasts fusion to myotube to myofibre). During this period, histological signs of regeneration are enlarged euchromatic nuclei, increased basophilic staining, internal nucleation of muscle fibres and apparent fibre splitting or fusion, and the appearance of numerous small basophilic fibres with prominent nuclei (Fig. 2.15). In mammalian muscles the nuclei may remain 'internalized' or eventually move to their normal peripheral or subsarcolemmal positions (Fig. 2.16). In avian muscles the situation is somewhat unclear due to the 'normal' presence of numerous internalized nuclei (Fig. 2.44). Histochemically, regenerating fibres show increased RNA content and intermediate or fetal types of myosin ATPase. Immunocytochemical staining for desmin is also revealing of developing and regenerating fibres which show excess amounts (Fig. 2.17). The regenerative capacity of the muscle may vary due to genetic, hormonal, neural and other factors such as age and vascular supply and is discussed later in this section under 'Control Factors in Growth and Regeneration, and Satellite Cells' as is the importance of the basal lamina as a scaffold for repair (Schmalbruch, 1985).

Altered Intracellular Composition

This may take many forms but in particular often involves changes in the ratio of the contractile (fibrillar) and metabolic (interfibrillar) components of the muscle fibre. Increases or decreases in aerobic structures such as mitochondria

Fig. 2.14.   **Fig. 2.15.**

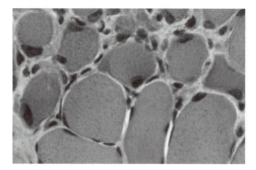

Fig. 2.16.   **Fig. 2.17.**

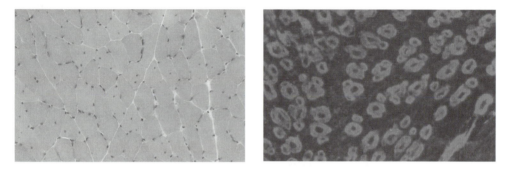

Fig. 2.14. Early stages of regeneration in which satellite cells are activated and fuse to the underlying overloaded or damaged muscle fibre. Electronmicrograph, × 10,000.
Fig. 2.15. Middle stages of regeneration in which numerous smaller regenerating basophilic muscle fibres are present. H&E, × 400.
Fig. 2.16. Late stages of regeneration in human muscle in which the repaired muscle fibres are now only visible due to their internalized nuclei. H&E, × 100.
Fig. 2.17. Antibody staining for desmin in developing fibres, × 200.

and their enzymes may lead to subsarcolemmal accumulations (ragged-red fibres), granularity or lobulation, or vacant areas as in core, moth-eaten, or target fibres (Fig. 2.18). Such changes can be brought about by enzyme defects, ischaemia, exercise, electrical stimulation, drugs, denervation, re-innervation or altered tension. Similarly, excess intracellular inclusions or vacuoles may portray increased storage of metabolites such as lipid or glycogen (Fig. 2.19), the latter reflecting disturbances or absence of anaerobic (glycolytic) enzymes. Sometimes vacuoles are rimmed or have membranous inclusions. Occasionally, non-specific proteinaceous inclusions (e.g. nemaline bodies), Z-band streaming, or absent myosin ATPase indicate disturbances in the filamentous contractile arrays and may be due to improper development or degeneration. Gross changes in the metabolic and contractile components of a muscle fibre can lead to fibre type conversion and hence predominance or *fibre type grouping* of either or both of the major fibre types within a muscle (Fig. 2.20). Such

Fig. 2.18.

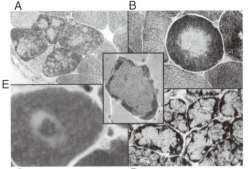

A   B

E

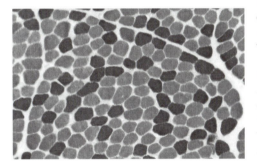

C   D

Fig. 2.19.

Fig. 2.20.

Fig. 2.18. Various alterations in intracellular composition are shown. (A) Multi- or minicores, NADHtr; (B) central core, NADHtr; (C) target fibre, ATPase; (D) lobulated fibres, NADHtr; (E) ragged-red fibre, Trichrome, × 200.

Fig. 2.19. The uneven staining shows excess storage of glycogen within the muscle fibres in a case of glycogen storage myopathy. PAS, × 200.

Fig. 2.20. Fibre type grouping of light (type 1) fibres is readily apparent in this biopsy. ATPase, × 100.

alterations are often a consequence of neural or endocrine disorders. Proliferation of the internal membranes (sarcoplasmic reticulum, t-tubules) into visible tubular aggregates is often non-specific but may also be associated with defects in their accompanying enzymes or receptors (see later). Defects in the external membrane are more serious and have already been alluded to above in relation to calcium-induced degeneration and are revisited in the section on Myopathies. Other architectural defects leading to apparent internal alterations are the splitting of fibres often seen in chronic overload (sometimes appearing as internal whorls in section), hyaline (or glassy) fibres where hypercontraction bands have occurred during degeneration, and the various placements and multiplicity of internalized nuclei which may be due to deficient development, degeneration or regeneration.

Other changes

Other changes that occur in skeletal muscles may involve the connective tissue, haemopoietic, vascular, or neural elements. Rapid proliferation of connective tissue (fibrosis) and fatty replacement is common following chronic atrophy, degeneration or loss of muscle fibres (Fig. 2.21) although it can also occur in specific connective tissue disorders. Muscle fibres tend to become rounded and

Fig. 2.21.   **Fig. 2.22.**

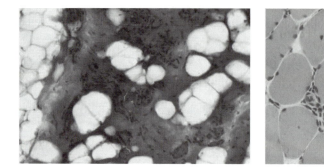

Fig. 2.23.   **Fig. 2.24.**

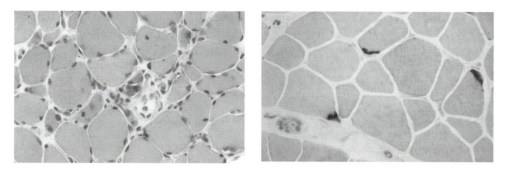

Fig. 2.21. Almost complete fibrosis in this specimen shows only the end-stage of a muscle disease. Trichrome, × 200.

Fig. 2.22. Excess white blood cells between the muscle fibres and phagocytosis by macrophages indicates an inflammatory response. H&E, × 200.

Fig. 2.23. This biopsy from an individual with an inflammatory myopathy shows blood vessels with thickened walls. H&E, × 200.

Fig. 2.24. The neuromuscular junctions are revealed by heavy staining with non-specific esterase, × 200.

separated from their neighbours by thickened endomysium which may lead to subsequent ischaemia. Invasion of excess white blood cells or macrophages between and within the muscle fibres is prominent in many of the inflammatory disorders as part of the immune response (Fig. 2.22) and can lead to subsequent muscle fibre destruction. Increased capillarization may result from increased metabolic demands on the muscle and a high capillary to muscle fibre ratio is usual with type 1 or aerobic muscle fibres. However, thickened vessel walls, especially where the basement membrane is involved (Fig. 2.23) is usually associated with inflammation, immune, or specific vascular disorders. Neural elements are rarely increased though there may be an apparent excess of fibres with neuromuscular junctions when sections are obtained from the motor point which occurs midway along the muscle fibre length (Fig. 2.24). More commonly there is a decrease or abnormality of the neural elements in denervating conditions as explained later.

Artefactual anomalies

Sometimes natural but rare occurrences within muscle samples such as myotendinous junctions or muscle spindles may be mistaken for splitting and fibrosis or muscle regeneration respectively. On other occasions poor preparative technique may induce apparently pathological features such as fibre splitting (cracks in the section), vacuoles (ice damage), enzyme loss (wrong pH or temperature, or fixation damage), or metabolite storage (incomplete washing). Most of these can be avoided with experience and the use of good control material and technique (Cumming *et al.*, 1994). Further useful references regarding pathological reactions of skeletal muscle may be found in Carpenter and Karpati (1984), Mastaglia and Walton (1992), Dubowitz (1985) and Walton *et al.* (1994).

NEUROMUSCULAR DISORDERS

Although each specific abnormality of muscle has been described above in isolation, they generally occur in combination and follow a specific spatial and temporal sequence according to the nature of the insult or defect. Therefore, in order to interpret muscle abnormalities found in poultry it is necessary to understand first the pattern of the major disease processes which affect skeletal muscle. To fully appreciate the range and nosology of those diseases it is important to realize that muscles are closely integrated with components of the nervous system (Fig. 2.25) and that their fibres work in conjunction with motor neurones as functional units (the *motor units*). Thus, muscle disorders are roughly divided into two main groups: those in which the muscle fibre bears the primary defect (*myopathic*) and those in which defects in the nervous system are the cause of the muscle disease (*neurogenic*). Of course, some changes are secondary to abnormalities in other systems and in others the primary cause is as yet unknown. Nevertheless a classification of muscle

Fig. 2.25.

Fig. 2.26.

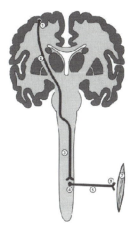

Myopathic	**Neurogenic**
• Congenital	• Central
• Dystrophic	• Peripheral
• Inflammatory	• Junctional
• Metabolic	
• Ion Channel	**Syndromes**
• Secondary	• LGD, FSH, SPD

Fig. 2.25. Diagrammatic representation of the relationship between components of the nervous and muscular systems.
Fig. 2.26. Classification of human neuromuscular disorders.

diseases for humans has evolved (Fig. 2.26) which forms a good basis for describing muscle disorders in other phylogenetically advanced vertebrates. Alternative classifications may be based on 'clinical' presentation or on the origin of the insult into 'acquired' or 'genetic' muscle disorders. More complete accounts may be found in Cumming *et al.* (1994); Walton *et al.* (1994) and Weller *et al.* (1997), and the latest updates are regularly published as an appendix to the journal *Neuromuscular Disorders* along with current genetic information.

Experimental pathology

It must also be emphasized that much of our present understanding of these myopathological mechanisms has been acquired from experimental situations in which cell cultures, animals, or human muscles have been subjected to altered physiological demand or insult. For example skeletal muscles have been subjected to exercise, altered gravity, disuse, tenotomy, overuse, stretch, myectomy of synergist or anatagonist, denervation, electrical stimulation, transplantation, temperature changes, perturbation of the endocrine or vascular system, altered nutrition, irradiation, application of drugs, toxins, metabolic inhibitors, growth factors, infectious agents, or genetic manipulation (see McComas, 1977; Bedi *et al.*, 1982; Goldspink, 1983; Florini, 1985; Pette, 1980, 1990; Saltin and Gollnick, 1983; Taylor *et al.*, 1985; Vrbova *et al.*, 1995 for references). It is also well understood that the end stages of myopathologies, whether originating from an experimental, myopathic or neurogenic basis, usually look very similar (essentially massive muscle fibre atrophy and loss, and extensive fibrosis and fatty replacement) thus making it difficult to elucidate the underlying cause.

Myopathic Muscle Diseases

In these disorders, where the primary lesions occur in the muscle fibres, muscles are usually equally and symmetrically affected. Onset is often in the more proximal and weight-bearing muscles but age of onset is variable. Symptoms may include weakness, wasting, fatigue, and pain associated with more severely affected muscles. Some may be described as the destructive myopathies where the muscles degenerate and achieve varying success at regeneration, others involve biochemical aberrations of enzymes or membranes and show altered intracellular composition with little muscle destruction. A 'myopathic muscle biopsy' is often recognizable microscopically by increased variation in fibre size, with degeneration and regeneration or altered internal fibre characteristics.

Congenital

These disorders are often due to arrested development of the muscle fibres and are distinguished by their morphological features such as arrest at the myotube stage (centronuclear or myotubular myopathy, Fig. 2.27), cessation of growth of a fibre type population (CFTD, congenital fibre type disproportion (Fig. 2.28), or type 1 fibre hypotrophy) and anomalies in the distribution of

Fig. 2.27.

A   B

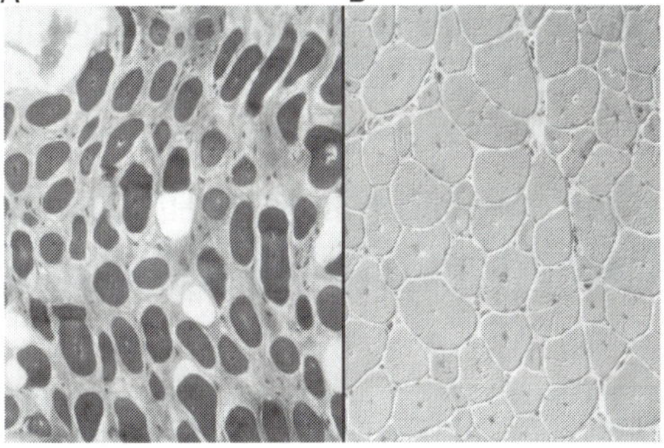

Fig. 2.28.

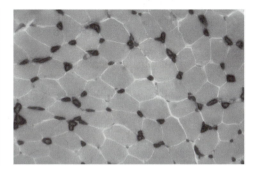

Fig. 2.29.

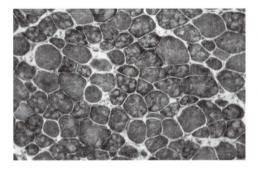

Fig. 2.27. Congenital muscle disorders showing arrested growth of muscle fibres at the myotubular stage in (A) an infant, Trichrome × 400; (B) an adult, H&E, × 100.
Fig. 2.28. Congenital muscle disorder showing differential growth and development of the different fibres types. ATPase, × 100.
Fig. 2.29. Multi- and minicores in a non-specific congenital myopathy. NADHtr, × 200.

various types of filament (e.g. desmin, tropomyosin (in nemaline myopathy), myotubularin, merosin) or organelle. In particular, disturbances in mitochondrial distribution may lead to the appearance of pale areas on enzyme staining known as central cores, multicores or minicores (Fig. 2.29). However, at least one of these disorders, central core disease, is known to involve a gene deletion affecting the ryanodine receptor located at the triad rather than the mitochondria directly (Zhang *et al.*, 1993). Muscle abnormalities in these disorders are often non-progressive and do not show destructive changes.

Dystrophies

These are progressive, destructive myopathies many of which arise due to faulty or deleted genes coding for membrane or membrane associated proteins (Emery, 1993; Partridge, 1993). The most well understood are Duchenne and Becker muscular dystrophy (DMD and BMD) which lack dystrophin (a rod-like protein attaching the contractile filaments to the plasma membrane; Matsumura and Campbell, 1994). In these disorders weakness and wasting is progressive through human childhood and death occurs in early adulthood. Early appearance of hyaline fibres, gross muscle degeneration and regeneration, with the former predominating in later stages and fibrosis, are the distinctive muscle abnormalities (Fig. 2.30). Due to the enormous muscle damage, vastly raised levels of muscle-specific CK are found in the bloodstream and provide a convenient diagnostic tool.[2] A variety of animal correlates have been associated with this disorder (mouse, hamster, mink, chicken and quokka) but only those showing similar gene deletions are now accepted as true models and include the mdx mouse, CMD cat, and GRMD dog. Similar to these dystrophinopathies in pathological mechanisms (i.e. damaged membranes and calcium-mediated destruction), but varying in clinical severity, are a number of disorders in which other components of the dystrophin glycoprotein complex (DGC) within the sarcolemma are abnormal. Many of the limb girdle dystrophies affecting primarily proximal muscles belong to this group.

Inflammatory

Inflammatory myopathies are a most common group of muscle disorders and many are completely treatable with steroids. They vary from mild myositis, where a limited invasion of white blood cells and a few degenerating/regenerating muscle fibres are observed through to a massive inflammatory response and muscle destruction with varying degrees of regeneration (often prominent around the edges of fascicles) as in polymyositis, dermatomyositis and inclusion body myositis (Fig. 2.31). In the latter, skin reactions also occur and their is also associated muscle pain. A likely cause of many of these muscle responses, particularly in non-human organisms, is infection (bacterial, viral, protozoal, or parasitic; see Pallis and Lewis, 1988) and often leads to a focal reaction which may not be present in every tissue sample making diagnosis difficult. There is presently little understanding of the causes of the non-infective inflammatory myopathies although some are thought to be due primarily to vascular pathology (vasculitides).

Fig. 2.30.   **Fig. 2.31.**

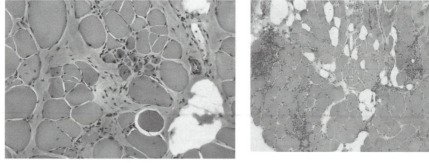

Fig. 2.30. Combination of histopathological changes in a biopsy from a patient with advanced Duchenne muscular dystrophy. H&E, × 200.
Fig. 2.31. Varying degrees of inflammation, degeneration, regeneration, and fibrosis in an inflammatory myopathy. H&E, × 100.

---

[2]Serum CK elevation is a non-specific indicator of muscle damage and may also be raised in other myopathies, obligate carriers of dystrophies, and in the normal ageing population (Keller *et al.*, 1996).

Metabolic

Myopathies due primarily to defective or missing enzymes or associated carrier molecules involved in metabolism often lead to accumulation of substrates creating vacuoles within the muscle fibre. Examples include disorders of glycolytic metabolism (glycogenoses, where glycogen is stored; Fig. 2.32), lipid storage disorders (Fig. 2.33), or the mitochondrial cytopathies (CPEO, MELAS, MERRF, MNGIE, NARP; see Weller *et al.*, 1997) in which both proliferation of abnormal mitochondria and lipid storage may occur (Fig. 2.34). The latter group of disorders have a complex aetiology and inheritance since part of the respiratory chain enzymes are encoded by myonuclear DNA and part by mitochondrial DNA. Such lesions may therefore occur in a mosaic manner within individual muscle fibres. The result of such myopathies is often decreased ability to exercise, rapid fatigue, lactic acid production, susceptibility to stress induced muscle damage, and eventually muscle degeneration, weakness and wasting. For obvious reasons muscles having different complements of the two major fibre types will show differing susceptibility to these diseases.

Fig. 2.32.

Fig. 2.33.

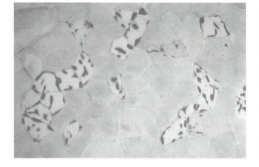

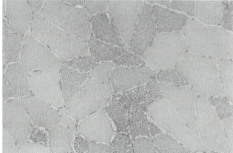

Fig. 2.34.

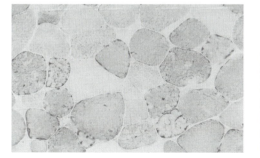

Fig. 2.32. Vacuolar glycogen storage disorder type IV. PAS, × 200.
Fig. 2.33. Lipid storage disorder. Oil Red O, × 200.
Fig. 2.34. Mitochondrial cytopathy showing disturbances and absences of enzyme activity. Cytochrome oxidase, × 200.

Ion channel

This grouping of muscle disorders has only recently become apparent since a number of differing clinical and pathological manifestations of muscle abnormality have succumbed to molecular genetic analysis (Lehmann-Horn and Rudel, 1996). These include disorders of chloride channels (leading to myotonia), sodium channels (hyperkalaemic periodic paralysis), calcium (or dihydropyridine receptor) channels (hypokalaemic periodic paralysis), and potassium (or calcium-release) channels (malignant hyperthemia). In the latter disorder (first described in 1960 by Denborough and Lovell) halothane anaesthesia can often precipitate muscle weakness, extensive muscle necrosis, CK elevation, myoglobinuria, raised serum potassium, raised temperature, and even death (Gronert, 1986; McLennan and Philips, 1992; McLennan et al., 1992). In man, the defective gene is co-localized with that for central core disease and is responsible for encoding the ryanodine receptor (calcium-release channel of the sarcoplasmic reticulum) within the triad (Gillard et al., 1991; Quane et al., 1993, 1994; Martin et al., 1998). Similar mutations in the ryanodine receptor gene have been reported for the pig where malignant hypothermia is associated with the porcine stress syndrome (Fujii et al., 1991). The excitability and contractility of muscle fibres is under the control of their external and internal membranes, thus functional deficits are wide and varied in these disorders from muscle weakness and intermittent paralysis to overactivity and damage. Increased fibre size variation, multiplicity of internal nuclei, and central cores are seen in myotonia. In other cases defective internal membranes proliferate and form tubular aggregates visible by light or electron microscopy, or no muscle myopathology is identifiable.

Secondary

These, often destructive myopathies, are reactions to externally applied or sourced toxins (venoms, alcohol), drugs, trauma, or infectious agents (Fig. 2.35). Basically, membrane damage induced by these agents leads to muscle degeneration, inflammation, and regeneration, the degree and distribution of which varies with the severity, locality and duration of the insult. Some agents, however, may merely disturb the metabolic apparatus leading to vacuolation (e.g. following chloroquine excess) and perhaps perturbation of mitochondrial enzymes (e.g. after barbiturate overdosage). Disorders of the endocrine system may also lead to a secondary myopathy (Kaminski and Ruff, 1994; Moxley, 1994). For example acromegaly (pituitary hypersecretion) leads to muscle weakness and lobulation of muscle fibres (Kinfu et al., 1989), hypothyroidism produces an excess of type 1 muscle fibres, hyperthyroidism and hyperparathyroidism give rise to non-specific muscle abnormalities. Chronic steroid excess (natural or iatrogenic) leads to type 2 fibre atrophy; although this non-specific change is also common during disuse and ageing. Some alterations may also be corrected by administration of synthetic hormones (Mahon et al., 1994).

Fig. 2.35.   **Fig. 2.36.**

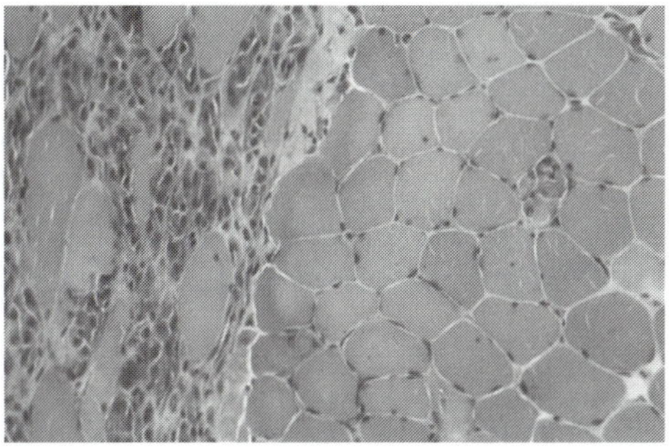

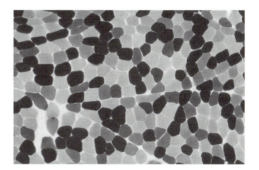

Fig. 2.37.

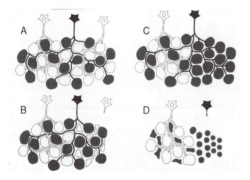

Fig. 2.35. Toxic induced myopathic (degenerative and regenerative) changes. H&E, × 200.

Fig. 2.36. Normal motor unit distribution showing checkerboard pattern of muscle fibre types. ATPase, × 150.

Fig. 2.37. Diagram of motor units undergoing denervation and re-innervation. (A) normal, (B) denervated, (C) reinnervated, (D) later wave of denervation.

Neurogenic Muscle Diseases

These disorders involve abnormalities of muscle structure or function due to lesions within the nervous system, particularly those involving the lower motor neurone, peripheral nerve, or the neuromuscular junction (Fig. 2.36). Onset of muscle pathology, weakness and wasting is often in the more distal muscles, asymmetric, and can vary with age. In many cases whole motor units are affected (Fig. 2.37). A 'neurogenic muscle biopsy' is therefore often recognizable microscopically by a bimodal variation in fibre size frequently including groups of small angulated fibres, fibre type grouping, and little sign of degeneration and regeneration or altered internal fibre characteristics.

Central

Disorders of the anterior horn cell (motor neurone disease/amyotrophic lateral sclerosis, spinal muscular atrophy, spinal cord injury) within the spinal cord lead to disturbance of the trophic and excitatory influences arriving at the muscle fibres belonging to that motor unit. These denervated muscle fibres atrophy and become squashed between fibres of healthy motor units (Fig. 2.38) and may later wither and degenerate or become re-innervated from collateral branches of healthy nerve fibres thus transforming their fibre type characteristics and forming fibre type groups (Fig. 2.39). Target fibres are often

Fig. 2.38. **Fig. 2.39.**

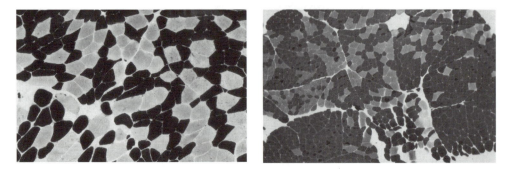

Fig. 2.38. Muscle biopsy showing denervation atrophy of type 2 (dark) motor units. ATPase, × 150.
Fig. 2.39. Large areas of fibre type grouping of both fibre types in a well-compensated denervating condition. ATPase, × 100.

associated with re-innervation. Subsequent denervation will, of course, lead to grouped atrophy, pyknotic fibres, and eventually muscular wasting and secondary myopathic changes as the muscle undergoes end-stage fibrosis and fatty replacement. Some compensatory hypertrophy of healthy muscle fibres will also be apparent. Therefore central neurogenic disorders depict as varying degrees of muscle weakness and wasting in the early stages (depending on the ratio of denervation to re-innervation) without fibre necrosis and consequently raised CK levels. Massive central denervation *in utero* can lead to collapse of the muscular system and early death of the individual. Recent molecular genetic studies suggest that some of these disorders are related to accelerated neuronal apoptosis (Rodrigues *et al.*, 1995; Roy *et al.*, 1995). Central neuronal disorders affecting upper motor neurones or the cerebellar system affect muscle functionally but usually show little muscle pathology.

Peripheral
Lesions of the peripheral nerve (e.g. trauma, pressure, peripheral neuropathy) or of its coverings (demyelinating disorders) lead to denervation and wholesale muscular atrophy regardless of motor unit type usually with accompanying sensory loss. End-stage atrophy or subsequent re-innervation may occur leading to fibre type grouping depending on the duration and severity of the lesion.

Junctional
The neuromuscular junction although affected in the previous two categories of disease is also subject to specific primary lesions whereby the motor end-plate region shows pathological change because of reduced acetylcholine release, or acetylcholine receptor, immunological or related anomalies (myasthenia gravis, myasthenic syndromes). However, muscle pathology is minimal in these disorders although function is disturbed, particularly initiation and maintenance of muscle contraction and is best detected electrophysiologically.

Miscellaneous Syndromes

Clinically and anatomically defined syndromes in man (limb girdle dystrophy, facio-scapulo-humeral dystrophy, scapulo-peroneal dystrophy) show a variety of myopathological changes which often differ between individuals (Mahon *et al.*, 1990). However, recent molecular genetic studies are beginning to redistribute aetiological subsets of these syndromes into the above disease classifications notwithstanding that some may remain multifactorial. It is also recognized that different genetic abnormalities may produce similar clinical phenotypes thus confusing diagnosis and treatment even further.

MUSCLE ABNORMALITIES IN TURKEYS AND OTHER SPECIES

Muscle abnormalities and neuromuscular disorders in other species have been described and include glycogenoses (in cattle, sheep, dogs, cats and quail), mitochondrial cytopathy (dog), myasthenia gravis (dog), myotonia (goat, dog, horse) and the muscular dystrophies already referred to in mink, dog, cat, hamster, mouse and chicken (Bradley *et al.*, 1988). Richards *et al.* (1988) also described a congenital progressive muscular dystrophy in merino sheep which show histopathological features of myotonic dystrophy and metabolic disorder. Numerous toxic and nutritional myopathies have been reported across a wide range of species, some attributable to toxic plants or metals (see Austic and Scott, 1984), others to selenium or vitamin E deficiency (see Bradley *et al.*, 1988; Cardona *et al.*, 1992). Lower motor neurone (neurogenic) disorders of viral, nutritional or hereditable origin are found in cattle, pigs, horses, dogs, cats, rabbits and mice (Bradley *et al.*, 1988). Unfortunately, the causes of many animal myopathies are unknown since epidemiological data are limited (ill animals are often left by their peers to die), and it is difficult to obtain accurate clinical data because active 'patient' cooperation is limited! Serum CK levels remain a good diagnostic test of assumed muscle necrosis in live animals (Hollands *et al.*, 1980). *Selective breeding* has lead to double muscling particularly in cattle and increased muscle yield in pigs and domestic poultry. Unfortunately, in the pig, this has often also selected for *porcine stress syndrome* (PSS) where increased stress due to transport, excitement, raised temperature, or anaesthesia gives rise to disease (muscle degeneration, hyaline fibres, internal nuclei, moth-eaten fibres; Sosnicki, 1987), watery meat (pale soft exudate, PSE), rapid rises in body temperature, and sudden death (Gronert, 1986). This porcine malignant hyperthermia (with a defective ryanodine receptor) has already been alluded to under 'Ion Channel Myopathies'. For an excellent review of muscle thermogenesis see Block (1994).

Avian myopathies are rare and have received limited attention except for chicken inherited muscular dystrophy which is known to involve progressive muscle weakness and degenerative changes and fibrosis, especially in white muscles (Wilson *et al.*, 1979; Bradley *et al.*, 1988). For further details of muscle abnormalities in chickens see Barnard *et al.* (1982) and Pizzey *et al.* (1983). There is also an acid maltase (glycogenosis) of quail, and a progressive myopathy with extensive fibrosis and necrosis in the duck (Bradley *et al.*, 1988).

TURKEY MUSCLE DISEASES

Compared to the work on general pathology, infection and toxicology of turkeys there has been relatively little research published on turkey muscle pathology. Most of the information that is available concerns degenerative muscle changes brought about by physical means particularly during capture, slaughter, or other stress. The general opinion is that many of these myopathies are growth-related, suggesting that some aspects of muscle growth have not kept pace with bird growth, and muscle degeneration has occurred leading to deep pectoral myopathy, focal myopathy, leg weakness and oedema (Sosnicki and Wilson, 1992). Many of the diseases and syndromes described below therefore overlap or are referred to under varying names by different authors. In the present review we have deliberately kept these descriptions separate since it would be unwise to clump together differing pathologies until a proper basis for their aetiology is established, a lesson well-heeded from the human neuromuscular literature. The majority of reports have arisen from the laboratories of Sosnicki, Wilson and Ferkut in the USA, Swatland and Barbut in Canada, Cherel and Wyers in France, and Siller in Scotland. Descriptions of incidental muscle abnormalities found in modern fast-growing commercial lines are discussed in the subsequent section.

Deep pectoral myopathy

First identified by Dickinson *et al.* (1968) and also known as Oregon disease, this is one of the most common muscle disorders of turkeys and is thought to be hereditable but requiring environmental modifiers to express it clinically (Harper *et al.*, 1975, 1983). For experimental purposes a specific deep pectoral myopathy selected line (DPMS), where the incidence is between 80% and 90%, has been raised in Oregon (Harper *et al.*, 1981). The disorder is limited to the supracoracoid muscle (supracoracoideus, pectoralis profundus, deep pectoral, or fillet[3]) which, in well muscled turkeys (particularly older breeders over 24 weeks), shows muscle hypercontraction, necrosis, fibrosis, elevated serum CK, and a reddish followed by greenish discoloration (Harper *et al.*, 1975; Henrichs *et al.*, 1979; Siller and Wight, 1978; Siller, 1985; Siller *et al.*, 1979a, b; Swash *et al.*, 1980; Hollands *et al.*, 1981; Fig. 2.40). Affected muscles occur in both sexes, unilaterally and bilaterally (Harper *et al.*, 1975) and give rise to dry, stringy meat. Harper and Helfer (1972) have shown that the disorder is not associated with dietary insufficiency or toxicity. It is generally thought that the disorder is due to ischaemia and muscle infarction brought about by excessive muscle growth within an inelastic sheath, possibly in a muscle with deficient arterial branching. The disorder has been compared to the human 'anterior tibial compartment syndrome'. Our own observations on five inbred sire lines of BUT stock confirm the tight muscle sheath from which the muscle extrudes following fascial incision (M. Mahon, S. Gilpin and J. Mills, unpublished data). Experimental studies have shown that the ischaemia and degeneration may be

---

[3]The reader is referred to Shufeldt (1890), Marshall (1960), George and Berger (1966), Harvey *et al.* (1968), Baumel *et al.* (1979) and Abourachid (1991a, b) for anatomical nomenclature of avian musculature.

Fig. 2.40.

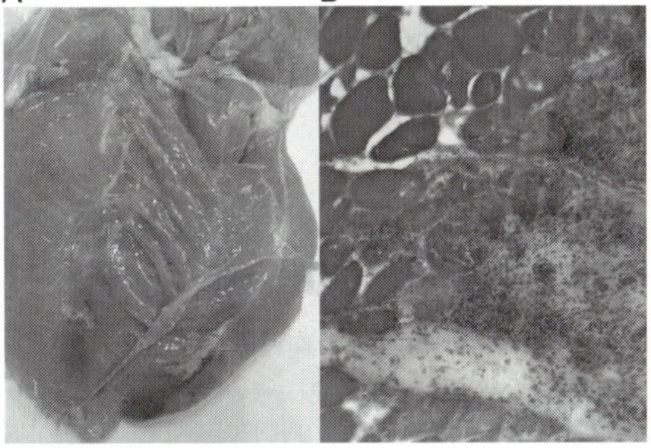

A   B

Fig. 2.40. Turkey muscle showing (A) green discoloration and (B) histopathological changes in Oregon disease. H&E × 200.

prevented by fasciotomy (Siller *et al.*, 1979b). Henrichs *et al.* (1979) suggest that overdevelopment of the supracoracoid is not matched by its vascular supply, and Orr and Riddell (1977) and Siller *et al.* (1978) have noted its similarity to experimentally induced infarct or vascular occlusion. In susceptible birds, exercise, excessive or forced wing-flapping or nervous stimulation may precipitate the myopathy or hasten its onset (Siller *et al.*, 1979a; Wight *et al.*, 1979; Hollands *et al.*, 1981, 1983; Harper *et al.*, 1983). Results from experimental aspirin feeding in an attempt to reduce the stroke-like effects are equivocal (Harper *et al.*, 1983). The disorder is also apparent in well muscled broiler chickens (Page and Fletcher, 1975). Precise quantitative data on the capillarization of turkey pectoralis and biceps muscles (Sosnicki *et al.*, 1991a; Sosnicki and Wilson, 1991) support the suggestion of limited vascular supply to explain these hypotheses. Interestingly, similar data are now becoming available for other avian muscles in providing a better understanding of structure–function correlations (Torrella *et al.*, 1998). A fuller account of the quantitative relationship between the respiratory, cardiovascular and muscular systems is given in Weibel (1984). Newer unbiased stereological methods (Artacho-Perula and Roldan-Villobos, 1995; Nyengaard *et al.*, 1996) have yet to be applied to the study of turkey muscle capillaries and may reveal interesting spatial data of functional significance. Our own observations of affected muscles support the hypothesis of reperfusion injury as described in other situations of muscle damage (Gute *et al.*, 1998; Rocca *et al.*, 1998).

Degenerative myopathy

This is synonymous with deep pectoral myopathy or 'green muscle disease' as described above, affecting specifically supracoracoideus muscle, and giving rise to muscle necrosis and elevated serum CK (Dickinson *et al.*, 1968; Harper *et al.*, 1969, 1975; Jones *et al.*, 1974; Grunder *et al.*, 1979; Hollands *et al.*, 1980). The disorder is also found in chickens (Grunder *et al.*, 1984).

Turkey leg oedema

This condition, also known as *transport myopathy* of turkeys, was systematically studied by Sosnicki and co-workers in 1988. It was generally noted that the condition occurred more commonly in selected turkey lines, was especially prominent in adductor muscles and may involve impaired circulation (Merck Veterinary Manual, 1986). Sosnicki *et al.* (1988a) showed the oedematous muscles to have excess connective tissue, fatty replacement and separation of fascicles, necrosis, hypercontracted fibres, pyknotic nuclei and mononuclear cells in vessel walls. Some alteration, particularly weakness and diffusion, of histochemical enzyme staining was also observed. Of major significance was their report of the same findings in non-oedematous muscles (both breast and leg) from the same and non-affected birds, suggesting a general occurrence of myopathic changes in commercial turkeys which may not always manifest clinically. This point is discussed further in the section on growth related changes below.

Focal myopathy

Maranopot *et al.* (1968) first reported a focal myopathy of turkey pectoral and cervical muscles typified by poor condition of the bird and lameness. Myopathological changes observed included hyaline fibres and segmental fibre necrosis which were more common in red than white muscles. Other workers (Sosnicki *et al.*, 1988a, b, 1989, 1991a, b; Wilson, 1990; Wilson *et al.*, 1990; Sosnicki and Wilson, 1992) have reported similar features in clinically normal commercial turkeys. Necrosis and phagocytosis have been described in pectoralis (breast) and iliofibularis (leg) muscles to include several adjacent muscle fibres and are accompanied by inflammation and fatty tissue replacement. Ultrastructural features show typical degenerative changes within the muscle fibres and serum CK is raised (Sosnicki *et al.*, 1991a; Sosnicki and Wilson, 1992). In the latter review the authors emphasize the excessive growth in muscle fibre diameter which outstrips the accompanying connective tissue and microcirculation as the primary cause of the disorder (see later). Furthermore, experimental studies on exercise-induced focal degeneration in rat muscles would seem to support this idea (Binkhorst *et al.*, 1989). The onset of rigor mortis and decline in meat quality, texture and colour connected with this disorder have been associated with handling conditions and suggest increased muscle excitability. Similar histopathological changes have been reported by Cherel *et al.* (1995) but were not restricted to deep pectoral muscles.

Relative-ischaemia syndrome

Because of the interest raised in studies of deep pectoral myopathy Sosnicki *et al.* (1991a) have studied the capillary bed in muscles from turkeys prone to ischaemic degenerative changes. Although there was no evidence of muscle fibre size differences in relative-ischaemia syndrome (RIS) birds compared with unaffected birds, there was a significant reduction in capillary density and capillary/muscle fibre ratios. The authors suggest that this may be due to the relative sedentary activity of the modern commercial turkey. As with many other descriptors of turkey muscle pathology RIS appears to be part of the spectrum of the focal myopathy described earlier.

Rear limb necrotizing myopathy

Cardona *et al.* (1992) have reported a myopathic syndrome (paresis or paralysis) in commercial turkeys with a rear-limb necrotizing myopathy. In their study the condition was found in 17 flocks, with a mean mortality of 2.3%. Onset of the symptoms was around 7 weeks and was accompanied by an approximate twofold elevation in CK and pale streaking of muscles. In some birds there was also myofibre degeneration but no fibrosis; some muscle fibres displayed a foamy cytoplasm and others showed signs of regeneration. There was also evidence of cell proliferation adjacent to the sarcolemma and their published micrographs are reminiscent of a toxic or inflammatory myopathy. The changes were found both in rear limb and abdominal muscles (predominantly slow-twitch muscles) including fibularis longus, flexor perforans, gastrocnemius, tibialis cranialis, tibialis caudalis, sartorius, tensor fascia lata, biceps femoris, semitendinosus, semimembranosus, quadriceps femoris, adductors, gracilis, and pectineus. The breast muscles (pectoralis superficialis and pectoralis profundus) and wing muscles appeared normal. No obvious cause of this myopathy was apparent, however, Cardona *et al.* suggested that the histopathological picture resembled monensin toxicity (although the antibiotic was present at normal levels), possibly aggravated by warm weather. These two factors (ionophores and heat stress) are further discussed below.

Capture and handling myopathy

Grey (1989) extensively reviewed the various factors in commercial processing affecting meat quality. Injuries, such as broken bones, bruising and blisters caused by the capture and caging process are frequent (Taylor and Helbecka, 1968; Mayes, 1980; Barbut *et al.*, 1990) and lead to a downgrading costing the US poultry industry alone around $90 million per year (Wesley, 1986). However, only few workers have reported on specific muscle damage due to the capture process (Spraker *et al.*, 1987). In this study, Spraker and colleagues noted that up to 48% of wild turkeys showed white streaks within breast and leg muscles and even higher occurrences of microscopic lesions (including basophilia, enlarged nuclei, necrosis). Although they attributed these finding to the stress of trapping, transportation and housing there is no evidence that such features were not previously present in the birds. Several controlled studies in the commercial industry have shown the effects of immediate pre-mortem (including struggle and heat stress (see below)) and early post-mortem processing in relation to colour, glycolysis, protein solubility and shear on turkey meat (Ma *et al.*, 1971; Ma and Addis, 1973; Froning *et al.*, 1978; van Hoof, 1979; Northcutt *et al.*, 1994, 1998a), but there is still a dearth of information on morphological changes of the muscle fibres themselves.

Hereditary muscular dystrophy

Inherited muscular dystrophy has been reported for the chicken (Wilson *et al.*, 1979, 1988; Bradley *et al.*, 1988). This disorder is exemplified by degenerative muscle changes, fibrosis, and an associated progressive weakness. A similar condition in the turkey, possibly involving a single autosomal recessive gene abnormality, primarily affects the pectoral muscles (Harper and Parker, 1964, 1967; Sutherland, 1974). Tripp and Schmitz (1982) have reported elevated serum CK levels in such turkeys both at rest and following exercise. However, confusion between this condition and degenerative, deep pectoral and focal myopathy arises when comparing further histopathological studies from the literature (Maranopot *et al.*, 1968; Jones *et al.*, 1974; see also Sosnicki *et al.*, 1988a, b).

Pale soft exudate

Several studies on the effect of pre-slaughter conditions (especially heat stress) on turkey meat have commented upon the pale colour, low pH, toughness and poor water-holding capacity of breast muscles in some birds (Babji *et al.*, 1982). Recently, a number of workers have described pale soft exudative (PSE) meat in chickens (Barbut, 1997b) and turkey hens analogous to the porcine disorder (Sosnicki, 1993; Ferket, 1995; Barbut, 1996, 1997a; Pietrzak *et al.*, 1997). Indeed, its incidence has been estimated as ranging from 5 to 30% in commercial turkey flocks (McCurdy *et al.*, 1996). Although post-mortem meat from PSE birds shows a rapid pH decline, Barbut (1996, 1997a, b) showed that PSE pectoralis muscles could be readily detected using a simple colour measurement in the processing plant in his studies of broilers and turkeys. Swatland (1987, 1991, 1993; Swatland and Barbut, 1995) has also reported extensively on the use of fibre-optic probes and spectrophotometry in assessing meat colour. Histopathological studies of PSE turkey muscles do not appear to have been carried out; however, many of the microscopic features observed in PSE pigs are similar to those observed in focal and other myopathies of turkeys. There is, however, histomorphometric muscle biopsy data for turkey breast muscles showing discoloured scallops (Wyers *et al.*, 1992) but these were no different to unaffected muscles except for their lower glycogen levels. Pietrzak *et al.* (1997) in an extensive biochemical study showed that irreversible myosin insolubility was a decisive factor in the early onset rigor-mortis associated with PSE in turkeys. Suggested causes include connective tissue maturation not keeping pace with muscle fibre growth thus allowing muscle rupturing, microvascular defects, limited tolerance to stressors, defective ryanodine receptor genes, and production of excess reactive oxygen metabolites (see review by Ferket, 1995). In respect of the latter, vitamin E supplements to the diet have been shown to reduce the incidence of pale meat (Sheldon *et al.*, 1997). Experimentally induced heat stress in turkeys has recently been shown to produce similar results (McKee and Sams, 1997, 1998) as described below (Experimental Pathology). Analogous findings in relation to heat stress and CK release have also been reported for the domestic fowl (Mitchell and Sandercock, 1995) and are discussed later in Chapter 3.

Ionophore induced myopathy

Ionophores or ion carriers (monensin, salinomycin, narasin, lasalocid) are used in the farming and poultry industry for their anticoccidial effects. From spontaneous and experimental intoxications it is well established that monensin toxicosis occurs in horses, cattle, sheep, pigs, dogs and birds and produces cardiac and skeletal muscle necrosis and elevated serum CK (see van Fleet *et al.*, 1983; Ficken *et al.*, 1989; Dowling, 1992; for references). In swine, damage was greatest in muscle with high proportions of type 1 fibres (van Fleet *et al.*, 1983). Stuart (1978, 1983) reported the toxic effects of monensin and salinomycin on adult turkeys and Halvorson *et al.* (1982) showed that even low levels of monensin and salinomycin caused mortality and clinical effects (dyspnoea, paresis, fever) in adult turkeys but did not affect growing turkeys. Halvorson *et al.* also carried out microscopic studies on the muscles of affected birds which showed extensive degeneration, hyaline fibres, nuclear proliferation and myofibre calcification. Further studies on turkeys (Wages and Ficken, 1988; Ficken *et al.*, 1989) confirmed these finding and also noted leg trembling and weakness, massive sarcolemmal nuclear proliferation in the muscles, and axonal degeneration. In a detailed experimental study of monensin feeding to turkeys (Cardona *et al.*, 1993) the above histopathological changes were confirmed and dose-related effects were observed in relation to the number of damaged myofibres in leg muscles. The relevance of ionophore effects on membrane permeability (particularly monensin to sodium transport) and muscle cell homeostasis are discussed in Chapter 3.

Nutritional myopathy

Nutritional deficiency diseases in poultry have been reviewed by Austic and Scott (1984). In particular, the authors noted that vitamin E and selenium deficiency may lead to pectoral myopathy. Shaptala (1973) also reported on the experimental production of 'white muscle disease' in the gut of turkeys fed oxidized fish oil and altered carotene and vitamin A levels. Gill *et al.* (1980) have also investigated the effects of selenium and vitamin E on this disorder.

Toxic myopathy

A number of workers have reported the weakening effects of coffee senna (*Cassia occidentalis*) on chicken muscles (Simpson *et al.*, 1971; Graziano *et al.*, 1983; Novilla, 1984). These workers also noted gross and microscopic lesions in pectoral and leg muscles similar to those for ionophore intoxication described above.

Other experimental pathologies

The effects of experimental vascular occlusion (Orr and Riddell, 1977; Siller *et al.*, 1978) and exercise of susceptible birds (Harper *et al.*, 1983) and their similarity to deep pectoral myopathy have already been mentioned above. For an excellent review of muscle damage produced by exercise the reader is referred to Salmons (1997).

The well-established response of the PSS animal to raised environmental temperature and the malignant hyperthermic response of patients with ryanodine receptor defects has led to the use of *heat stress* as an experimental model to investigate suspect turkey flocks. Babji *et al.* (1982) showed that holding pre-slaughter turkeys for only 4 h at 38°C produced meat that was paler, and had a lower pH, water-holding capacity, cooking yield and a higher shear value than muscles from birds held at 21°C or 5°C. Many of these findings are in accord with an earlier study on the combined effects of several pre-slaughter conditions (Froning *et al.*, 1978). However, in the latter study meat colour became darker rather than paler. More recently McKee and Sams (1997) reported pale breast meat, increased drip loss, and rapid pH decline following sustained (4 week) exposure to raised (+15°C) temperatures in Nicholas tom turkeys. They found no difference in mortality compared with a control group but attributed this to an acclimatization programme. Most significantly, however, the heat stress increased the percentage of birds which would be classified as PSE-like. Unfortunately no microscopic studies of the stressed muscles were carried out in this study. Recent acute heat stress experiments in our laboratories suggest increased occurrence of muscle fibre abnormalities in turkey muscles (J. Mills, M. Mitchell and M. Mahon, unpublished data) and increased CK leakage in broilers when the latter were also exposed to oxygen deprivation or calcium ionophores (Sandercock, 1998).

Chicken and turkey muscles have also been used as an experimental model for a number of studies directly investigating the effects of altering the physical load or nerve supply on muscle morphology or investigating developmental regulatory factors (Feng *et al.*, 1963; Cullen *et al.*, 1975; Gordon and Vrbova, 1975; Holly *et al.*, 1980; Ashmore and Summers, 1981; McFarland, 1992; Bakou *et al.*, 1996). Both overuse and stretch can cause wing muscle hypertrophy and increases in oxidative enzyme profiles and if acute may lead to muscle damage and attempted regeneration (Sola *et al.*, 1973; Holly *et al.*, 1980). In the turkey, muscle repair following denervation has been studied by Bakou *et al.* (1996) who showed initial atrophy and necrosis and activation of satellite cells and hypertrophy of slow-twitch and slow-tonic fibres. Variability in NADH-TR enzyme staining also occurred. These authors also reported greater satellite cell activation in heavy strains as compared to light-weight strains. McFarland *et al.* (1993) have also reported differential responses of satellite cells from different turkey strains to mitogenic stimuli. The latter experiments could have significant implications to future regimes for muscle growth promotion and treatment therapies in the turkey industry.

Turkey Muscle Abnormalities in Relation to Rapid Postnatal Growth and Selection

Ever since the seminal work of Joubert (1956) on rabbits, sheep and cattle, significant differences in muscle structure and muscle fibre size have been recognized in different breeds. A great deal of data has now accumulated for poultry muscles such that it is difficult to draw the line between normal variability and abnormality. Furthermore, a caveat on variability due to technique and sample site within a muscle should be heeded (Mahon *et al.*, 1984; Smith and Fletcher, 1988). The reader is referred to Hess (1961), Dutson and Carter (1985) and Swatland (1989a, b, 1995) for a general overview of avian myology, to Aberle *et al.* (1979), Ashmore *et al.* (1973), Barnard *et al.*

(1982), George and Berger (1966), Iwamoto *et al.* (1984, 1992), Remignon *et al.* (1994, 1995), Sams and Janky (1990), Smith and Fletcher (1988) and Sosnicki and Cassens (1988a, b) for data on chicken histomorphology and to George and Berger (1966), Kiessling (1977), Swatland (1981) and Torrella *et al.* (1998) for other avian species; the following account is restricted to turkeys.

Normal (wild) turkeys

There is a dearth of literature on unselected (WILD) turkey muscle (Ricklefs, 1983) and data are limited to relatively unselected slow-growing lines (SMALL) that reach body weights of around 12 kg (male) or 10 kg (female) at 20 weeks posthatching. Our data on the Nebraska Spot line raised in small groups in an experimental rather than commercial environment show a good correlation between body and muscle weight, and muscle fibre size (J. Mills, L. Wylie, M. Mahon, M. Mitchell and P. Hocking, unpublished data; Figs 2.41-2.43). Body and breast muscle weights reached 5.4 kg and 0.5 kg respectively, connective tissue accounted for 10% of the muscle mass, and fibre diameters averaged around 70 μm in the superficial pectorals at 25 weeks of age. Leg muscle fibres were slightly smaller and connective tissue slightly higher. There was, however, a bimodal distribution of muscle fibre diameters even in the breast muscle where only one major fibre type (fast glycolytic) was present (Fig. 2.48a).[4] In many birds, between 8 and 25 weeks of age, muscle abnormalities were recorded which included hyaline fibres, occasional necrotic fibres, basophilia, angular fibres, and inflammatory cell infiltrates (Figs 2.44-2.46 and 2.48). In all muscles examined, internalized myonuclei were found in addition to the subsarcolemmal nuclei typical of mammalian muscle. Electron microscopical examination of these nuclei in commercial turkeys identified them as typical myonuclei rather than belonging to invading mononuclear cells (M. Mahon and S. Gilpin – unpublished data, Fig. 2.44). Centralized nuclei have been reported in avian muscle by other workers (George and Berger, 1966; Shepherd, 1988; Cherel *et al.*, 1995) although their incidence does not seem to have been recorded and most workers ignore their existence altogether.

Rapid growth

The significant increases in growth and development of poultry species and the associated increase in skeletal anomalies have been discussed recently by Lilburn (1994). In the last 20–30 years chicken and turkey body weights have doubled, with slightly larger increases in breast weight (see also Swatland, 1979d; Nixey and Grey, 1989). Grey (1989), in his extensive review on commercial turkey meat, noted that the 'influence of breeding on muscle structure, the response of the bird to stress and the consequent effects of these factors on muscle texture should receive more attention'. Here we turn this attention to the effects on muscle before processing and cooking. Commercial

---

[4]A summary of fibre type populations in poultry musculature is given in Wiskus *et al.* (1976).

Fig. 2.41.   **Fig. 2.42.**

Fig. 2.43.   **Fig. 2.44.**

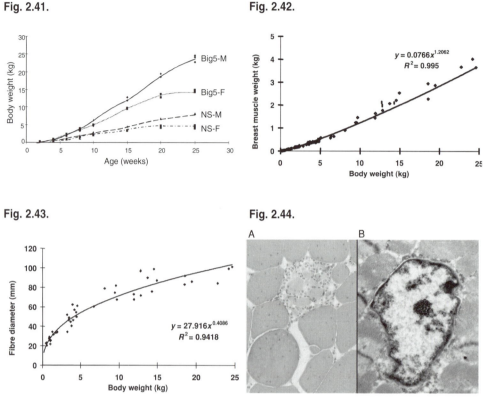

Fig. 2.41. Comparative growth curves (body weights in kg) for large commercial (upper two lines, males and females respectively) and unselected (lower two lines, males and females respectively) turkeys. Data in conjunction with Jo Mills.

Figs. 2.42 & 2.43. Relationship between (2.42) breast muscle weight and (2.43) muscle fibre diameter and body weight in commercial and unselected turkey lines. Data in conjunction with Jo Mills.

Fig. 2.44. Excess internalized myonuclei (and a necrotic fibre) in turkey pectoralis muscle. Age 16 weeks. (A) H&E, × 200. (B) Electronmicrograph, × 8000.

turkey breeding has produced significant enhancements in breast muscle mass compared with leg muscles both in terms of final mass (Lilburn and Nestor, 1991), reaching up to one-third of body weight (Summers and Spratt, 1990), and in allometric growth relationships (Maruyama *et al.*, 1993). The latter authors showed that all the major muscles studied matured later than the whole body with the breast muscles showing an initial spurt which exceeded that of the leg muscles. Hurwitz *et al.* (1991) studying BUT flocks also favoured biphasic growth curves suggesting the late increase in muscle growth resulted from the increase in circulating androgens. A number of workers have set out to determine whether this growth is due to changes in muscle fibre girth, length or number or combinations of all three. Swatland (1979a, b, c) showed that muscle growth in the turkey pennate supracorocoideus was by greater radial than longitudinal hypertrophy of muscle fibres whereas the opposite was true for the leg sartorius. In a more recent study on male and female meat and egg lines (commercial hybrid turkeys), although he showed the meat line to have an enhanced pectoral growth rate and breast length, no differences were found in muscle depth, muscle fibre number or girth (Swatland, 1989a). Swatland's data show that fibre sizes reach about 80 μm diameter in the pectorals and 50 μm in the sartorius with little difference between males and females. Our data (M. Mahon and S. Gilpin, unpublished data) for BUT T42 commercial breeding birds (body weight 22 kg at 25 weeks) showed sizes for pectorals of around 70 μm and 97 μm narrow diameter, and for leg muscles of around 50 μm and 75 μm at 16 and 29 weeks of age, respectively (Fig. 2.47). However, in the older birds a number of smaller (undifferentiated, or damaged, or split?) fibres were present thus lowering the mean. A significant number of very large fibres were also present reaching up to 160 μm in pectorals and 140 μm diameter in leg muscles. Whether the latter should be considered abnormally hypertrophic or just part of the growth spectrum is difficult to evaluate but such fibres would surely have difficulty in maintaining normal oxygen and metabolite supplies at their core. In another study, using BUT BIG5 birds (J. Mills, M. Mahon and M. Mitchell, unpublished data) values reached 20 kg for body weight, 3.0 kg left pectoral weight, 90 μm fibre diameter (Figs 2.41-2.43) and 10% connective tissue. We found slightly lower values in a study of birds used for the consumer market (T8 and BIG6) killed at 11 weeks of age and weighing approximately 4–6 kg (S. Jamdar, M. Mahon, S. Gilpin and S. Tullet). In this study pectoral muscle fibre sizes reached 40–60 μm with those from the deep (profundus) muscle being significantly larger than those from the superficialis. Connective tissue content varied from 9% to 13%. There was no significant difference between sexes or the two strains.

Cherel et al. (1994) compared postnatal muscle development in the slow-tonic anterior latissimus dorsi (ALD) from light and heavy turkey lines showing hypertrophy in the former and hypertrophy and hyperplasia in the latter. However, Maruyama et al. (1993) found that myosin isoform transitions (embryonic to adult) were complete by 28 days posthatching. Wilson et al. (1990) have provided data for male and female bird and muscle weights and for changes in muscle fibre size in turkey lines selected for rapid growth up to 16 weeks of age. Except for pectoralis superficialis, muscle weights (deep pectoral, medial lateral adductor, gastrocnemius) were proportional to body weight. Pectoralis superficialis was relatively larger and showed rapid increases in muscle fibre calibre up to 83 μm. These authors also reported on shape and packing changes in the muscle fibres and noted the presence of fibres with either peripheral or subsarcolemmal myonuclei. Similar findings have been noted by the present authors (Mahon et al., 1995; J. Mills, S. Gilpin, M. Mahon and M. Mitchell, unpublished results) for 11 muscles of the BUT lines T42, BIG5, BIG6 and T8 (Fig. 2.45). In particular we found differential growth and maturity between breast and leg muscles (Fig. 2.47). Both Wilson et al. (1990) and the present authors also noted a number of muscle abnormalities (see later). Comparative data for chicken muscles (Remignon et al., 1994, 1995) showed that selection for rapid growth increased the number (+20% in ALD) and size (+30% in pectoralis) of muscle fibres without changing their typing or myosin isoforms.

Fig. 2.45.   Fig. 2.46.

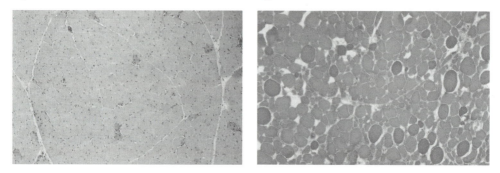

Fig. 2.45. Basophilic (dark) fibres are frequent in this specimen from an 8 week old commercial turkey line. H&E, × 50.

Fig. 2.46. Hyaline, atrophic, necrotic, split, vacuolar and regenerating muscle fibres amidst fibrosis and oedema are commonplace in this leg muscle sample from a 16 week old commercial line turkey. H&E, × 100.

Another approach to analysing turkey muscle growth was taken by Kang and co-workers (1985). These authors measured protein turnover, and DNA and RNA levels in both breast and leg muscles from a LARGE (Nicholas) strain during the first 8 weeks posthatching. They found that muscle growth involved increases in total DNA and RNA but decreased concentrations, thus suggesting that growth was due to cellular hypertrophy which was in part due to decreased protein degradation. Final muscle size was determined by total DNA but the growth rate was determined by the efficiency of protein disposition, ruled mainly by the protein degradation rate.

A number of workers have reported on the increased incidence of myopathological features in turkey lines selected for rapid growth (LARGE) compared to slower growing counterparts (SMALL). We propose to refer to these conditions as *growth-induced myopathy* (GIM) as distinct from the disorders described above where gross degenerative muscle changes, observable alterations in muscle or meat quality, and clinical symptoms are usually observed. However, it would not be unreasonable to include most of the above pathologies as part of the spectrum of GIM and add their characteristics to those included in this section. The title of Siller's (1985) review 'Deep pectoral myopathy: a penalty of successful selection for muscle growth' reflects this view. Wilson *et al.* (1990) have noted more frequent focal myopathy (hyaline, degenerating and irregularly shaped fibres, and loose packing) without inflammation, and raised serum CK in LARGE versus SMALL lines. Further supporting data is given by Sosnicki and Wilson (1991). Cherel *et al.* (1995) in a careful histomorphometric study reported that up to 75% of commercial slaughter turkeys showed some muscle abnormalities (hyaline fibres, necrosis, fibre splitting, and fatty infiltration). Sosnicki *et al.* (1989, 1991b) have reported similar findings for two pectoral and three 'leg' muscles using light and electron microscopy and have noted the changes to occur both segmentally and over widespread portions of the fibre length. These authors also provide semi-quantitative data and have noted fibrosis and fatty replacement, mononuclear infiltration and increased staining for free calcium. Motor end-plates were normal. In our own studies of 11 muscles in fast-growing turkey lines (BUT T42, BIG 5, BIG 6, and T8) we have shown an increased incidence of muscle abnormalities coincident with the rapid growth phase in both breast and leg muscles (Mahon *et al.*, 1995; M. Mahon, T. Ford, S. Gilpin, S. Jamdar and J. Mills, unpublished data; Figs 2.45 and 2.46). Comparative muscle studies of fast-growing selected birds to the unselected traditional strain (Nebraska Spot) have confirmed these findings (Mills *et al.*, 1998a, b; J. Mills, S. Gilpin, M. Mahon and M. Mitchell, unpublished data; Fig. 2.48). We have also found a coincident massive rise in serum CK in the LARGE turkeys around 15 weeks posthatching (Fig. 2.49). The histopathological features include hyaline fibres (often at the corners of fascicles), loose packing and oedematous connective tissue, necrosis, phagocytosis, inflammation, enzyme changes (decreased central or increased peripheral staining with SDH), increased esterase, regeneration and extensive basophilia, and multinucleation. We also found the number of internalized myonuclei per muscle fibre cross-section to increase with age for both leg muscles (from about 0.5 per fibre at hatching to 2–4 per fibre at 20 weeks) and pectoral muscles (3.5–4.5 per fibre respectively). It is not known whether this has any significance to the enhanced growth characteristics or myopathology of these muscles at the present time. Swatland also reported 'growth' related differences in muscle histology and histochemistry in different turkey lines

Fig. 2.47.

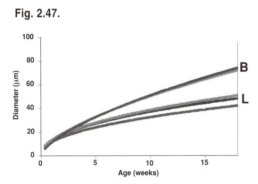

Fig. 2.48.

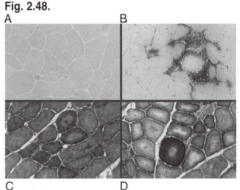

Fig. 2.49.

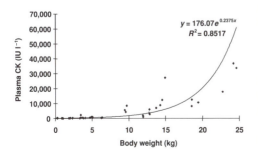

$$y = 176.07e^{0.2375x}$$
$$R^2 = 0.8517$$

Fig. 2.47. Muscle fibre growth in breast muscles (line B) exceeds that in the leg muscles (line L). Data from a BUT commercial line.

Fig. 2.48. Breast muscle samples from commercial line turkeys showing (A) bimodal distribution of fibre sizes, H&E; (B) localized inflammatory infiltrate, H&E; (C) and (D) target, targetoid, core, and stain accumulation fibres, NADHtr. All × 100.

Fig. 2.49. Relationship between plasma creatine kinase (CK) levels in growing commercial turkeys. Data courtesy of Jo Mills.

(Swatland, 1980, 1985). Sosnicki *et al.* (1988b) reported an increased incidence and random occurrence of hypercontracted (giant, hyaline) fibres in both breast and leg muscles of about 50% of birds sampled from large white male turkey lines. Although morphometric analysis was not performed to determine their exact occurrence or distribution, the histological and histochemical staining characteristics of these fibres indicated increased hydrolytic enzyme activity. The authors favoured a calcium influx aetiology due to possible mitochondrial or sarcoplasmic reticulum defects to explain their observations. Increased incidence of hyaline fibres was also a significant finding in our analysis of several commercial flocks. Sosnicki and Wilson (1991, 1992) have reviewed these findings and suggested a number of possible aetiologies to explain them, in summary stating that 'selection for rapid growth led to muscles that outgrow their life-support systems and bring about muscle damage when coupled with the conditions used to grow turkeys'. Their data from muscles showing ischaemic change (focal myopathy) in which the capillary bed was reduced appear to support these hypotheses (Sosnicki *et al.*, 1991a; Sosnicki and Wilson, 1991).

Sosnicki and Wilson (1991) also comment that in turkeys selected for rapid growth, the growth of the muscle fibre outstrips that of the connective tissue which may lead to loss of muscle integrity. This may adversely affect cohesiveness and juiciness of processed turkey breast meat (Grey, 1989). Swatland (1990) measured the thickness of endomysial and perimysial connective tissue bands within turkey pectoralis muscles and showed that it failed to keep pace with radial muscle fibre growth. He also noted that excess muscle fibre growth leads to fragmentation and poor cohesion and this may help explain the shear values reported by Babji *et al.* (1982). Our current histomorphometric data show no significant differences in the amounts of connective tissue between different commercial lines and in Nebraska Spot turkeys.

Overview

In general, our observations agree with the literature reports on the association of increased myopathy with selection for enhanced growth in that they show greater incidence of muscle abnormalities in commercial lines than in non-selected turkey lines, both from histomorphological and serum CK studies, and the incidence was age/weight related. Furthermore the incidence of histopathological features was much greater in leg than in breast muscles, perhaps indicating the greater functional demand in the support structures of big-breasted birds. The possibility of such selection also selecting for inherent muscle fibre defects (e.g. defective ryanodine receptors), or developmental defects (insufficient capillary or fascial growth) which then lead to myopathy when the birds are stressed is discussed in Chapter 3. Indeed, serendipitous selection of a single gene leading to a defect in the metabolism of the muscle fibre in commercial turkeys could explain the overlap of myopathies (deep pectoral, focal, PSE, etc.) and reactions to environmental stress described above. Treatment strategies could include either, altered pre-slaughter housing and transport, appropriate exercise conditioning of the muscles during the rapid growth phase (Siller, 1985), or genetic deselection of specific harmful muscle genes (Sosnicki and Wilson, 1991). A breed in which leg muscle growth was ahead of breast muscle growth during the rapid growth phase would also be beneficial in terms of reducing overload and leg muscle pathology.

CALCIUM-BASED MUSCLE DAMAGE

It has already been mentioned that their is much experimental and clinical evidence to suggest that degenerative changes in muscle fibres following a variety of insults are triggered by calcium influx. Intracellular calcium accumulation, due to metabolic imbalance or damaged muscle membranes, leading to muscle cell death has an extensive literature (Jackson *et al.*, 1991; Jackson, 1993; McArdle and Jackson, 1997; Salmons, 1997). It is thought that the eventual damage may be due to excess calcium activating intracellular proteases, lysosomal proteases or lipases thus leading to muscle fibre breakdown and increased calcium influx and hence initiating a vicious circle of damage, or to disturbance of mitochondrial function leading to decreased energy supplies and another vicious circle whereby calcium cannot be pumped out of the cell sufficiently. The disturbed energy supply and excess calcium are also thought to cause hypercontraction (seen as hyaline fibres) and tearing of the fibres followed by influx of macrophages to remove the debris and eventual necrosis (Cullen and Fulthorpe, 1975). Most of the observed features in human myopathies (for example in Duchenne muscular dystrophy where the defective gene leads to a weak muscle membrane lacking its structural protein dystrophin) or in the turkey myopathies (where ischaemic damage, physical overload of the legs, ionophore effects, or heat damage insult the muscle fibre integrity) can bring about a common pathological response involving calcium, usually signified by raised serum CK from the leaky muscles. What is not obvious from these descriptions and many of the explanatory hypotheses is whether there is an integral problem with calcium homeostasis in turkey muscle *per se* as a result of selective breeding which may lead to muscle damage. There is now increasing evidence that this may be the case. For example Tripp and Schmitz (1982) reported elevated serum CK levels in normal healthy turkeys and in birds following exercise. Hocking *et al.* (1998) and Mitchell *et al.* (1996) noted increased CK in a commercial sire line compared to traditional turkeys and we (J. Mills, S. Gilpin and M. Mahon) and others (see above) have noted frequent hyaline (hypercontracted) fibres and other myopathic features commensurate with calcium-related degeneration in commercial turkeys showing no overt clinical signs of myopathy. In our studies we also noted a prevalence of muscle fibre anomalies during the rapid growth phase simultaneous with the extensive calcification of leg tendons. Reiner *et al.* (1995) have also implicated defective calcium regulation and muscle hyperactivation as responsible for sudden death syndrome in broiler chickens. The enhanced sensitivity of commercial turkeys and muscle changes similar to those of the PSS pig also implicates the ryanodine receptor (calcium-release channel of the sarcoplasmic reticulum) as a common factor. In our investigations one interesting likeness was the presence of pale muscle fibre cores on oxidative enzyme staining which is also found in human central core disease, a disorder also due to a defective ryanodine receptor gene. The involvement of calcium in muscle fibre homeostasis and possible involvement of the ryanodine receptor and related ion channels is discussed in Chapter 3.

CONTROL FACTORS IN GROWTH AND REGENERATION, AND SATELLITE CELLS

Much of the molecular and cellular events involved in myogenesis, development and growth are now understood (El Haj, 1992; Kelly and Blau, 1992; Swatland, 1995; Dauncey and Gilmour, 1996; Goldspink, 1977, 1996; see also Chapter 1). Skeletal muscle cells and connective tissues arise from the somites and surrounding mesoderm; the former divide, fuse, differentiate, mature and grow under the influence of the MyoD gene family, growth factors, innervation, hormones, nutrition, tension and temperature. Turkey muscle is astonishing for its rapid and sustained growth and provides a useful model for studying regulatory factors during growth and development (McFarland *et al.*, 1991, 1993; McFarland, 1992; Sun and McFarland, 1993; Bakou *et al.*, 1996; Barbour and Lilburn, 1996; see also Chapter 1). It would be plausible to suggest that it may also have excellent regenerative powers since satellite cells (potential muscle myoblasts) are involved in both processes (Atherton *et al.*, 1981; Schultz and McCormick, 1993; Grounds and Yablonka-Reuveni, 1993; Bischoff, 1994; Brotchie *et al.*, 1995; Lawson-Smith and McGeachie, 1998). The work from South Dakota (McFarland *et al.*, 1993; showing the enhanced response of satellite cells from a commercial strain to mitogenic stimuli) and from Nantes (Bakou *et al.*, 1996; showing greater satellite cell responses to denervation in heavy turkey strains versus light strains) supports this hypothesis. Indeed, recent *in vivo* and *in vitro* work (Merly *et al.*, 1998) suggests that variations in postnatal muscle growth between heavy and light strains may be related to differences in the capacity of their satellite cell proliferation. Perhaps much of the myopathy inherent in commercial turkey lines is therefore masked by successful regeneration since basophilic (regenerating) fibres are frequently observed, thus we are only seeing the tip of the iceberg with respect to the amount of abnormality really present. Thus, are *all* commercial turkey muscle fibres defective and only reveal problems when regeneration cannot keep pace or their is some environmental overload such as heat stress? Current experiments being performed in our laboratories are studying the combination of these phenomena (commercial versus traditional turkeys, myopathy versus regeneration, and heat stress) with the aim of elucidating the exact mechanisms involved in turkey muscle abnormalities. The possibilities of treating myopathies with growth factors to enhance regeneration is already becoming a possibility in human neuromuscular disorders (Lefaucheur and Sebille, 1997) and is likely to circumvent the difficulties associated with myoblast transfer therapy (Morgan and Watt, 1993). Finally, a study of satellite cell activity, myonuclei–cytoplasmic ratios, and relative growth performance in leg versus breast muscles in different commercial turkey lines would be beneficial for reasons stated previously.

The key role played by basement membrane laminins (Aumailley and Smyth, 1998) and other connective tissue elements in the regulation of muscle structure also requires further study. Physiological and biochemical aspects of turkey muscle abnormalities, including the triggering of the contractile apparatus, the generation and management of energy, and the regulation of internal calcium stores, are covered in Chapter 3.

FUTURE STUDIES

Future studies of turkey muscle pathology are likely to involve further elucidation of the turkey genome and related phenotypes to help determine inheritance patterns and possible alterations to breeding programmes (P. Hocking and J. Bentley, personal communications), and the use of transgenic birds to test hypotheses concerning ryanodine receptor involvement, or studies of pharmacological treatments for calcium-induced muscle damage such as calmodulin antagonist therapies (Beitner and Lilling, 1993). More work is necessary on the regenerative as well as the growth capacities of muscle fibres from commercial species. Further work on animal welfare and environmental factors affecting turkey myopathy are also of immense importance as should be the application of modern imaging methods and clinical function tests. In particular, tracking down the exact locations of muscle damage and CK release (primarily breast or thigh–leg?) would be of benefit to the commercial turkey industry. Our laboratories and other studies (Northcutt *et al.*, 1998b) already favour more extensive involvement of the thigh and leg. Some of these issues are elucidated upon further in Chapter 3.

ACKNOWLEDGEMENTS

My grateful thanks to co-workers in Manchester (Sally Gilpin, Tamsin Ford, Saurabh Jamdar, Jo Mills, Chris Philips, Mark Seddon), Chester (Cliff Nixey, Nick French, James Bentley), Norwich (Steve Tullet) and Edinburgh (Malcolm Mitchell, Paul Hocking, Dale Sandercock, Lynne Wylie) for their expert technical and academic contributions to this work. A special thanks to Jo Mills for pushing forward the work and providing some of her own unpublished material for this chapter. The valued financial support from British United Turkeys (Tarvin), Bernard Matthews PLC (Norfolk) and the British Turkey Federation is also acknowledged.

REFERENCES

Aberle, E.D., Addis, P.B. and Shoffner, R.N. (1979) Fiber types in skeletal muscles of broiler- and layer-type chickens. *Poultry Science* 58, 1210–1212.
Abourachid, A. (1991a) Myology of the pelvis limb of the domestic turkey *Meleagris gallopavo*. *Anatomia Histologia Embryologia* 20, 75–94.

Abourachid, A. (1991b) Comparative gait analysis of two strains of turkey, *Meleagris gallopavo. British Poultry Science* 32, 271–277.

Artacho-Perula, E. and Roldan-Villobos, R. (1995) Estimation of capillary length density in skeletal muscle by unbiased stereological methods: 1. Use of vertical slices of known thickness. *Anatomical Record* 241, 337–344.

Ashmore, C.R. and Summers, P.J. (1981) Stretch-induced growth in chicken wing muscles: myofibrillar proliferation. *American Journal of Physiology* 51, C93–C97.

Ashmore, C.R., Addis, P.B., Doerr, L. and Stokes, H. (1973) Development of muscle fibers in the complexus muscle of normal and dystrophic chicks. *Journal of Histochemistry and Cytochemistry* 21, 266–278.

Atherton, G.W., James, N.T. and Mahon, M. (1981) Studies on muscle fibre splitting in skeletal muscle. *Experientia* 37, 308–310.

Aumailley, M. and Smyth, N. (1998) The role of laminins in basement membrane function. *Journal of Anatomy* 193, 1–21.

Austic, R.E. and Scott, M.L. (1984) Nutritional deficiency diseases. In: Hofstad, M.S., Barnes, H.J., Calnek, B.W., Reid, W.M. and Yoder, H.W. (eds) *Diseases of Poultry*, 8th edn. Iowa State University Press, Iowa, pp. 47–49.

Babji, A.S., Froning, G.W. and Ngoka, D.A. (1982) The effect of preslaughter environmental temperature in the presence of electrolyte treatment on turkey meat quality. *Poultry Science* 61, 2385–2389.

Bakou, S., Cherel, Y., Gabinaud, B., Guigand, L. and Wyers, M. (1996) Type-specific changes in fibre size and satellite cell activation following muscle denervation in two strains of turkey (*Meleagris gallopavo*). *Journal of Anatomy* 188, 677–691.

Bar, P.R., Reijneveld, J.C., Wokke, J.H.J., Jacobs, S.C.J.M. and Bootsma, A.L. (1997) Muscle damage induced by exercise: nature, prevention and repair. In: Salmons, S. (ed.) *Muscle Damage*. Oxford University Press, Oxford, pp. 1–27.

Barbour, G.W. and Lilburn, M.S. (1996) Comparative growth and development of Nicholas and hybrid toms from 16 to 82 days and effects of protein restriction from 0–59 days on growth of hybrid toms through 125 days of age. *Poultry Science* 75, 790–796.

Barbut, S. (1996) Estimates and detection of the PSE problem in young turkey breast meat. *Canadian Journal of Animal Science* 76, 455–457.

Barbut, S. (1997a) Occurrence of pale soft exudative meat in mature turkey hens. *British Poultry Science* 38, 74–77.

Barbut, S. (1997b) Problem of pale soft exudative meat in broiler chickens. *British Poultry Science* 38, 355–358.

Barbut, S., McEwen, S.A. and Julian, R.J. (1990) Turkey downgrading: effect of truck cage location and unloading. *Poultry Science* 69, 1410–1413.

Barnard, E.A., Lyles, J.M. and Pizzey, J.A. (1982) Fibre types in chicken skeletal muscles and their changes in muscular dystrophy. *Journal of Physiology* 331, 333–354.

Baumel, J.J., King, A.S., Lucas, A.M., Breazile, J.E. and Evans, H.E. (1979) *Nomina Anatomica Avium*. Academic Press, London.

Bedi, K.S., Birzgalis, A.R., Mahon, M., Smart, J.L. and Wareham, A.C. (1982) Early life undernutrition in rats. 1 Quantitative histology of skeletal muscles from underfed young and refed adult animals. *British Journal of Nutrition* 47, 417–431.

Beitner, R. and Lilling, G. (1993) Treatment of muscle damage induced by high intracellular Ca^{2+} with calmodulin antagonists. *General Pharmacology* 24, 847–855.

Binkhorst, F.M.P., Kuipers, H., Heymans, J., Frederik, P.M., Slaaf, D.W., Tangelder, G.J. and Reneman, R.S. (1989) Exercise-induced focal skeletal muscle fiber degeneration and capillary morphology. *Journal of Applied Physiology* 66, 2857–2865.

Bischoff, R. (1994) The satellite cell and muscle regeneration. In: Engel, A.G. and Franzini-Armstrong, C. (eds) *Myology*, 2nd edn. McGraw-Hill, New York, pp. 97–133.

Block, B.A. (1994) Thermogenesis in muscle. *Annual Review of Physiology* 56, 535–577.

Bradley, R., McKerrell, R.E. and Barnard, E.A. (1988) Neuromuscular disease in animals. In: Walton, J. (ed.) *Disorders of Voluntary Muscle*, 5th edn. Churchill Livingstone, Edinburgh, pp. 910–980.

Brotchie, D., Davies, I., Ireland, G. and Mahon, M. (1995) Dual-channel laser scanning microscopy for the identification and quantification of proliferating skeletal muscle satellite cells following synergist ablation. *Journal of Anatomy* 186, 97–102.

Cardona, C.J., Bickford, A.A., Galey, F.D., Charlton, B.R. and Cooper, G. (1992) A syndrome in commercial turkeys in California and Oregon characterized by a rear-limb necrotizing skeletal myopathy. *Avian Diseases* 36, 1092–1101.

Cardona, C.J., Galey, F.D., Bickford, A.A., Charlton, B.R. and Cooper, G.L. (1993) Skeletal myopathy produced with experimental dosing of turkeys with monensin. *Avian Diseases* 37, 107–117.

Carpenter, S. and Karpati, G. (1984) *Pathology of Skeletal Muscle*. Churchill Livingstone, New York.

Cherel, Y., Hurtrel, H., Gardahaut, M.F., Merly, F., Magras-Resch, C., Fontaine-Perus, J. and Wyers, M. (1994) Comparison of postnatal development of anterior latissimus dorsi (ALD) muscle in heavy- and light-weight strains of turkey (*Meleagris gallopavo*). *Growth, Development and Aging* 58, 157–165.

Cherel, Y., Wyers, M. and Dupas, M. (1995) Histopathological alterations of turkey skeletal muscle observed at the slaughterhouse. *British Poultry Science* 36, 443–453.

Cullen, M.J. and Fulthorpe, J.J. (1975) Stages in fibre breakdown in Duchenne muscular dystrophy. An electron microscopic study. *Journal of Neurological Sciences* 24, 179–200.

Cullen, M.J., Harris, J.B., Marshall, M.W. and Ward, M.R. (1975) An electrophysiological and morphological study of normal and denervated chicken latissimus dorsi muscles. *Journal of Physiology* 245, 371–385.

Cumming, W.J.K., Fulthorpe, J.J., Hudgson, P. and Mahon, M. (1994) *Color Atlas of Muscle Pathology*. Mosby-Wolfe, London.

Dauncey, M.J. and Gilmour, R.S. (1996) Regulatory factors in the control of muscle development. *Proceedings of the Nutrition Society* 55, 543–559.

Denborough, M.A. and Lovell, R.R.H. (1960) Anaesthetic deaths in a family. *The Lancet* ii, 45.

Dickinson, E.M., Stevens, J.O. and Helfer, D.H. (1968) A degenerative myopathy in turkeys. *Proceedings of the 17th Western Poultry Diseases Conference*, University of California, Davis, p. 6.

Dowling, L. (1992) Ionophore toxicity in chickens: a review of pathology and diagnosis. *Avian Pathology* 21, 355–368.

Dubowitz, V. (1985) *Muscle Biopsy A Practical Approach*, 2nd edn. Baillière-Tindall, London.

Dutson, T.R. and Carter, A. (1985) Microstructure and biochemistry of avian muscle and its relevance to meat processing industries. *Poultry Science* 64, 1577–1590.

El Haj, A. (ed.) (1992) *Molecular Biology of Muscle*. Company of Biologists, Cambridge.

Emery, A.E.H. (1993) *Duchenne Muscular Dystrophy*, 2nd edn. Oxford Monographs on Medical Genetics: 24. Oxford University Press, Oxford.

Engel, A.G. and Franzini-Armstrong, C. (1994) *Myology*. McGraw-Hill, New York.

Feng, Tp., Jung, H.W. and Wu, W.Y. (1963) The contrasting trophic changes of the anterior and posterior latissimus dorsi of the chick following denervation. In: Gutmann, E. and Hnik, P. (eds) *The Effect of Use and Disuse on Neuromuscular Functions*. Czech Academy of Science, Prague, pp. 431–442.

Ferket, P.R. (1995) Pale, soft, and exudative breast meat in turkeys. *Turkeys* August, 19–21.

Ficken, M.D., Wages, D.P. and Gonder, E. (1989) Monensin toxicity in turkey breeder hens. *Avian Diseases* 33, 186–190.

Florini, J.R. (1985) Hormonal control of muscle cell growth. *Journal of Animal Science* 61, (Suppl. 2), 21–38.

Froes, M.M.Q., Kristmundsdottir, F., Mahon, M. and Cumming, W.J.K. (1987) Muscle morphometry in motor neuron disease. *Neuropathology and Applied Neurobiology* 13, 405–419.

Froning, G.W., Babji, A.S. and Mather, F.B. (1978) The effect of pre-slaughter temperature, stress, struggle, and anaesthetization on color and textural characteristics of turkey muscle. *Poultry Science* 57, 630–633.

Fujii, J., Otsu, K., Zorzato, F., De Leon, S., Khanna, V.K., Weller, J.E., O'Brien, P.J. and MacLennan, D.H. (1991) Identification of a mutation in porcine ryanodine receptor associated with malignant hyperthermia. *Science* 253, 448–451.

George, J.C. and Berger, A.J. (1966) *Avian Myology*. Academic Press, New York.

Gill, T.A., Sundeen, G.B., Richards, J.F. and Bragg, D.B. (1980) The effects of dietary selenium and vitamin E on avian white muscle disease as measured by both chemical and physical parameters. *Poultry Science* 59, 2088–2097.

Gillard, E.F., Otsu, K. and Fujii, J., Khanna, V.K., Leon, S.D., Derdemezi, J., Britt, B.A., Duff, C.L., Worton, R.G. and MacLennan, D.H. (1991) A substitution of cysteine for arginine 614 in the ryanodine receptor is potentially causative of human malignant hyperthermia. *Genomics* 11, 751–755.

Goldspink, G. (1977) The growth of muscles. In: Boorman, K.N. and Wilson, B.J. (eds) *Growth and Poultry Meat Production*. British Poultry Science Ltd, Edinburgh.

Goldspink, G. (1983) Alterations in myofibril size and structure during growth, exercise, and changes in environmental temperature. In: Peachey, L.D. (ed.) *Skeletal Muscle*. Handbook of Physiology, 10. American Physiological Society, Bethesda.

Goldspink, G. (1996) Muscle growth and muscle function: a molecular biological perspective. *Research in Veterinary Science* 60, 193–204.

Gordon, T. and Vrbova, G. (1975) The influence of innervation on the differentiation of contractile speeds of developing chick muscles. *Pfluger's Archives* 360, 199–218.

Graziano, M.J., Flory, W., Seger, C.L. and Henert, C.D. (1983) Effects of a *Cassia occidentalis* extract in the domestic chicken (*Gallus domesticus*). *American Journal of Veterinary Research* 44, 1238–1244.

Grey, T.C. (1989) Turkey meat texture. In: Nixey, C. and Grey, T.C. (eds) *Recent Advances in Turkey Science*. Butterworths, London, pp. 289–311.

Gronert, G.A. (1986) Malignant hyperthermia. In: Engel, A.G. and Banker, B.Q. (eds) *Myology*. McGraw-Hill, New York, pp. 1763–1784.

Grounds, M.D. and Yablonka-Reuveni, Z. (1993) Molecular and cell biology of skeletal muscle regeneration. In: Partridge, T. (ed.) *Molecular and Cell Biology of Muscular Dystrophy*. Chapman & Hall, London, pp. 210–256.

Grunder, A.A., Hollands, K.G. and Gavora, J.S. (1979) Incidence of degenerative myopathy among turkeys fed corn or wheat based rations. *Poultry Science* 58, 1321–1324.

Grunder, A.A., Hollands, K.G., Gavora, J.S., Chambers, J.R. and Cave, N.A.G. (1984) Degenerative myopathy of the musculus supracoracoideus and production traits in strains of meat-type chickens. *Poultry Science* 63, 781–785.

Gute, D.C., Ishida, T., Yarimizu, K. and Korthuis, R.J. (1998) Inflammatory responses to ischaemia on reperfusion in skeletal muscle. *Molecular and Cellular Biochemistry* 179, 169–187.

Halvorson, D.A., Van Dijk, C. and Brown, P. (1982) Ionophore toxicity in turkey breeders. *Avian Diseases* 26, 634–639.

Harper, J.A. and Helfer, D.H. (1972) The effect of vitamin E, methionine and selenium on degenerative myopathy in turkeys. *Poultry Science* 51, 1757–1759.

Harper, J.A. and Parker, J.E. (1964) Hereditary muscular dystrophy in the domestic turkey, *Meleagris gallopavo*. *Poultry Science* 43, 1326

Harper, J.A. and Parker, J.E. (1967) Hereditary muscular dystrophy in the domestic turkey. *Journal of Heredity* 58, 189–193.

Harper, J.A., Bernier, P.E., Stevens, J.O. and Dickinson, E.M. (1969) Degenerative myopathy in the domestic turkey. *Poultry Science* 48, 1816.

Harper, J.A., Bernier, P.E., Helfer, D.H. and Schmitz, J.A. (1975) Degenerative myopathy of the deep pectoral muscle in the turkey. *Journal of Heredity* 66, 362–366.

Harper, J.A., Bernier, P.E. and Thompson-Cowley, L.L. (1981) Incidence of deep pectoral myopathy in turkeys due to breeding and altered expression from forced exercise. *Poultry Science* 60, 1667.

Harper, J.A., Bernier, P.E. and Thompson-Cowley, L.L. (1983) Early expression of hereditary deep pectoral myopathy in turkeys due to forced wing exercise. *Poultry Science* 62, 2303–2308.

Harvey, W.R., Kaiser, H.E. and Rosenberg, L.E. (1968) Atlas of the domestic turkey (*Meleagris gallopavo*). US Atomic Energy Commission, Maryland.

Henrichs, K.J., Jones, J.M., Berry, C.L. and Swash, M. (1979) Pathogenesis of ischaemic pectoral myopathy in the domestic turkey. *British Veterinary Journal* 135, 286–290.

Hess, A. (1961) Structural differences of fast and slow extrafusal fibres and their nerve endings in chicken. *Journal of Physiology* 157, 221–231.

Hocking, P.M., Mitchell, M.A., Bernard, R. and Sandercock, D.A. (1998) Interaction of age, strain, sex and food restriction on plasma creatine kinase activity in turkeys. *British Poultry Science* 39, 360–364.

Hollands, K.G., Grunder, A.A., Williams, C.J. and Gavora, J.S. (1980) Plasma creatine kinase as an indicator of degenerative myopathy in live turkeys. *British Poultry Science* 21, 161–169.

Hollands, K.G., Grunder, A.A. and Gavora, J.S. (1981) Induction by exercise of deep pectoral myopathy and associated changes in plasma creatine kinase levels in female turkeys. *Poultry Science* 60, 1669.

Hollands, K.G., Grunder, A.A. and Gavora, J.S. (1983) Plasma creatine kinase as an indicator of degenerative myopathy of the *M. supracoracoideus* (DMS) in exercised chickens. *Poultry Science* 62, 1435.

Holly, R.G., Barnett, J.G., Ashmore, C.R., Taylor, R.G. and Mole, P.A. (1980) Stretch-induced growth in chicken wing muscles: a new model of stretch hypertrophy. *American Journal of Physiology* 238, C62–C71.

Hurwitz, S., Talpaz, H., Bartov, I. and Plavnik, I. (1991) Characterization of growth and development of male British United Turkeys. *Poultry Science* 70, 2419–2424.

Iwamoto, H., Morita, S., Ono, Y., Takahara, H., Higashiuwatoko, H., Kukimoto, T. and Gotoh, S. (1984) A study on the fiber composition of breast and thigh muscles in Sanatsumadori crossbred broilers. *Japanese Journal of Zoological Science* 55, 87–94.

Iwamoto, H., Morita, S., Ono, Y. and Takahara, H. (1992) Breed differences in the histochemical properties of M iliotibialis lateralis myofibre of domestic cocks. *British Poultry Science* 33, 321–328.

Jackson, M.J. (1993) Molecular mechanisms of muscle damage. In: Partridge, T. (ed.) *Molecular and Cell Biology of Muscular Dystrophy*. Chapman & Hall, London, pp. 257–282.

Jackson, M.J., McArdle, A. and Edwards, R.H.T. (1991) Free radicals, calcium and damage in dystrophic and normal skeletal muscle. In: Duncan, C.J. (ed.) *Calcium*

Free Radicals and Tissue Damage. Cambridge University Press, Cambridge, pp. 139–148.

Jones, J.M., King, N.R. and Mulliner, M.M. (1974) Degenerative myopathy in turkey breeder hens: a comparative study of normal and affected muscle. *British Poultry Science* 15, 191–196.

Joubert, J.M. (1956) An analysis of factors influencing postnatal growth and development of the muscle fibre. *Journal of Agricultural Sciences* 47, 59–102.

Kaminski, H.F. and Ruff, R.L. (1994) Endocrine myopathies. In: Engel, A.G. and Franzini-Armstrong, C. (eds) *Myology*, 2nd edn. McGraw-Hill, New York, pp. 1726–1753.

Kang, C.W., Sunde, M.I. and Swick, R.W. (1985) Characteristics of growth and protein turnover in skeletal muscle of turkey poults. *Poultry Science* 64, 380–387.

Keller, H., Emery, A.E.H., Spiegler, A.W.J., Apacik, C., Muler, C.R. and Grimm, T. (1996) Age effects on serum creatine kinase (SCK) levels in obligate carriers of Duchenne muscular dystrophy (DMD) and Becker muscular dystrophy (BMD) and its implication on genetic counselling. *Acta Cardiomyologica* 8, 27–34.

Kelly, A.M. and Blau, H.M. (eds) (1992) *Neuromuscular Development and Disease.* Raven Press, New York.

Kiessling, K.K. (1977) Structure and function of pectoralis major in the broiler chicken during growth. *Swedish Journal of Agricultural Research* 7, 115–119.

Kinfu, Y., Brain, N.D., Cumming, W.J.K., Harris, P.F., Kristmundsdottir, F. and Mahon, M. (1989) A qualitative histological, histochemical and ultrastructural study of muscle in acromegaly. *Journal of Anatomy* 167, 262.

Kristmundsdottir, F., Mahon, M., Froes, M.M.Q. and Cumming, W.J.K. (1990) Histomorphometric and histopathological study of the human cricopharyngeus muscle: in health and in motor neuron disease. *Neuropathology and Applied Neurobiology* 16, 461–475.

Lawson-Smith, M.J. and McGeachie, J.K. (1998) The identification of myogenic cells in skeletal muscle, with emphasis on the use of tritiated thymidine autoradiography and desmin antibodies. *Journal of Anatomy* 192, 161–171.

Lefaucheur, J.P. and Sebille, A. (1997) What is the future for intramuscular administration of basic fibroblast growth factor in muscular diseases? *Muscle Nerve* 20, 119–120.

Lehmann-Horn, F. and Rudel, R. (1996) Molecular pathophysiology of voltage-gated ion channels. *Reviews of Physiology, Biochemistry and Pharmacology* 128, 195–268.

Lilburn, M.S. (1994) Skeletal growth of commercial poultry species. *Poultry Science* 73, 897–903.

Lilburn, M.S. and Nestor, K.E. (1991) Body weight and carcass development in different lines of turkeys. *Poultry Science* 70, 2223–2231.

Loughlin, M. (1993) *Muscle Biopsy. A Laboratory Investigation.* Butterworth-Heinemann, Oxford.

Ma, R.T.I. and Addis, P.B. (1973) The association of struggle during exanguination to glycolysis, protein solubility and shear in turkey pectoralis muscle. *Journal of Food Science* 38, 995–997.

Ma, R.T.I., Addis, P.B. and Allen, E. (1971) Response to electrical stimulation and post-mortem changes in turkey pectoralis major muscle. *Journal of Food Science* 36, 125–129.

MacLennan, D.H. and Philips, M.S. (1992) Malignant hyperthermia. *Science* 256, 789–794.

MacLennan, D.H., Otsu, K., Fujii, J., Zorzato, F., Phillips, S., O'Brien, P.J., Archibald, A.L., Britt, B.A., Gillard, E.F. and Worton, R.G. (1992) The role of the skeletal muscle ryanodine receptor gene in malignant hyperthermia. In: El Haj, A. (ed.) *Molecular Biology of Muscle.* Company of Biologists, Cambridge.

McArdle, A. and Jackson, M.J. (1997) In: Salmons, S. (ed.) *Muscle Damage.* Oxford University Press, Oxford, pp. 90–106.

McComas, A.J. (1977) *Neuromuscular Function and Disorders.* Butterworths, London.

McCurdy, R., Barbut, S. and Quinton, M. (1996) Seasonal effects on PSE in young turkey breast meat. *Food Research International* 29, 363–366.

McFarland, D.C. (1992) Cell culture as a tool for the study of poultry skeletal muscle development. *Journal of Nutrition* 122, 818–829.

McFarland, D.C., Pesall, J.E., Gilkerson, K. and Ferrin, N.H. (1991) Comparison of the proliferation and differentiation of myogenic satellite cells and embryonic myoblasts derived from the turkey. *Comparative Biochemistry and Physiology* 100A, 439–443.

McFarland, D.C., Pesall, J.E. and Gilkerson, K.K. (1993) Comparison of the proliferation and differentiation of myogenic satellite cells derived from Merriam's and commercial varieties of turkeys. *Comparative Biochemistry and Physiology* 3, 455–460.

McKee, S.R. and Sams, A.R. (1997) The effect of seasonal heat stress on rigor development and the incidence of pale, exudative turkey meat. *Poultry Science* 76, 1616–1620.

McKee, S.R. and Sams, A.R. (1998) Rigor mortis development at elevated temperatures induces pale exudative turkey meat characteristics. *Poultry Science* 77, 169–174.

Mahon, M. (1996) Muscle Pathology, Muscle Biopsy Service, and Bibliography. http://www.biomed.man.ac.uk/ns/mm/mushome.html

Mahon, M., Toman, A., Willan, P.L.T. and Bagnall, K.M. (1984) Variability of histochemical and morphometric data from needle biopsy specimens of human quadriceps femoris. *Journal of Neurological Sciences* 63, 85–100.

Mahon, M., Kristmundsdottir, K. and Cumming, W.J.K. (1990) Pathological heterogeneity within the facioscapulohumeral syndrome. *Neuropathology and Applied Neurobiology* 16, 273.

Mahon, M., Cumming, W.J.K. and Shalet, S. (1994) Effects on skeletal muscle of treatment with recombinant somatotropin in adults with growth hormone deficiency. *Muscle Nerve Supplement* 1, S257.

Mahon, M., Ford, T., Gilpin, S., Nixey, C. and French, N.A. (1995) Does your Christmas dinner (*Meleagris gallopavo*) show muscle pathology? *Neuropathology and Applied Neurobiology* 21, 163.

Maranopot, R.R., Bucci, T.J. and Stedham, M.A. (1968) Focal degenerative myopathy in turkeys. *Avian Diseases* 12, 96–103.

Marshall, A.J. (ed.) (1960) *Biology and Comparative Physiology of Birds.* Vol. 1. Academic Press, London.

Martin, C., Chapman, K.E., Seckl, J.R. and Ashley, R.H. (1998) Partial cloning and differential expression of ryanodine receptor/calcium-release channel genes in human tissues including the hippocampus and cerebellum. *Neuroscience* 85, 205–216.

Maruyama, K., Kanemaki, N., Potts, W. and May, J.D. (1993) Body and muscle growth of domestic turkeys (*Meleagris gallopavo*) and expression of myosin heavy chain isoforms in breast muscle. *Growth, Development and Aging* 57, 31–43.

Mastaglia, F.L. and Walton, J.N. (eds) (1992) *Skeletal Muscle Pathology,* 2nd edn. Churchill Livingstone, Edinburgh.

Matsumura, K. and Campbell, K.P. (1994) Dystrophin–glycoprotein complex: its role in the molecular pathogenesis of muscular dystrophies. *Muscle Nerve* 17, 2–15.

Mayes, F.J. (1980) The incidence of bruising in broiler flocks. *British Poultry Science* 21, 505–509.

Merck Veterinary Manual (1986) *A Handbook of Diagnosis, Therapy, and Disease Prevention and Control,* 6th edn. Merck & Co, Inc., Rahway, New Jersey.

Merly, F., Magras-Resch, C., Rouaud, T., Fontaine-Perus, J. and Gardahaut, M.F. (1998)

Comparative analysis of satellite cell properties in heavy- and lightweight strains of turkey. *Journal of Muscle Research and Cell Motility* 19, 257–270.

Mills, L.J., Mahon, M. and Mitchell, M.A. (1998a) Incidence of skeletal muscle damage in selected and unselected strains of turkey. *British Journal of Poultry Science* (abstract, in press).

Mills, L.J., Mahon, M. and Mitchell, M.A. (1998b) Growth characteristics and incidence of damage in the breast muscle of selected and unselected strains of turkey. *Poultry Science* (abstract, in press).

Mitchell, M.A. and Sandercock, D.A. (1995) Creatine kinase isoenzyme profiles in the plasma of the domestic fowl (*Gallus domesticus*). *Research in Veterinary Science* 59, 30–34.

Mitchell, M.A., Hocking, P.M., Hunter, R.R. and Sandercock, D.A. (1996) A relationship between growth and plasma creatine kinase activity in sire line and traditional turkeys. *British Poultry Science* 37, Suppl. 586–587.

Morgan, J.E. and Watt, D.J. (1993) Myoblast transplantation inherited myopathies. In: Partridge, T. (ed.) *Molecular and Cell Biology of Muscular Dystrophy*. Chapman & Hall, London, pp. 303–331.

Moxley, R.T. (1994) Metabolic and endocrine myopathies. In: Walton, J.N., Karpati, G. and Hilton-Jones, D. (eds) *Disorders of Voluntary Muscle*, 6th edn. Churchill Livingstone, Edinburgh, pp. 647–716.

Nixey, C. and Grey, T.C. (1989) *Recent Advances in Turkey Science*. Butterworths, London.

Northcutt, J.K., Foegeding, E.A. and Edens, F.W. (1994) Water-holding properties of thermally preconditioned chicken breast and leg meat. *Poultry Science* 73, 308–316.

Northcutt, J.K., Buhr, R.J. and Young, L. (1998a) Influence of preslaughter stunning on turkey breast muscle quality. *Poultry Science* 77, 487–492.

Northcutt, J.K., Pringle, T.D., Dickens, J.A., Buhr, R.J. and Young, L.L. (1998b) Effects of age and tissue type on the calpain proteolytic system in turkey skeletal muscle. *Poultry Science* 77, 367–372.

Novilla, M.N. (1984) Diagnosis and differential diagnosis of monensin toxicity. In: *Monensin Diagnostic Manual*. Elanco Products Co, Indianapolis.

Nyengaard, J.R., Bendtsen, T.F., Bjugn, R., Lokkegaard, A., Tang, Y. and Gunderson, H.J.G. (1996) A stereological approach to capillary networks. In: Sharma, A.K. (ed.) *Morphometry: Applications to Medical Sciences*. Macmillan, New Delhi, pp. 217–231.

Orr, J.P. and Riddell, C. (1977) Investigation of the vascular supply of the pectoral muscles of the domestic turkey and comparison of experimentally produced infarcts with naturally occurring deep pectoral myopathy. *American Journal of Veterinary Research* 38, 1237–1242.

Page, R.K. and Fletcher, O.J. (1975) Myopathy of the deep pectoral muscle in broiler breeder hens. *Avian Diseases* 19, 814–821.

Pallis, C.A. and Lewis, P.D. (1988) Involvement of human muscle by parasites. In: Walton, J. (ed.) *Disorders of Voluntary Muscle*, 5th edn. Churchill Livingstone, Edinburgh.

Partridge, T. (1993) *Molecular and Cell Biology of Muscular Dystrophy*. Chapman & Hall, London.

Pette, D. (ed.) (1980) *Plasticity of Muscle*. Walter de Gruyter, Berlin.

Pette, D. (ed.) (1990) *The Dynamic State of Muscle Fibers*. Walter de Gruyter, Berlin.

Pietrzak, M., Greaser, M.L. and Sosnicki, A.A. (1997) Effect of rapid rigor mortis processes on protein functionality in pectoralis major muscle of domestic turkeys. *Journal of Animal Science* 75, 2106–2116.

Pizzey, J.A., Barnard, E.A. and Barnard, P.J. (1983) Involvement of fast and slow twitch muscle fibres in avian muscular dystrophy. *Journal of Neurological Sciences* 61, 217–233.

Quane, K.A., Healy, J.M.S., Keating, K.E., Manning, G.M., Couch, F.J., Palmucci, L.M., Doriguzzi, C., Fagerlund, T.H., Berg, K., Ording, H., Bendixen, D., Mertier, W., Linz, U., Muller, C.R. and McCarthy, T.V. (1993) Mutations in the ryanodine receptor gene in central core disease and malignant hyperthermia. *Nature Genetics* 5, 51–55.

Quane, K.A., Keating, K.E., Manning, B.M., Healy, J.M.S., Monsieurs, K., Heffron, J.J.A., Lehane, M., Heytens, L., Krivasic-Horber, R., Adnet, P., Ellis, F.R., Monnier, N., Lunardi, J. and McCarthy, T.V. (1994) Detection of a novel common mutation in the ryanodine receptor gene in malignant hyperthermia: implications for diagnosis and heterogeneity studies. *Human Molecular Genetics* 3, 471–476.

Reiner, G., Hartman, J. and Dzapo, V. (1995) Skeletal muscle sarcoplasmic calcium regulation and sudden death syndrome in chickens. *British Journal of Poultry Science* 36, 667–675.

Remignon, H., Lefaucheur, L., Blum, J.C. and Ricard, F.H. (1994) Effects of divergent selection for body weight on three skeletal muscles characteristics in the chicken. *British Poultry Science* 35, 65–76.

Remignon, H., Gardahaut, M.F., Marche, G. and Ricard, F.H. (1995) Selection of rapid growth increases the number and the size of muscle fibres without changing their typing in chickens. *Journal of Muscle Research and Cell Motility* 16, 95–102.

Richards, R.B., Passmore, I.K. and Dempsey, E.F. (1988) Skeletal muscle pathology in ovine congenital progressive muscular dystrophy. *Acta Neuropathologica* 77, 161–167.

Ricklefs, R.E. (1983) Avian postnatal development. In: Farner, D.S., King, J.R. and Parkes, K.C. (eds) *Avian Biology* VII. Academic Press, New York, pp. 1–83.

Rocca, M., Giavaresi, G., Fini, M., Orienti, L. and Giardino, R. (1998) Laser Doppler evaluation of microcirculation behaviour during an ischaemia-reperfusion injury. *European Surgical Research* 30, 108–114.

Rodrigues, N.R., Owen, N., Talbot, K. *et al.* (1995) Deletions in the survival motor neuron gene on 5q13 in autosomal recessive spinal muscular atrophy. *Human Molecular Genetics* 4, 631–634.

Roy, N., Mahadevani, M. and McLean *et al.* (1995) The gene for neuronal apoptosis inhibitory protein is partially deleted in individuals with spinal muscular atrophy. *Cell* 80, 167–178.

Rushton, J.L., Davie, I., Horan, M.A., Mahon, M. and Williams, R. (1997) Production of consistent crush lesions of murine skeletal muscle *in vivo* using an electro-mechanical device. *Journal of Anatomy* 190, 417–422.

Salmons, S. (1997) *Muscle Damage*. Oxford University Press, Oxford.

Saltin, B. and Gollnick, P.D. (1983) Skeletal muscle adaptability: significance for metabolism and performance. In: Peachey, L.D. (ed.) *Skeletal Muscle*. Handbook of Physiology, 10. American Physiological Society, Bethesda.

Sams, A.R. and Janky, D.M. (1990) Simultaneous histochemical determination of three fiber types in single sections of broiler skeletal muscles. *Poultry Science* 69, 1433–1436.

Sandercock, D.A. (1998) Biochemical and physiological mechanisms of creatine kinase release from avian skeletal muscle during acute stress. PhD Thesis, University of Edinburgh.

Schmalbruch, H. (1985) *Skeletal Muscle*. Springer-Verlag, Berlin.

Schultz, E. and McCormick, K.M. (1993) Cell Biology of the satellite cell. In: Partridge, T. (ed.) *Molecular and Cell Biology of Muscular Dystrophy*. Chapman & Hall, London, pp. 190–209.

Shaptala, I. (1973) Experimental production of white muscle disease in turkey poults. *Ptitsevodstvo* 2, 46–47.

Sheldon, B.W., Curtis, P.A., Dawson, P.L. and Ferket, P.R. (1997) Effect of dietary vitamin

E on the oxidative stability, flavor, color and volatile profiles of refrigerated and frozen turkey breast meat. *Poultry Science* 76, 634–641.

Shepherd, G.M. (1988) *Neurobiology*, 2nd edn, Oxford University Press, Oxford.

Shufeldt, R.W. (1890) *The Myology of the Raven*. Macmillan & Co., London.

Siller, W.G. (1985) Deep pectoral myopathy: a penalty of successful selection for muscle growth. *Poultry Science* 64, 1591–1595.

Siller, W.G. and Wight, P.A.L. (1978) The pathology of deep pectoral myopathy of turkeys. *Avian Pathology* 7, 583–618.

Siller, W.G., Wight, P.A.L., Martindale, L. and Bannister, D.W. (1978) Deep pectoral myopathy: an experimental simulation in the fowl. *Research in Veterinary Science* 24, 267–268.

Siller, W.G., Wight, P.A.L. and Martindale, L. (1979a) Exercise-induced deep pectoral myopathy in broiler fowls and turkeys. *Veterinary Science Communications* 2, 331–336.

Siller, W.G., Martindale, L. and Wight, P.A.L. (1979b) The prevention of experimental deep pectoral myopathy of the fowl by fasciotomy. *Avian Pathology* 8, 301–307.

Simpson, C.F., Damron, B.L. and Harms, R.H. (1971) Toxic myopathy of chicks fed *Cassia occidentalis* seeds. *Avian Diseases* 15, 284–290.

Smith, D.P. and Fletcher, D.L. (1988) Chicken breast muscle fiber type and diameter as influenced by age and intramuscular location. *Poultry Science* 67, 908–913.

Sola, O.M., Christensen, D.L. and Martin, A.W. (1973) Hypertrophy and hyperplasia of adult chicken latissimus dorsi muscles following stretch with and without denervation. *Experimental Neurology* 41, 76–100.

Sosnicki, A. (1987) Histopathlogical observation of stress myopathy in *M. longissimus* in the pig and relationships with meat quality, fattening, and slaughter traits. *Journal of Animal Science* 65, 584–596.

Sosnicki, A.A. (1993) PSE in turkey. *Meat Focus International* 2, 75–78.

Sosnicki, A. and Cassens, R.G. (1988a) Determination of fibre types of chicken skeletal muscles based on reaction for actomyosin, calcium^{+2}, magnesium^{+2}-dependent adenosine triphosphate. *Poultry Science* 67, 973–978.

Sosnicki, A. and Cassens, R.G. (1988b) Metachromatic procedure for fiber typing in chicken skeletal muscle. *Poultry Science* 67, 982–985.

Sosnicki, A.A. and Wilson, B.W. (1991) Pathology of turkey skeletal muscle: Implications for the poultry industry. *Food Structure* 10, 317–326.

Sosnicki, A.A. and Wilson, B.W. (1992) Relationship of focal myopathy of turkey skeletal muscle to meat quality. *Turkey* 1, 43–47.

Sosnicki, A., Cassens, R.G., McIntyre, D.R. and Vimini, R.G. (1988a) Structural alterations in oedematous and apparently normal skeletal muscle of domestic turkey. *Avian Pathology* 17, 775–791.

Sosnicki, A., Cassens, R.G., McIntyre, D.R., Vimini, R.J. and Greaser, M.L. (1988b) Characterization of hypercontracted fibres in skeletal muscle of domestic turkey (*Meleagris gallopavo*). *Food Microstructure* 7, 147–152.

Sosnicki, A., Cassens, R.G., McIntyre, D.R., Vimini, R.J. and Greaser, M.L. (1989) Incidence of microscopically detectable degenerative characteristics in skeletal muscle of turkey. *British Poultry Science* 30, 69–80.

Sosnicki, A.A., Cassens, R.G., Vimini, R.J. and Greaser, M.L. (1991a) Distribution of capillaries in normal and ischemic turkey skeletal muscle. *Poultry Science* 70, 343–348.

Sosnicki, A.A., Cassens, R.G., Vimini, R.J. and Greaser, M.L. (1991b) Histopathological and ultrastructural alterations of turkey skeletal muscle. *Poultry Science* 70, 349–357.

Spraker, T.R., Adrian, W.J. and Lance, W.R. (1987) Capture myopathy in wild turkeys (*Meleagris gallopavo*) following trapping, handling and transportation in Colorado. *Journal of Wildlife Diseases* 23, 447–453.

Stuart, J.C. (1978) An outbreak of monensin poisoning in adult turkeys. *Veterinary Record* 102, 303–304.

Stuart, J.C. (1983) Salinomycin poisoning in turkeys. *Veterinary Record* 113, 597.

Summers, J.D. and Spratt, D. (1990) Weight gain, carcass yield, and composition of large white male turkeys reared at 28 weeks of age on growing and finishing diets with varying levels of dietary protein. *Poultry Science* 69, 584–591.

Sun, S.S. and McFarland, D.C. (1993) Interaction of fibroblast growth factor with turkey embryonic myoblasts and myogenic satellite cells. *Comparative Biochemistry and Physiology* 105A, 85–89.

Sutherland, I.R. (1974) Hereditary pectoral myopathy in the domestic turkey. *Canadian Veterinary Journal* 15, 77–81.

Swash, M., Henrichs, K.J., Berry, C.L. and Jones, J.M. (1980) Deep pectoral myopathy (Oregon disease) in the turkey. In: Rose, F.C. and Behan, P.O. (eds) *Animal Models of Neurological Disease*. Pitman Medical, Tunbridge Wells, p. 3.

Swatland, H.J. (1979a) Allometric radial growth in muscle, comparing fibres with strong and with weak adenosine triphosphatase activity. *Journal of Anatomy* 129, 591–596.

Swatland, H.J. (1979b) Differential growth in the sartorius muscles of male and female turkeys. *Zentralblatt für Veterinarmedizin A* 26, 159–164.

Swatland, H.J. (1979c) Differential growth in the supracoracoideus muscles of male and female turkeys. *Zentralblatt für Veterinarmedizin C Anat Histol Embryol* 8, 227–232.

Swatland, H.J. (1979d) Development of shape in turkey carcasses. *Journal of Agricultural Sciences* 93, 1–6.

Swatland, H.J. (1980) A histological basis for differences in breast meat yield between two strains of white turkeys. *Journal of Agricultural Sciences* 94, 383–388.

Swatland, H.J. (1981) Allometric growth of histochemical types of muscle fibers in ducks. *Growth* 45, 58–65.

Swatland, H.J. (1985) Growth related changes in the intracellular distribution of succinate dehydrogenase activity in turkey muscle. *Growth* 49, 409–416.

Swatland, H.J. (1987) Fiber optic spectrophotometry of color intensity problems in raw and cooked turkey breasts. *Poultry Science* 66, 679–682.

Swatland, H.J. (1989a) Morphometry of pectoral development in turkey breeding stock. *British Poultry Science* 30, 785–795.

Swatland, H.J. (1989b) Physiology of muscle growth. In: Nixey, C. and Grey, T.C. (eds) *Recent Advances in Turkey Science*. Butterworths, London, pp. 167–182.

Swatland, H.J. (1990) A note on the growth of connective tissues binding turkey muscle fibers together. *Canadian Institute of Food Science and Technology Journal* 23, 239–241.

Swatland, H.J. (1991) Spatial and spectrophotometric measurements of light scattering in turkey breast meat using lasers and a xenon arc. *Canadian Institute of Technology Journal* 24, 27–31.

Swatland, H.J. (1993) Developing a fiber-optic probe to combine subcutaneous fat depth and meat quality measurements. *Journal of Animal Science* 71, 2666–2673.

Swatland, H.J. (1995) Physiology of growth and development. In: Hunton, P. (ed.) *Poultry Production*. Elsevier, Amsterdam, pp. 23–51.

Swatland, H.J. and Barbut, S. (1995) Optical prediction of processing characteristics of turkey meat using UV fluorescence and NIR birefringence. *Food Research International* 28, 227–232.

Taylor, C.R., Weibel, E. and Bolis, L. (eds) (1985) *Design and Performance of Muscular Systems.* Company of Biologists, Cambridge.

Taylor, M.W. and Helbecka, N.V.L. (1968) Field studies of bruised poultry. *Poultry Science* 47, 1166–1169.

Torrella, J.R., Fouces, V., Palomeque, J. and Viscor, G. (1998) Comparative skeletal muscle fibre morphometry among wild birds with different locomotor behaviour. *Journal of Anatomy* 192, 211–222.

Tripp, M.J. and Schmitz, J.A. (1982) Influence of physical exercise on plasma creatine kinase activity in healthy and dystrophic turkeys and sheep. *American Journal of Veterinary Research* 43, 2220–2223.

Van Fleet, J.F., Amstutz, H.E., Weirich, W.E., Rebar, A.H. and Ferrans, V.J. (1983) Clinical, clinicopathologic, and pathological alterations of monensin toxicosis in swine. *American Journal of Veterinary Research* 44, 1469–1475.

Van Hoof, J. (1979) Influence of ante- and peri-mortem factors on muscle biochemical and physical characteristics of turkey breast muscle. *Vet* 1, 29–36.

Vinken, P.J., Bruyn, G.W. and Klawans, H.L. (eds) (1992) *Handbook of Clinical Neurology; 18 v. 62 Myopathies.* Elsevier Science Publishers, Amsterdam.

Vrbova, G., Gordon, T. and Jones, R. (1995) *Nerve–Muscle Interactions,* 2nd edn. Chapman & Hall, London.

Wages, D.P. and Ficken, M.D. (1988) Skeletal muscle lesions in turkeys associated with the feeding of monensin. *Avian Diseases* 32, 583–586.

Walton, J.N., Karpati, G. and Hilton-Jones, D. (eds) (1994) *Disorders of Voluntary Muscle,* 6th edn. Churchill Livingstone, Edinburgh.

Weibel, E.R. (1984) *The Pathway to Oxygen.* Harvard University Press, Cambridge, Massachussetts.

Weller, R.O., Cumming, W.J.K. and Mahon, M. (1997) Diseases of muscle. In: Graham, D. I. and Lantos, P.L. (eds) *Greenfield's Neuropathology,* 6th edn. Arnold, London, pp. 489–581.

Wesley, R.L. (1986) How to avoid 99% of your downgrading. *Turkey World* 6, 24.

Wight, P.A.L., Siller, W.G., Martindale, L. and Filshie, J.H. (1979) The induction by muscle stimulation of a deep pectoral myopathy in the fowl. *Avian Pathology* 8, 115–121.

Wilson, B.W. (1990) Developmental and maturational aspects of inherited avian myopathies. *Proceedings of the Society of Experimental Biology and Medicine* 194, 87–96.

Wilson, B.W., Randall, W.R., Patterson, G.T. and Entrikin, R.K. (1979) Major physiologic and histochemical characteristics of inherited dystrophy of the chicken. *Annals of the New York Academy of Sciences* 317, 224–246.

Wilson, B.W.H., Abplanalp, R.J., Buhr, R.K., Entrikin, R.K., Hooper, J. and Nieberg, P.S. (1988) Inbred and inherited muscular dystrophy of the chicken. *Poultry Science* 67, 367–374.

Wilson, B.W., Nieberg, P.S., Buhr, R.J., Kelly, B.J. and Shultz, F.T. (1990) Turkey muscle growth and focal myopathy. *Poultry Science* 69, 1553–1562.

Wiskus, K.J., Addis, P.B. and Ma, R.T.I. (1976) Distribution of βR, αR and αW fibers in turkey muscles. *Poultry Science* 55, 562–572.

Wyers, M., Tapie, S., Hurtrel, M. and Cherel, Y. (1992) Histomorphometric study of the superficial pectoral muscle of the turkey. Relationship with the meat discoloration syndrome. *Annales de Recherches Veterinaires* 23, 49–58.

Zhang, Y., Chen, H.S., Khanna, V.K., De Leon, S., Phillips, M.S., Schapperty, K., Britt, B.A., Browell, A.K. and MacLennan, D.H. (1993) A mutation in the human ryanodine receptor gene associated with central core disease. *Nature Genetics* 5, 46–50.

CHAPTER 3
Muscle abnormalities: pathophysiological mechanisms

M.A. Mitchell
Roslin Institute (Edinburgh), Roslin, Midlothian EH25 9PS, UK

INTRODUCTION

Chapter 2 describes the anatomical, morphological and histological character-istics of normal and abnormal skeletal muscle. The changes occurring in trauma, myopathies and dystrophies of various aetiologies have been detailed. It has been proposed recently that the incidence of such muscle abnormalities has increased in response to genetic selection for improved growth rate and other production traits in modern commercial poultry (Soike, 1995; Rémignon *et al.,* 1996) and that this may underlie a deterioration in meat and eating quality (Henckel, 1996). In order to confirm or refute this assertion it is necessary to develop a precise definition and standards of poultry meat quality and objective criteria for its assessment. In turn, to provide a sound scientific basis for these procedures it is essential to fully elucidate the physiological mechanisms and morphological characteristics pertaining to normal and deranged muscle function in the appropriate commercial birds. Ultimately, problems with meat quality are caused by changes in the biochemistry and morphology of muscle as well as post-mortem events (Sosnicki and Wilson, 1991). To facilitate assessment of the effects of ante-mortem factors on meat quality, such as genetic selection, pathology, nutrition, environment and stress, including handling and transport, it is necessary vastly to expand current knowledge of live muscle physiology and to identify and characterize those cellular systems which may determine or mediate post-mortem changes in the tissue (Ngoka *et al.,* 1982; Ming-Tsao *et al.,* 1991; Sosnicki and Wilson, 1991; Henckel, 1996). A prerequisite for the characterization of the pathophysio-logical mechanisms, which may produce muscle abnormalities associated with genetic factors or environmental stress, is an understanding of the normal physiological function of muscle tissue. This facilitates identification of those changes or derangements in function which result in the develop-ment of myopathic states and overt muscle pathologies.

SKELETAL MUSCLE FORM AND FUNCTION

Avian skeletal muscle is fundamentally similar in structure and function to the more extensively studied mammalian tissue (Bowman and Marshall, 1971; Harvey and Marshall, 1983; 1986). Clearly the major function of skeletal muscle is the generation of force or the performance of work in the form of movement or support of the skeletal structures (Best and Taylor, 1965). The outstanding property of muscle is therefore contractility. Avian skeletal muscles contain the same types of contractile proteins as their mammalian counterparts. Actin and myosin filaments are arranged in the classical interdigitated pattern, giving rise to the 'striated' appearance, and contain the same regulatory contractile proteins troponins I, C and T, tropomyosin and α-actinin (Harvey and Marshall, 1986; Obinata, 1993; Yao *et al.,* 1994a, b; Szczesna *et al.,* 1996; Watanabe *et al.,* 1997). Skeletal muscle contraction is generally initiated by the arrival of an excitatory electrical signal at the neuromuscular junction which is transduced into the physical interactions between the contractile proteins. This process, by which muscle membrane depolarization is linked to contraction, is known as 'excitation–contraction' (EC) coupling and the mechanisms involved have been extensively studied and reviewed (Martonosi, 1984; Rios and Pizarro, 1988, 1991; Rios *et al.,* 1992; Schneider, 1994; Franzini-Armstrong and Jorgensen, 1994; Tsugorka *et al.,* 1995).

EXCITATION–CONTRACTION (EC) COUPLING

The mechanochemical reaction between actin and myosin can only take place in the presence of myoplasmic free calcium concentrations exceeding a threshold of 50–150 nM (Rios and Pizarro, 1988). This is achieved by the regulated release of calcium from intracellular stores, specifically in the sarcoplasmic reticulum (SR). As a result of more detailed elucidation of the mechanisms involved in this process, EC coupling is now regarded as the coupling between the depolarization of the T-tubule membrane and channel-mediated calcium release from the SR, a transduction which occurs with a millisecond to submillisecond time course (Rios and Pizarro, 1991; Rios *et al.,* 1992; Schneider, 1994; Franzini-Armstrong and Jorgensen, 1994). Three distinct components of the EC coupling have been identified and occur at the 'triads', specialized regions of junctional contact between the T-tubule and the SR. The first stage is voltage sensing which then triggers the second phase which is regarded as 'transmission' and involves charge movement within the voltage sensor and mechanical or chemical linking to the activation of the third phase of calcium release into the myoplasm (Rios and Pizarro, 1991; Rios *et al.,* 1992). The first phase voltage-sensing process, the study of which began with the recognition and measurement of intramembrane charge movement (Schneider and Chandler, 1973), consists of membrane-sensitive conformational changes of a charged sensor molecule located within the T-tubule membrane (Schneider, 1994). The intramembrane 'tetrads', identified by ultrastructural examination of the triadic regions, are thought to represent the sensors and are functionally areas of high 'dihydropyridine binding activity' (Rios *et al.,* 1992; Franzini-Armstrong and Jorgensen, 1994.). The properties of these dihydropyridine receptors (DHPRs) suggest their possible roles in the mechanism of the transmission phase. DHPRs are regarded as slowly activating calcium channels, a specialized form of the voltage gated L-type channel ubiquitous in both excitable and many non-excitable tissues (Bean, 1989; Tsien and Tsien, 1990), and are responsible for most of the charge movement associated with depolarizations to the contractile threshold (Franzini-Armstrong and Jorgensen, 1994). The receptors or channel proteins are composed of one each of four or five distinct subunits which have been sequenced and expressed in mammals (Bean, 1989; Tsien and Tsien, 1990). The available evidence suggests that one or more preliminary voltage-dependent charge-moving transitions, involving conformational changes in and interactions between the subunits, may precede the final transition which mediates transmission to the final calcium release event, i.e. appreciable voltage sensor charge movement precedes the actual channel opening step (Schneider, 1994). Considerable controversy still surrounds the precise molecular mechanism involved. The concepts of direct mechanical coupling, involving contact of the structures in the T-tubule and SR membranes (although there appears to be a 12–17 nm gap between the membranes), and an indirect mediation by diffusible channel modulators, both receiving substantial support (Rios *et al.,* 1992; Franzini-Armstrong and Jorgensen, 1994; Schneider, 1994; Sutko and Airey, 1996). It has been speculated that the DHPR may act as a channel containing a 'restricted space' in which a calcium ion is resident and that during depolarization-induced conformational changes this cation is afforded privileged access to another intracellular calcium-activated calcium channel which is responsible for release of calcium from the SR (Schneider, 1994). This is an example of the possible involvement of a 'diffusible mediator or modulator' in the interaction between the DHPR and the SR release channel but does not exclude the possibility of an alternative or concurrent voltage regulated, more mechanical or molecular mechanism of coupling (Rios *et al.,* 1992; Franzini-Armstrong and Jorgensen, 1994; Schneider, 1994; Sutko and Airey, 1996). In addition to calcium ions other putative chemical mediators of transmission include inositol 1,4,5-triphosphate (InsP$_3$), G-proteins and protein kinase stimulated DHPR phosphorylation (Schneider, 1994). Magnesium ions may exert an inhibitory effect on transmission (Meissner, 1994; Schneider, 1994).

RELEASE OF CALCIUM FROM THE SARCOPLASMIC RETICULUM

The third or final stage of EC coupling is the calcium release process involving efflux of the ion from the SR through a different type of calcium channel and the consequent elevation of myoplasmic calcium concentration. There are at least two categories of intracellular calcium channels in all vertebrate cells mediating the release of calcium from internal stores (Tsien and Tsien, 1990;

Pozzan *et al.*, 1994; Berridge, 1994, 1997; Ashley, 1995). These can be broadly defined as ryanodine receptors (RyRs), so called because they bind the plant alkaloid ryanodine and $InsP_3$ receptors ($InsP_3Rs$) (Berridge, 1997), which bind the phosphoinositide. Both receptor types are homotetrameric protein structures (Ashley, 1995). There are at least three subtypes of RyRs (RyR1, RyR2 and RyR3) and four types of $InsP_3Rs$ (Ashley, 1995; Berridge, 1997). All these receptors share considerable structural and physiological similarities and it is proposed that they have evolved from a common ancestor. RyRs and $InsP_3Rs$ are located in the membranes of the major intracellular calcium stores, i.e. the endoplasmic and sarcoplasmic reticulum. These receptor proteins exhibit some cell and tissue specific expression (Ashley, 1995). In mammals, different isoforms of both broad categories of intracellular calcium channel are distributed across excitable and non-excitable tissues but skeletal muscle is thought to possess only type-1 RyR and no $InsP_3R$ (Ashley, 1995). All the receptors have a membrane-spanning region in their C-terminal which acts as the calcium channel and stabilizes the intramembrane location of the protein. The very large and bulbous N-terminals represent the 'control region' which integrates the various signals and regulates channel opening. *In vitro* vesicle preparations of sarcoplasmic reticulum membranes have been employed to determine many of the characteristics of the calcium release channel. Ryanodine can either stimulate or inhibit calcium efflux dependent upon conditions (Meissner, 1986), but the predominant physiological stimulatory effect of the alkaloid is mediated by a conformational change induced by binding which prevents complete closure of the channel. RyRs can be activated by calcium ions, Ins $1,4,5-P_3$, adenine nucleotides, caffeine, cADP-ribose and voltage whereas $InsP_3Rs$ share sensitivity to only the first three of these stimuli (Ashley, 1995). Channel function may also be influenced by calmodulin and redox state (Sutko and Airey, 1996). The most significant of this range of properties of the receptors is that of sensitivity to calcium activation and therefore calcium-induced calcium release (CICR) which accounts for their ability to generate 'calcium spikes and waves'. Calcium ions play a central role in the control of a vast number of cellular activities and metabolic processes and in many pathways may be regarded as the final messenger in physiological signalling. For this reason the precise spatio-temporal regulation of calcium release and cytoplasmic concentration is essential and the intracellular calcium release channels constitute a major component of this system. In mammalian skeletal muscle, the SR membrane contains type 1 ryanodine receptors and this is the calcium release channel mediating the final phase of EC coupling (Tsien and Tsien, 1990; Rios *et al.*, 1992; Franzini-Armstrong and Jorgensen, 1994; Coronado *et al.*, 1994; Meissner, 1994; Pozzan *et al.*, 1994; Schneider, 1994; Ashley, 1995; Sutko and Airey, 1996; Berridge, 1994, 1997). Regardless of the precise mechanism of transmission, T-tubule depolarization and DHPR activation initiates the opening of the RyR calcium channels in the SR membrane, the release of calcium into the myoplasm and ultimately skeletal muscle contraction. By tight coupling of the calcium release through the RyRs to the depolarization of the T-tubule membrane, synchronization of the release event throughout a large muscle fibre can be achieved allowing rapid and repeated contraction. Not only does DHPR activity open the RyR channel during depolarization but in the membrane repolarization phase it is responsible for closure of the release channel (Berridge, 1997). It is suggested that RyR–DHPR association occurs at discrete sites or clusters in skeletal muscle known as 'calcium release units' (Franzini-Armstrong, 1995). RyRs, however, greatly outnumber DHPRs and some morphological evidence suggests that only a subpopulation of RyRs is mechanically or positionally linked to the T-tubule voltage sensors (Meissner, 1994; Berridge, 1997). The elementary unit mediating EC coupling may therefore be considered to be a DHPR–RyR pair together with some neighbouring unlinked RyRs which are activated by the calcium released from the linked channel (Rios et al., 1992; Meissner, 1994; Berridge, 1997). This would serve to amplify the initial signal considerably. This model of dual regulation of SR calcium release is consistent with the observations of spontaneous unitary release of calcium, apparently from a single RyR, a fundamental event the frequency of which increases when myoplasmic calcium concentration is raised or in the presence of caffeine (Klein et al., 1996; Berridge, 1997). These calcium 'sparks' are thought to be the elementary unit of calcium release which summate to produce the myoplasmic calcium transiently occurring during contraction. The frequency of these calcium 'sparks' is also increased during membrane depolarization and as DHPR–RyR pairs are recruited evoked sparks with multiple amplitudes can be observed (Tsugorka et al., 1995). It has been argued that the non-unitary nature and quantal growth of evoked sparks reflects the recruitment of neighbouring non-linked RyRs by calcium-induced calcium release (CICR). Although the actual magnitude of calcium release constituting the fundamental or elementary calcium release event (do sparks consist of quarks ?) has recently been questioned (Eisner and Trafford, 1996; Berridge, 1997), in response to reports of smaller but constant units of calcium efflux from the SR (Parker et al., 1996), the proposed basic mechanism of EC coupling remains the same. A T-tubule membrane depolarization activates a DHPR–RyR linked pair resulting in calcium release, which in turn activates or opens adjacent but unlinked RyRs through CICR thus leading to a global calcium signal for contraction in skeletal muscle. This is derived from both depolarization and ligand activated events (Meissner, 1994; Klein et al., 1996; Berridge, 1997). There is, thus, a direct functional and structural interaction between the DHPR and the related RyRs. This process may be stabilized by other proteins such as 'triadin' (Meissner and Lu, 1995). The efflux of calcium from intracellular stores by such a mechanism allows for 'localized release' at the site of action far from the plasma membrane of the cell and does not require direct influx of extracellular calcium (Pozzan et al., 1994).

RYANODINE RECEPTORS

Vertebrate RyRs are homotetramers composed of polypeptide subunits with molecular masses of 500–600 kDa encoded by mRNAs of 15 kb (Dulhunty et al., 1996; Sutko and Airey, 1996). cDNA sequences from RyRs in human and rabbit skeletal muscle demonstrate that the protein consists of 5032 or 5076 amino acid residues with molecular masses of 563,584 Da or 565,223 Da (Coronado et al., 1994). All the RyR proteins studied are very similar in their overall topology and have highly conserved C-terminals in which resides the channel forming—membrane spanning region (Sutko and Airey, 1996). The large N-terminal part of the RyR, comprising approximately 80% of the protein mass, forms the cytoplasmic 'foot' domain and appears to act as the integrator of activation signals (see above). In mammals, mRNAs for the three recognized main classes of RyRs have been cloned and sequenced and have been found to be encoded by separate genes. These do not exhibit complete tissue specificity (the receptors having been isolated from over thirty tissues (Sutko and Airey, 1996) but are predominantly found in certain locations, ryr 1 being associated with skeletal muscle, ryr 2 with cardiac muscle and ryr 3 in brain (Dulhunty et al., 1996; Schmoelzl et al., 1996; Sutko and Airey, 1996). The expression of ryr 1 is regulated by at least two novel transcription factors RYREF-1 and RYREF-2 (Schmoelzl et al., 1996). Non-mammalian RyRs are often designated α, β and cardiac corresponding to RyR1, RyR3 and RyR2 (Sutko and Airey, 1996). RyRs can be detergent solubilized, isolated and purified and the general properties of RyR and the characteristics of the mammalian isoforms RyR1 and RyR2 have been examined (Coronado et al., 1994; Meissner, 1994; Dulhunty et al., 1996; Sutko and Airey, 1996). The binding of radiolabelled ryanodine has proved a powerful tool in the study of the calcium release channel. It appears that [^{3}H]ryanodine binds preferentially to the open state of the channel and this property has been used to examine the effects of ligands which open the channel (e.g. calcium and ATP) and close the channel (ruthenium red). Ryanodine is thus an important conformational probe which will indicate the gating state of the calcium release channel (Coronado et al., 1994). The RyR calcium release channel is cation selective exhibiting an unusually high conductance (600–750 pS) for monovalent cations, e.g. sodium and potassium, and for divalent cations (100–170 pS), e.g. calcium and barium (Coronado et al., 1994; Meissner, 1994; Dulhunty et al., 1996). The dissociation constant for Ca^{2+} was 3 mM. Although the conductances measured in isolated channels in lipid bilayers appear to favour translocation of the monovalent ions the findings are a consequence of the experimental conditions. Thus, although the conductance ratio for $K^+:Ca^{2+}$ was six the actual corresponding permeability ratio, in the presence of mixed salts, was 0.14 indicating that under physiological conditions the channel is highly calcium selective (Coronado et al., 1994).

More recently it has been proposed that, on the basis of both functional and structural criteria, there may be up to nine RyR isoforms expressed in vertebrate tissue and that more than one form may be expressed in a tissue including skeletal muscle (Sutko and Airey, 1996). Indeed, different muscles may express different combinations of isoforms. It is, as yet, unclear if the different isoforms subserve contrasting muscle cell functions but the use of one or more RyR types, with different functional properties, alone or in combination, may permit more sophisticated and precise control and regulation of the calcium release and signal amplification process. It may be suggested that, as investigation reveals increasingly complex but specific expressions or distributions of the isoforms of the ryanodine receptor-SR calcium release channel and the differential sensitivity of the various forms to the growing list of putative effector molecules, it is essential to characterize the role of each channel type and relate these to both normal and pathological muscle function in different species.

INTRACELLULAR CALCIUM

The regulated and compartmentalized release of calcium through intracellular calcium channels is essential not just for muscle contraction but for the control of a vast number of metabolic pathways and cellular activities including protein–protein interactions, phosphorylation cycles, release of neuro-transmitters, secretion, exocytosis, synaptic plasticity, gene expression, cell proliferation, cell growth and apoptosis (Carafoli, 1987; Williamson and Monck, 1989; Tsien and Tsien, 1990; Ashley, 1995; Berridge, 1997). Calcium is the most abundant cation in the vertebrate body but most of it is immobilized in the skeleton which acts as a reservoir from where Ca^{2+} can be mobilized as required by the organism to support dietary input (Pozzan et al., 1994). To a first approximation, individual cells mirror this distribution in that cytosolic calcium represents only 10–20% of cell content of the cation and is mostly bound to both soluble cytosolic proteins and membrane surfaces. The reason for this lies in the fact that calcium is a paradoxical 'choice' for a second messenger for cell signalling as it is remarkably toxic and unlike other biological messengers, e.g. cyclic nucleotides, $InsP_3$ or diacylglycerol, its concentration cannot be readily regulated by metabolic synthesis and degradation (Carafoli, 1987; Berridge, 1994). It may, of course, be argued that the 'toxicity' of calcium is a consequence of its regulatory role and that overstimulation of multiple calcium-sensitive pathways explains the pathological effects of raised intracellular calcium. Another source of calcium toxicity is the evolution of a phosphate-based cell metabolism. As phos-phorylated compounds are continuously hydrolysed to release energy and re-synthesized to store it, the intracellular concentrations of phosphate are high. If the free calcium concentration was elevated, calcium phosphate precipita-tion would occur (Carafoli, 1987). This phenomenon has been reported in mitochondria when cytoplasmic calcium is greatly raised and, in addition to direct inhibition of oxidative phosphorylation, will contribute to the observed mitochondrial dysfunction and overt physical damage to the organelle (Pozzan et al., 1994). The duality between functionality and toxicity has resulted in very precise regulation of intracellular free calcium through a number of mechanisms. In the resting state, cells maintain a cytosolic free calcium concentration which is 10^4-fold less than extracellular $[Ca^{2+}]$ by having a very low plasma membrane permeability to the cation and controlling release, uptake and extrusion, buffering by relatively mobile proteins and storage of the cation in membrane-bound compartments (Ashley, 1995).

Despite the major barrier to entry of external calcium into cells presented by the plasma membrane, there is still a requirement for controlled calcium influx to fill the internal stores. Currently, there appear to be three main entry channels involved which have been classified on the basis of their regulatory mechanism (Berridge, 1997). Hence, there are the voltage-operated channels (VOCs), receptor-operated channels (ROCs) and store-operated channels (SOCs). VOCs and ROCs provide brief high-intensity bursts of calcium influx whereas SOCs are involved in much smaller but sustained uptakes. The SOC activity appears to be controlled by the state of filling of internal stores through a mechanism known as 'capacitive calcium entry'. Therefore, when stores are full there is no entry but if stores empty then influx across the plasma membrane is activated (Berridge, 1997). It has been proposed that capacitive entry involves the $InsP_3$ receptor, as described previously, but that the information flow is in the opposite direction. Thus, depletion of calcium stores causes a conformational change in the $InsP_3R$ (type 3 isoform; Berridge, 1995) which is transmitted to the SOCs in the plasma membrane, which open and allow calcium entry. This mechanism is clearly analogous to the coupled release of calcium from the SR by the DHPR–RyR release units.

CALCIUM 'PUMPS'

Some of the diverse mechanisms mediating release of calcium from intracellular stores have been discussed above, e.g. intracellular calcium channels. These may mediate highly localized brief bursts of calcium (sparks) or longer and more sustained global elevations (waves) of cytosolic calcium (Berridge, 1997). It is apparent that the precise spatiotemporal organization of calcium signalling and cytosolic free calcium concentrations is crucial to normal metabolic regulation and that derangements in this process may have dire consequences for cell function resulting in pathology (Berridge, 1994). The 'normal' concentration of cytosolic ionized calcium is about 100 nM in the basal or 'unstimulated' state. Following stimulation, this concentration may rise 100-fold to approximately 10 mM (Ashley, 1995). Although Ca^{2+} release and thus signalling may be frequency encoded through calcium spikes, and thus tightly matched to the stimulus (Berridge, 1994) following cessation of stimulation, the general or local cytoplasmic calcium concentrations must be returned to base line. Prolonged exposure to elevated calcium would prove toxic and calcium stimulation must be confined to 'brief bursts'. The plasma membrane of eukaryotic cells contains specific extrusion mechanisms capable of reducing cytoplasmic calcium (Carafoli, 1987). These include a calmodulin-dependent calcium-ATPase and an electrogenic sodium–calcium (Na^+/Ca^{2+}) exchanger. The plasmalemmal Ca^{2+}-ATPase has an M_r of about 140,000 and shares many properties with its smaller counterpart found in the SR (Schatzmann, 1989; Carafoli, 1991). The ATPase is a high affinity enzyme which transports calcium with a $K_m < 1.0$ mM, but which has a low total transport capacity (< 0.5 nmol per mg protein^{-1} s^{-1}) and with a turnover rate of 10^3 min^{-1} (Carafoli, 1987, 1991; Schatzmann, 1989). Such values may be adequate for some cell types but not for excitable tissues such as striated or smooth muscle. An important feature of the enzyme is a direct interaction with calmodulin which increases the affinity for Ca^{2+} and the maximal transport rate (Carafoli, 1987). The reaction cycle is of the E_1–E_2 type involving phosphorylation and a magnesium-dependent component (Schatzmann, 1989; Carafoli, 1991). H^+ ions can compete with Ca^{2+} at both the *cis* and *trans* side of the membrane and a possible $Ca^{2+} - H^+$ transport function is proposed with a stoichiometry of $1:1$ and net charge movement (Schatzmann, 1989).

In cells where the calcium-ATPase cannot satisfy the extrusion require-ments, the Na^+–Ca^{2+} exchanger may operate in parallel as a bulk Ca^{2+} extruding system. This exchange mechanism behaves as a high capacity, low affinity system which is dependent on the sodium electrochemical gradient and the transmembrane potential (V_m) and has a coupling ratio of $3Na^+ : 1Ca^{2+}$ (Eisner and Lederer, 1985; Carafoli, 1987; Hoya and Venosa, 1995). The exchanger is thus electrogenic and generally operates in forward mode extruding calcium from the cell but may also act in the reverse direction. In many cells the exchanger may be inhibited by amiloride and nickel (Ni^{2+}).

CALCIUM UPTAKE INTO INTRACELLULAR COMPARTMENTS

Gross adjustments of cytosolic $[Ca^{2+}]$ may thus be achieved through the plasmalemmal extrusion mechanisms. An early event following stimulation of cells by a calcium-mobilizing signal is an increase in calcium efflux and fall in total calcium content (Williamson and Monck, 1989) but the time course is relatively slow (seconds) and is not consistent with the regulatory precision required. A more efficient mechanism for the removal of locally released calcium is re-uptake into those intracellular stores which are in rapid equilibrium with the cytosol (Pozzan *et al.*, 1994). Thus, both sarcoplasmic and endoplasmic reticulum (ER) possess calcium pumps or SERCAs (sarcoplasmic and endoplasmic reticulum Ca^{2+}-ATPases) which can translocate calcium into the organelle against a high concentration gradient. It has long been known that SR fractions can accumulate Ca^{2+} at the expense of ATP and that this explains their 'muscle relaxing activity'. SERCAs are members of the same group of E_1–E_2 type ATPase enzymes as those found in the plasma membrane (Carafoli, 1987; Schatzmann, 1989). The ATPase content of the ER is quite low but in the SR the enzymes are extremely abundant and may constitute up to 90–95% of the SR protein in skeletal muscle. The protein has an M_r of about 110,000 and the purified enzyme interacts with ionized calcium with high affinity ($K_m = 0.1$–1.0 mM). The maximum influx rates of Ca^{2+} into fast skeletal muscle SR through this system ranges from 14 to 70 nmol mg protein^{-1} s^{-1} (Carafoli, 1987). The properties and function of the Ca^{2+}-ATPases of the surface membrane or plasmalemma and the SR have been compared and contrasted by Schatzmann (1989). The isolation of cDNAs and more recently the genes of SERCAs has revealed a complex family of proteins whose distribution varies with tissue and species but which share many biochemical and molecular properties (Pozzan *et al.*, 1994). Sequestration of calcium by the

SR plays a vital role in the initiation of muscle relaxation. In this context the regulation of SERCA activity by hormonal or other chemical mediators (Carafoli, 1987) may be of major importance. SR from cardiac, smooth and slow skeletal muscle contains a low molecular mass phosphoprotein (25–28 kDa) called phospholamban (PLB), consisting of five similar subunits, in an approximate 1:1 stoichiometry with the Ca^{2+}-ATPase (Carafoli, 1987; Slack et al., 1997). Dephosphorylated PLB is an inhibitor of the ATPase (Hughes et al., 1996) but phosphorylation by cAMP and Ca^{2+}-calmodulin (CaM)-dependent protein kinases relieves this inhibitory effect (Slack et al., 1997). Thus PLB is a key determinant of relaxation in some muscle types (Slack et al., 1997) and may constitute an important means of endocrine regulation of muscle function.

In summary, the SERCAs represent a family of highly conserved proteins whose activities are regulated by a number of mechanisms. Contrasting activities in different cell types are probably attributable to the differential expression, the different levels and the molecular diversity of the various isoforms. In addition, there may be tissue specific expression of regulators such as phospholamban and the influences of highly controlled signals such as CaM-dependent phosphorylation (Pozzan et al., 1994). Together, these and other mechanisms provide the means of finely tuning SERCA activity and thus constitute a major component of cellular calcium homeostasis at the step of organellar Ca^{2+} accumulation or uptake.

SERCAs are not the only mechanism for the uptake of Ca^{2+} into intracellular stores or buffer compartments. In particular, mitochondria and some other acidic medium organelles can utilize the H^+ electrochemical gradient created by H^+-ATPases as the driving force for Ca^{2+} accumulation (Pozzan et al., 1994). Under physiological conditions, the mitochondrial electrochemical gradient is largely dominated by the electrical component – about 180 mV negative inside. The very low permeability of the inner mitochondrial membrane to cations prevents massive fluxes of Na^+ and K^+ which otherwise might occur. Calcium, on the other hand, possesses a very active electrogenic transport system that permits its rapid accumulation, driven by the membrane potential (Pozzan et al., 1994). It has long been known that energized mitochondria can take up large amounts of calcium, a process which was believed to have an important role in regulation of intracellular calcium concentrations (Carafoli, 1987). The physiological significance of the mechanism has been questioned on the grounds that the affinity of the mitochondrial uptake system was too low (K_m = 10 mM) to operate at the calcium concentrations found in the cytosol (0.1–1.0 mM) and that uptake rates were at least an order of magnitude less than those of the SR system (Carafoli, 1987; Pozzan et al., 1994). Under optimum experimental conditions, however, the maximum rate attained by mitochondria can be as high as 10 nmol mg protein^{-1} s^{-1} which compares favourably with values for the SERCAs reported above. In fact, if the uptake of calcium was driven by the powerful H^+ electrochemical gradient and was allowed to reach electrochemical equilibrium then mitochondrial matrix Ca^{2+} concentrations could exceed those in the cytosol by a factor of 10^6, which would not be compatible with normal mitochondrial function. The attainment of this electrochemical equilibrium is prevented by the presence of mitochondrial antiporters which exchange Na^+ and H^+ for Ca^{2+} which is extruded into the medium thus offsetting the influx of the divalent cation through the uniporter uptake system (Pozzan *et al.,* 1994). Work with isolated mitochondria and damaged cells indicates that, although the very high theoretical rates of mitochondrial calcium accumulation may not occur when cytosolic free calcium is at normal levels (0.1–1.0 mM), if large excursions in intracellular calcium (5–10 mM) do occur then this may result in an uptake so fast that oxidative phosphorylation may be uncoupled and calcium phosphate precipitation may impair mitochondrial integrity (Pozzan *et al.,* 1994). These observations may have significance in relation to abnormal states and the development of pathology and will be discussed in this context in a subsequent section.

CALCIUM BINDING PROTEINS

Many hundreds of intracellular proteins are known to bind calcium. Changes in cytosolic Ca^{2+} concentrations evoke a wide range of cellular responses and the binding proteins are the key molecules in the tranduction of Ca^{2+} signal via enzymic reactions or modulation of protein–protein interactions (Niki *et al.,* 1996). To catalogue the full range of proteins involved and their functions and mechanisms is obviously beyond the scope of the present review but the binding proteins may be broadly divided into two types. The calcium storage proteins are located in the main intracellular storage compartments, the endoplasmic and sarcoplasmic reticulum and provide the high Ca^{2+} capacity of these stores. The second category contains the cytosolic proteins which may be subdivided into the EF-hand proteins like calmodulin and S100, which are considered to exert their actions at the nucleus or in the cytoplasm (Zimmer *et al.,* 1995), and the cytoplasmic Ca^{2+}-phospholipid-binding proteins which translocate to the plasma membrane in response to increased intracellular calcium and exert their action in the vicinity of the membrane (Niki *et al.,* 1996). This latter group contains the annexins and the C2-region proteins.

CALCIUM-BINDING PROTEINS IN STORAGE COMPARTMENTS

Calcium ions taken up by organelles cannot remain in free solution in the lumen but must be stored in an appropriate complex form. This should allow large accumulations of the cation without risk of calcium phosphate precipitation but supply easily and quickly released Ca^{2+} when the store release mechanisms are activated, e.g. when channels are opened. In the case of the SR and ER two specific protein types have evolved which are segregated in the lumen and fulfil these operational criteria (Pozzan *et al.,* 1994). These calcium storage or binding proteins are known as calsequestrin (CSQ) and calreticulin (CR) and exhibit both similarities in their physical and chemical properties including molecular masses of 43–46 kDa, a single oligosaccharide chain, K_ds in the 1–4 mM range and a high content of acidic amino acid residues (about 30%) particularly in the carboxyl-terminal domain (about 60%) (Pozzan *et al.*, 1994). Calreticulin is the major luminal binding protein of the ER (Michalak *et al.*, 1992) and calsequestrin predominates in the SR of skeletal and cardiac muscle (Yano and Zarainherzberg, 1994) although they may be co-expressed in skeletal muscle SR (Tharin *et al.*, 1996). In the latter study, using a rat model myogenic system, differential control of the expression of CSQ and CR was demonstrated. Calsequestrin has been purified and cloned from skeletal and cardiac muscle in mammalian, amphibian and avian species and two different CSQ gene products have been identified, 'fast' and 'cardiac' (Yano and Zarainherzberg, 1994). The CSQ proteins bind calcium with high capacity (25–50 mol mol^{-1}) and moderate affinity (K_d approximately 1.0 mM) and in addition to their luminal roles as a Ca^{2+} store can be found associated with the calcium release channel complex of the SR through protein–protein interactions (Pozzan *et al.*, 1994; Yano and Zarainherzberg, 1994). Ultimately calsequestrin must play an important role in regulation of calcium stores in skeletal muscle and cation efflux following coupled opening of the ryanodine receptor–calcium release channel.

HIGH AFFINITY CYTOSOLIC CALCIUM-BINDING PROTEINS

Cytosolic proteins have evolved which exhibit exquisite selectivity in their cationic binding characteristics. Thus the calcium-binding proteins have high affinities and capacities for Ca^{2+} whilst apparently rejecting Mg^{2+} and other cations (Carafoli, 1987). It is suggested that the proteins subserve two distinct but complementary functions. The first and perhaps primary function is as mediators in the processing of a calcium signal which involves a conformational change on calcium binding which allows them to interact with other proteins including enzymes. The family of Ca^{2+}-modulated proteins exhibit a number of common properties and characteristics. They tend to have relatively low molecular masses (10,000–20,000 Da), are negatively charged at neutral pH, contain unusually high amounts of acidic amino acid residues and bind two to four Ca^{2+} with high affinity (Carafoli, 1987). The earliest studies of cytosolic calcium-binding proteins focused on troponin C (TnC) and parvalbumin. TnC is found in skeletal and cardiac muscle and forms one subunit of the ternary troponin complex which, through its association with actin and tropomyosin on the thin filament, inhibits the actomyosin interaction at submicromolar calcium concentrations and stimulates the interaction at higher concentrations (Farah and Reinach, 1995). TnC is thus a major mediator in the transduction of the calcium release from the SR into initiation of muscle contraction. The precise mechanism by which this occurs by a conformational change and interaction with troponins I and T has recently been elucidated (Gagne *et al.*, 1997). Parvalbumins are highly soluble, low-molecular-mass proteins (11 kDa) and are also found in muscles (Carafoli, 1987; Rall, 1996). There may be a number of isoforms of the protein dependent upon the species examined. It was the study of parvalbumin that led to the discovery of the 'EF-hand' calcium-binding motif common to more than 150 calcium-binding proteins which have been characterized (Rall, 1996). These molecules contain a loop-helix-loop structure associated with their calcium-binding properties. The mechanisms involved in EF-hand protein action, including the nature of the conformational change taking place during calcium binding, have been elucidated and described recently (Kawasaki and Kretsinger, 1995; Ikura, 1996). The EF-hand protein family includes calmodulin, the S100 proteins, of which 16 have been identified, troponin C and parvalbumin. These binding proteins generally appear to act as part of the signalling system by further interactions with other proteins and cell components. Parvalbumin, however, appears primarily to fulfil the second function of calcium-binding proteins which is to buffer changes in intracellular calcium. Indeed, it now appears that parvalbumin sequesters calcium rapidly from the myoplasm, but at a rate determined by the dissociation of magnesium from the protein, promoting relaxation of skeletal muscle (Rall, 1996). The cytosolic calcium-binding protein calbindin-D-9k is generally regarded as occurring in mammalian smooth muscle (Miller et al., 1994) but some studies suggest that it is present in rat (Toury et al., 1994) and chick (Drittanti et al., 1994) skeletal muscle where it may have an important regulatory function. This calcium-binding protein may be vitamin D dependent (Toury et al., 1990, 1994) and a calbindin-D-9k-like protein can be induced in avian muscle cells by 1:25-dihydroxy vitamin D_3 (Drittanti et al., 1994). It is not currently known if vitamin deficiencies lead to reduced production of calcium-binding proteins and thus decreased calcium buffering capacity, but this area merits further investigation particularly in rapidly growing poultry. It is apparent, however, that it is essential to consider the Ca^{2+} buffer function of the whole range of cytosolic calcium-binding proteins in the general control of cytosolic free calcium.

It is likely that all the calcium-binding proteins, both organellar and myoplasmic, that have been characterized in mammalian cells or their analogues, will exist in avian muscle. Calmodulin, the calsequestrins, the troponins and calreticulin have all recently been studied in muscle from the domestic fowl (Yano and Zarainherzberg, 1994; Yao et al., 1994a, b; Satyshur et al., 1994; Szczesna et al., 1996; Filipek and Wojda, 1996).

VARIATIONS IN INTRACELLULAR 'FREE' CALCIUM CONCENTRATIONS

The ubiquitous nature of the calcium ion, its multifarious roles in metabolic and biochemical control and the complex and numerous systems for the regulation of its unbound concentration, indicate the importance of maintaining intracellular free calcium homeostasis. In active muscle tissue the controlled release, buffering and re-uptake of calcium require tight regulation in order to avoid sustained increases in myoplasmic calcium and only transient 'calcium spikes' should be associated with the contractile process (Schneider et al., 1987; Konishi et al., 1991; Vergara et al., 1991). The potentially toxic effects and catastrophic consequences of failure of this system are central to any consideration of muscle cell pathology, myopathies and muscle tissue properties.

Elevated intracellular calcium has long been implicated in the aetiology of cell injury and tissue necrosis (Schanne et al., 1979; Nicotera et al., 1990). In muscular dystrophies, elevated myoplasmic calcium is associated with the development of muscle damage (Bodenstein and Engel, 1978; Duncan, 1978; Jackson et al., 1985). If cytosolic calcium is increased outwith the normal limits then a cascade is initiated which may result in severe membrane disruption, metabolic disturbance and activation of self-degradative processes setting in train a vicious cycle resulting in cell death (Jackson et al., 1984; Trump et al., 1989; Nicotera et al., 1992). Thus, increased uptake of calcium by mitochondria may cause decreased energy production coupled to stimulated energy usage by increased calcium pumping and will result in ATP depletion (Wrogemann and Pena, 1976; Armstrong, 1990; Tani, 1990). In parallel, increased cytoplasmic calcium will stimulate the activity of calcium dependent lipases and proteases causing degradation of cellular and membrane elements (Tani, 1990). Increased activity of phospholipase A_2 (Jackson et al., 1984; Jackson, 1993) will produce changes in membrane structure and prompt eicosanoid production and calcium-induced stimulation of free radical production will precipitate membrane lipid peroxidation (Jackson, 1993) and therefore changes in sarcolemmal integrity. These alterations in cell energy metabolism and membrane structure will lead to a loss of control of ion balance including further perturbations in intracellular calcium homeostasis and, if unchecked, will lead to cell death (Trump et al., 1989). In muscle cells in which myoplasmic calcium undergoes sustained elevation, there will be losses of intracellular constituents such as enzymes and metabolites (Jones et al., 1984; Claremont et al., 1984; Jackson et al., 1984; Phoenix et al., 1989) and morphological changes ranging from disturbances in myofilament structure (Duncan and Jackson, 1987) to fibre death.

Elevations in intracellular free calcium may occur by one or both of two fundamental mechanisms. Calcium may enter the cell via the sarcolemma at a rate which exceeds extrusion capacity and buffering or excessive amounts of the cation may be released from intracellular stores, e.g. the sarcoplasmic reticulum. During periods of excessive contractile activity, calcium release is increased and if energy depletion ensues then extrusion is limited and a net gain of free calcium may result causing exercise-induced myopathy (Jackson, 1993). Any deficiency in any of the components of the calcium regulatory systems may predispose to such problems even in inactive muscle. In Duchenne muscular dystrophy, failure to regulate entry of external calcium, due to the absence of the protein dystrophin, has been implicated (Jackson, 1993). Several other recognized pathologies will predispose animals to muscle damage due to elevated myoplasmic calcium. Excessive exercise will cause extensive muscle damage (rhabdomyolysis) and conditions such as tissue hypoxia or ischaemia may lead to calcium accumulation via the Na^+–Ca^{2+} exchange system due to an initial loss of cell sodium balance (Piper, 1989). Monensin and other drug-induced myotoxicities may be mediated by a similar mechanism (Sandercock and Mitchell, 1995). Perhaps one of the most widely studied aberrations of intracellular calcium control, however, is a group of conditions containing the malignant hyperthermias including the porcine stress syndrome. In the latter the muscle pathology is associated with major changes in the quality of the meat obtained from the pigs affected.

MALIGNANT HYPERTHERMIA AND THE PORCINE STRESS SYNDROME

Exposure of some mammals, including humans, pigs and dogs, to halothane anaesthesia alone or in conjunction with muscle relaxants, may induce malignant hyperthermia (MH) (O'Brien, 1987; O'Brien *et al.*, 1990a; Fay and Gallant, 1990; MacLennan and Phillips, 1992). This is a pharmacogenetic hypermetabolic disorder attributed to inherited defects in the sarcoplasmic reticulum RyR or calcium release channel and a resulting abnormal and sustained elevation of sarcoplasmic ionized calcium in the skeletal muscle cell (MacLennan *et al.*, 1990; Fujii *et al.*, 1991; Rosenberg *et al.*, 1992; MacLennan, 1992; MacLennan and Phillips, 1992; Fletcher *et al.*, 1993; Decanniere *et al.*, 1993; Bull and Marengo, 1994; Mickelson and Louis, 1996). The clinical state is characterized by uncontrolled muscle contracture, greatly elevated muscle metabolism, hyperthermia, lactacidosis, hyperkalaemia and disruption of sarcolemmal integrity and consequent release of intracellular muscle enzymes into the circulation (Britt, 1977; O'Brien *et al.*, 1990b; MacLennan, 1992; Rosenberg *et al.*, 1992). The hypermetabolism is a consequence of the heat production associated with muscle contraction including the enormous expenditure of energy in an attempt to remove calcium from the cytoplasm by pumping (ATPases) into the SR, mitochondria and by extrusion across the sarcolemma (Block, 1994). Skeletal muscle is thus the site of a lesion involved in the mechanism producing malignant hyperthermia and of tissue damage resulting from the syndrome. In pigs, malignant hyperthermia may be triggered by a number of factors other than anaesthesia including physical activity and 'stress' and frequently proves fatal (O'Brien, 1987; Gallant and Goettl, 1989; O'Brien *et al.*, 1990a; MacLennan and Phillips, 1992) and the 'Porcine Stress Syndrome' (PSS) is a source of major economic losses to the pig industry. The presence of defects in sarcoplasmic calcium homeostasis may render pigs, both homozygous and heterozygous for the 'halothane gene' mutation proposed to be responsible for the syndrome, more susceptible to stress-induced muscle dysfunction and damage and reduced meat quality than normal animals (Rempel *et al.*, 1993; Klont *et al.*, 1994; Backstrom and Kaufmann, 1995; Shibata, 1996).

The ryanodine receptor (RYR1) or the sarcoplasmic reticulum ryanodine-sensitive calcium release channel (SR-RSCRC) is the main mediator of calcium release from storage in the process of excitation–contraction coupling (vide infra) and thus is a major determinant of myoplasmic free calcium. PSS is an excellent example of a condition in which a defect in the control of intra-cellular free calcium concentration, due to excessive and inappropriate release from intracellular stores, causes changes in sarcolemmal permeability, extensive muscle damage, potentially fatal metabolic disturbances and major alterations in ante-mortem muscle quality and post-mortem meat quality. Human MH is a more complex disorder than that observed in pigs and may involve derangements in control of free calcium in a number of tissues through not only calcium release in deranged excitation–contraction coupling but in calcium transport, uptake and storage and exhibits considerable genetic heterogeneity (Mickelson and Louis, 1996). Thus although the function of the RYR1 or SR-RSCRC is central to myoplasmic calcium regulation and may be involved in the aetiology of a number of muscle pathologies, lesions in other components of the calcium control system may be equally important causes of muscle damage and dysfunction (Jackson, 1993; Mickelson and Louis, 1996).

It is therefore pertinent to examine the role that myoplasmic calcium homeostasis might play in recognized muscle pathologies in poultry and to consider how this might relate to changes in poultry meat quality. Clearly changes in the function of any of the components of the calcium regulatory systems might underlie damage found in skeletal muscle and alterations in post-mortem properties of the meat derived therefrom. It is important to recognize that inherent dysfunction of calcium regulation, perhaps as a consequence of genetic selection as in the PSS affected pigs, is a possible source of problems but that other factors such as nutritional and environmental stressors or disease may disrupt sarcoplasmic calcium homeostasis leading to equivalent muscle pathology.

THE AVIAN RYANODINE RECEPTOR

Before considering the pathophysiological basis of the known common muscle abnormalities in poultry in detail, the current knowledge relating to the avian ryanodine receptor or SR-RSCRC should be reviewed. From the evidence available in mammals, particularly pigs, it may be proposed that this component of the sarcoplasmic calcium regulatory system might constitute an important source of functional variability or lesions leading to muscle dysfunction and damage.

All vertebrates possess the ryanodine receptor or SR-RSCRC, a calcium release channel protein and three distinct genes express different isoforms (RyR1, RyR2 and RyR3) in specific tissue locations (Coronado *et al.*, 1994; Ogawa, 1994; Ashley, 1995). In avians, three corresponding ryanodine receptor isoforms have been identified in striated muscle (Airey *et al.*, 1993a). The two predominating isoforms have been categorized as alpha (α) and beta (β) and are homologous with mammalian RyR1 and RyR3 (Ottini *et al.*, 1996). Although only one isoform (RyR1) is expressed in mammalian skeletal muscle, both the alpha and beta isoforms (α-Ryr and β-Ryr or Ryr1 and RyR3) are found in developing avian muscle (Percival *et al.*, 1994). This co-existence may be related to differentiation or specialization but the biological significance remains to be clarified (Ogawa, 1994) and may have important implications for muscle cell function, calcium homeostasis and perhaps ultimately meat quality. An autosomal recessive mutation in chicken, crooked Neck Dwarf, causes a failure to produce normal α-Ryr and results in skeletal muscle dysgenesis, muscle dysfunction, myodegeneration and death (Airey *et al.,* 1993b, c). The absence of the α isoform prevents the development of calcium-independent calcium release from the SR and contractions and failure to sustain calcium-dependent calcium release (Ivanenko *et al.,* 1995). The contributions of the α isoform to the development of chick muscle cannot be duplicated by the β isoform alone. The sequential expression of such proteins during embryonic (Sutko *et al.,* 1991) and postnatal (Damiani *et al.,* 1992) development in chicks and the control of these processes may have major implications for myoplasmic calcium homeostasis and muscle cell integrity and function in modern poultry. The effects of commercial genetic selection for production traits in broiler birds upon ryanodine receptor expression and isoform distribution are unknown.

INDICATORS OF MUSCLE CELL DAMAGE

In studies of the aetiology of muscle abnormalities and pathologies it is essential to develop clinical indicators of the type, extent and origin of the lesions. Muscle biopsy is of course useful once overt morphological changes have occurred but more easily assessed and less invasive analyses are more desirable perhaps involving the taking of simple blood samples. If sarcolemmal integrity or permeability is altered then there will be losses of intracellular constituents such as enzymes and metabolites (Jones *et al.,* 1984, 1986; Claremont *et al.,* 1984; Jackson *et al.,* 1984, 1991; Phoenix *et al.,* 1989). Muscle cell enzymes are particularly useful indicators of membrane disruptions and can be readily determined in plasma and correlate well with morphological or histological changes (Jones *et al.,* 1984, 1986). The circulating activities of a number of enzymes are raised in muscle injury or myopathy including lactate dehydrogenase (LDH), aspartate aminotransferase (AST) and aldolase but by far the most commonly employed indicator of muscle pathology is creatine (phospho)kinase (CK or CPK) due to the very high activity which is present in muscle tissue (Dawson and Boston, 1966; Suarez-Kurtz and Eastwood, 1981; Jones *et al.,* 1983; Mitchell and Sandercock, 1995a). In mammals it has been shown that CK is a dimeric molecule composed of two immunologically distinct subunits CK-M and CK-B (Oguni *et al.,* 1992). Thus, three fundamental isoenzymes, resulting from the possible permutations of dimerization, have been demonstrated in a number of tissues and designated MM-CK, BB-CK and MB-CK and identified as the skeletal muscle, brain and cardiac muscle types due to their apparent differential distribution among, and predominant forms in, these tissues (Eppenburger *et al.,* 1967; Hamburg *et al.,* 1991). Measurements of CK activity and isoenzyme profiles in human plasma or serum samples are well established as an important diagnostic technique of major clinical significance in a number of pathologies including myopathies and dystrophies, myocardial infarction, central nervous system lesions and neoplastic disease (DeLuca *et al.,* 1981; Capocchi *et al.,* 1987; Vretou-Jockers and Vassilopoulos, 1989; el Mallakh *et al.,* 1992; Karkela *et al.,* 1993). The diagnostic interpretation is based on the assumption of the efflux of the relatively tissue specific and distinguishable isoenzymes in response to cellular damage resulting in characteristic blood profiles (Kenyon and Reed, 1983; Hamburg *et al.,* 1991). In a number of avian species, changes in total plasma CK activity, in response to various pathologies (Siller *et al.,* 1978; Hollands *et al.,* 1980; Tripp and Schmitz, 1982; Lumeij *et al.,* 1988a, b; Itoh, 1993), acute heat stress (Ostrowski-Meissner, 1981) and transportation (Mitchell *et al.,* 1992) have been reported but without reference to the associated isoenzyme profiles. Although the MM-CK and BB-CK isoenzymes in the skeletal and nervous tissues of birds may be truly analogous to those identified in mammals, it has been suggested that the CK-M monomer is not expressed in postembryonic, avian cardiac muscle and therefore the MB-CK dimer does not appear in this tissue which exclusively contains BB-CK (Schafer and Perriard, 1988; Quest *et al.,* 1990). The work of Mitchell and Sandercock (1995a) demonstrated that the muscle isoenzyme (MM-CK) was the predominant form in chicken plasma and was exclusively raised by stressful stimuli likely to cause muscle damage. Thus, measurements of plasma CK activities in poultry are a very useful index of the extent and nature of muscle cell damage induced by a range of treatments, environments and challenges.

MUSCLE ABNORMALITIES IN POULTRY

Details of the morphological characteristics and changes occurring in a number of recognized muscle pathologies in poultry are described in a preceding section. The common muscle abnormalities may be conveniently divided into five groups.

Deep Pectoral Myopathy

Deep pectoral myopathy (DPM), Oregon disease or green muscle disease is a degenerative myopathy of the m. supracoracoideus (a wing levator) in broilers and turkeys (Siller and Wight, 1978; Siller *et al.,* 1979a, b; Siller, 1980; Harper *et al.,* 1983; Hollands *et al.,* 1986; Wilson, 1990). Affected birds have extremely elevated plasma CK activities (Hollands *et al.,* 1980). At post-mortem examination the muscle is inflamed and oedematous with localized haemorrhages, pigmented green and may exhibit large central areas of tissue necrosis (Siller and Wight, 1978). The problem is attributed to ischaemia during exercise due to raised intramuscular pressure within an osteofascial space of limited size (Martindale *et al.,* 1979; Siller *et al.,* 1979a, b) and can be simulated by forced exercise and arterial occlusion which produce similar lesions and large increases in the plasma activity of CK and AST (Siller *et al.,* 1978; Wight *et al.,* 1979; Harper *et al.,* 1983). The defect is inherited as a polygenic recessive trait (Harper *et al.,* 1983) but is associated with desirable production features such as rapid growth rate and body conformation (Hollands *et al.,* 1986) and thus complex multitrait selection programmes are required for its efficient reduction in commercial populations. It has been proposed that DPM is a direct consequence of selection for improved muscle growth rate but that selection against birds with elevated plasma CK activities might represent a strategy for reductions in the incidence of the disorder (Siller, 1985). An exercise-induced subgastrocnemial ischaemic myopathy leading to marked lameness has been reported in broiler breeders and is thought to have a similar aetiology to DPM (Christensen, 1986). The cellular changes mediating the predisposition to exercise-induced pathology are not known but the final common mechanism leading to the myonecrosis probably involves depletion of cell energy reserves and loss of ion balance leading to raised intracellular calcium.

Progressive Muscular Dystrophy

Progressive muscular dystrophy or genetic muscular dystrophy (GMD) is another inherited abnormality of muscle growth in poultry and presents as obvious weakness and disability with muscle degeneration and atrophy (Wilson, 1990; Hudecki et al., 1995). Symptoms appear during late embryogenesis and neonatal muscle maturation. Muscle fibre composition is altered in dystrophic birds and fast twitch α-white fibres are most affected, e.g. superior pectoralis and biceps, whereas slow or tonic 'red' fibres appear to be unaffected (Barnard et al., 1982; Wilson, 1990). The precise mechanisms leading to avian muscular dystrophy have not been fully elucidated (Hudecki et al., 1995) but it is thought to be a useful model of the human disease in which failure to produce the membrane protein dystrophin leads to membrane instability, increased calcium entry and cell damage (Jackson, 1993). In avian GMD a dystrophin protein is present but it is not known if it is the same as the one in normal chickens (Wilson, 1990; Fabbrizio et al., 1992). It has recently been proposed that the dihydropyridine receptor content of dystrophic chicken muscle is higher than that of normal tissue and that this elevation in L-type calcium channels may underlie the calcium overload which is such a fundamental pathogenic event in the condition (Moro et al., 1995).

Dietary Deficiency Myopathies

The most common dietary deficiency muscle abnormality in poultry is that associated with an inadequate supply of the antioxidants vitamin E (α-tocopherol) and selenium (Cheville, 1966; Hassan et al., 1990; McDowell, 1989; Jenkins et al., 1992). Imbalance of sulphur amino acids, vitamin E and selenium will also produce this condition (Wilson, 1990).

Deficient birds exhibit a wide range of clinical symptoms from a number of systemic lesions other than the muscular dystrophy or myopathy. Affected muscles show degenerative changes including calcium deposits, vascular lesions and haemorrhages (Hassan et al., 1990). Some flavonoids and phenolics offer a degree of protection against nutritional myopathy or nutritional muscular dystrophy (NMD) in chicks receiving vitamin E-deficient diets (Jenkins *et al.*, 1992). The cellular mechanisms mediating NMD await elucidation but the existing evidence suggests a role for free radical generation and membrane lipid peroxidation which may implicate changes in sarcolemmal permeability and subsequent altered ion balance.

Toxic Myopathies

A number of agents may be responsible for toxic myopathies in poultry but the most frequently described is probably that associated with the use of the anticoccidial ionophore antibiotic or growth promoter monensin (Dowling, 1992). In monensin toxicity there are signs of weakness, depression and paralysis and histological examination of affected muscle reveals hyalinization, myofibre degeneration and necrosis (Julian, 1991; Barragry, 1994). There are numerous reports of the incidence of muscle lesions and necrotizing myo-pathies following monensin administration in broilers (Hanrahan *et al.*, 1981), laying hens (Weisman *et al.*, 1994) and growing (Wages and Ficken, 1988; Cardona *et al.*, 1992) and breeder turkeys (Ficken *et al.*, 1989). A dose-dependent myopathy assessed from plasma CK activity has been reported in growing broilers even in the therapeutic range of monensin administration (Sandercock and Mitchell, 1996; Mitchell and Sandercock, 1998). Ionophore myotoxicity is generally indicated by extreme increases in the plasma activity of the intracellular enzymes CK and AST (Dowling, 1992; Barragry, 1994) reflecting the disruptions in membrane integrity. It has been proposed that monensin, which is a sodium ionophore (Hoya and Venosa, 1992), disrupts sodium–potassium balance across the sarcolemma which results in increases in intracellular calcium and thus would cause the cellular damage (Trump *et al.*, 1989; Barragry, 1994).

A toxic mitochondrial myopathy in chickens fed seed from the plant *Senna occidentalis* has recently been reported in which skeletal and cardiac muscles exhibited floccular degeneration, proliferation of sarcolemmal nuclei and necrosis (Cavaliere *et al.*, 1997). The mechanism of this toxic action is unknown.

Myopathies of Other Origins

Another muscle abnormality has been described in turkeys and has been termed 'focal myopathy' (Wilson, 1990). It occurs in young rapidly growing birds and several muscle groups appear to be affected including the superficial pectoralis and gastrocnemius which exhibit degenerative changes such as hypercontracted fibres, fatty infiltration, fragmentation of the sarcoplasm, infiltration by mononuclear cells and areas of focal necrosis (Wilson *et al.*, 1990; Sosnicki *et al.*, 1989; 1991a; Cherel *et al.*, 1995). Although muscles may be swollen, rounded and opaque and plasma CK activities (Wilson, 1990) are greatly elevated, the birds may not show any overt signs of impaired mobility or posture (Sosnicki *et al.,* 1991a). It is suggested that the rapidly growing muscle may outpace the growth of the connective tissue elements and blood supply (Wilson, 1990; Sosnicki *et al.,* 1991b) and that localized ischaemia might therefore mediate the pathology particularly when birds are exposed to stress (Wilson, 1990). During catching, handling and transport the stress imposed may accelerate glycogen utilization and cause changes in muscle blood flow and cell pH exacerbating the effects of the inadequate blood supply. This would result in the degenerative changes observed in turkey muscle at the slaughterhouse (Cherel *et al.,* 1995). It is not known if focal myopathy is related to other problems in turkeys such as the 'shaky leg syndrome' (Wilson, 1990) or the apparent increased incidence of 'pale, soft, exudative' meat (PSE) in turkeys (Ferket, 1995; van der Sluis, 1996; Barbut, 1996). It may be proposed that a predisposition to 'focal myopathy' and susceptibility to 'stress-induced myopathy' may have a strong genetic component as in PSS and the associated high incidence of PSE in affected pigs (van der Sluis, 1996). This area is currently under investigation in the authors' laboratories. Generalized myopathy, perhaps similar to the focal myopathy in turkeys, has been reported in broiler breeders (Randall, 1981) but may be alleviated if birds are transferred to feeding *ad libitum* from their restriction programmes (Perelman and Avidar, 1994).

The concept of stress-induced myopathy has developed from the observations that modern poultry may exhibit elevated levels of muscle damage associated with their genetic selection for high growth rates (e.g. Wilson, 1990; Soike, 1995) and that, in response to stressful stimuli, plasma muscle enzyme activities may be further elevated indicating altered permeability of the muscle cell membrane (Ostrowski-Meissner, 1981; Mitchell *et al.,* 1992; Mitchell and Sandercock, 1995a). Clearly the cellular mechanisms which may mediate such myopathy are of importance in relation to both productivity and welfare. The effects of current selection programmes on muscle function and cell stability are poorly understood. If parallels with the selection of pigs may be drawn then there must be a risk of producing undesirable changes in systems such as the regulation of myoplasmic calcium with the consequent effects on muscle activity, metabolism, meat quality and survival. Some evidence of such problems has been provided by the work of Reiner *et al.* (1995) which demonstrated a decreased calcium transport rate and efficiency in the SR of rapidly growing broiler chickens compared to a more traditional laying line. It was proposed that a similar lesion in cardiac muscle might underlie the sudden death syndrome in modern broilers.

MECHANISMS OF MYOPATHY IN POULTRY

Although it seems likely that the fundamental mechanisms mediating muscle cell damage which are characterized in mammals will pertain in birds, there has, until recently, been little work examining these processes in relation to genetic selection programmes and modern poultry production practices and problems. It has been demonstrated, using plasma CK activity as an indicator of muscle cell membrane integrity, that the degree of myopathy increases with age in commercial lines of broilers (Mitchell and Sandercock, 1994a) and turkeys (Mitchell et al., 1996; Hocking et al., 1997) and that in both species there is significantly greater muscle damage in modern lines selected for rapid growth rate than in their genetic predecessors or more traditional lines. In addition, the muscle damage caused by acute exposure to heat stress (Mitchell and Sandercock, 1995a) is greater in highly selected broilers than in control lines and is associated with a larger heat stress-induced increase in metabolic heat production in the more rapidly growing birds (Mitchell and Sandercock, 1995b; Sandercock et al., 1995). In vitro preparations of isolated skeletal muscle from broilers have been used to elucidate the mechanisms of both stress-induced myopathy and monensin myotoxicity (Mitchell and Sandercock, 1994b, 1995c, 1997; Sandercock and Mitchell, 1995, 1996). These studies have examined both the uptake of radioisotopic calcium (^{45}Ca) and the efflux of CK. The results demonstrate that elevating intracellular calcium either by increased entry of external calcium (by calcium specific ionophores) or release from sarcoplasmic stores results in altered membrane integrity and efflux of enzymes particularly CK. Both sodium and calcium overload will induce enzyme efflux and membrane disruption (Sandercock and Mitchell, 1995, 1996; Sandercock et al., 1996). The mechanism of membrane damage involves activation of phospholipase A_2 (PLA$_2$) probably as a direct consequence of the raised intracellular calcium as described for mammalian muscle (Jackson et al., 1984). CK efflux following raised intracellular calcium can be reduced by inhibitors of PLA$_2$ (Sulieman et al., 1992) and vitamin E (Mitchell et al., 1994; Sandercock and Mitchell, 1995; 1996; Mitchell and Sandercock, 1995c). In response to monensin treatment increased entry of sodium, by sodium-proton exchange (Hoya and Venosa, 1992), into muscle cells promotes calcium entry by the sodium–calcium exchange mechanisms in the sarcolemma in addition to releasing calcium into the myoplasm via the SR calcium channel or ryanodine receptor (Mitchell and Sandercock, 1995c, 1997; Sandercock and Mitchell, 1995, 1996). Monensin-induced CK efflux from isolated muscle can be inhibited by dantrolene which is specific for the ryanodine receptor confirming the role of this channel in the process (Sandercock and Mitchell, 1995, 1996; Mitchell and Sandercock, 1997). These findings offer a complete explanation for the myotoxic effects of monensin in broilers and it is suggested that similar mechanisms involving altered ion balance and calcium release through the SR-RSCRC may mediate the myopathy induced by stress and thermal challenge (Mitchell and Sandercock, 1997). The disturbances in ion balance underlying the myopathies in poultry are consistent with the mechanisms proposed in mammals (Trump et al., 1989). A further insight into mechanisms involved in muscle abnormalities in poultry may be gained from recent work indicating reduced CK loss from muscle in female broiler chickens at sexual maturity or following the administration of oestrogen (Mitchell and Sandercock, 1996; Carlisle et al., 1997). This response is mediated by the oestrogen receptor and appears to improve intracellular calcium homeostasis or inhibit the calcium-induced degenerative process. An understanding of this action may help identify the lesions mediating the predisposition of modern rapidly growing birds to spontaneous or stress-induced muscle damage. The evidence suggests that the influence of genetic selection for production traits upon muscle cell calcium homeostasis should be further investigated and correlated to susceptibility to the recognized myopathies and stress-induced muscle dysfunction and injury.

PATHOPHYSIOLOGICAL MECHANISMS, MYOPATHIES AND MEAT QUALITY

Some of the commercial procedures and environmental challenges known to induce muscle damage or myopathy in poultry have been linked with alterations in meat quality. It has been proposed that artificial genetic selection may have induced changes in muscle cell structure and function resulting in alterations in histological characteristics which may have implications for meat quality (Soike, 1995; Rémignon *et al.*, 1996). In turn, the underlying changes in muscle function may predispose the tissue to stress-related damage and further effects upon meat quality. Thus, preslaughter heat stress negatively affects meat shrink loss, colour and toughness in broilers (Holm and Fletcher, 1997). Acute pre-slaughter heat stress accelerates the rate of pH decline in turkey meat and increases the likelihood of PSE and may thus explain the higher incidence of this condition during the summer (McKee and Sams, 1997). Chronic heat stress has similar effects in ducks (Kunst *et al.*, 1996). Breast and leg meat colour and other meat quality variables may be adversely affected by pre-slaughter holding conditions and transportation (Ngoka *et al.*, 1982; Moran and Bilgili, 1995; Kannan *et al.*, 1997). The physiological basis of these problems and the relationship between muscle cell function, myopathic change and meat quality are poorly understood. Thus, although numerous instances of altered meat quality in poultry have been described any pathophysiological characteristics or responses in live muscle directly responsible for changes in the post-mortem attributes of the tissue have not been identified. For example, in the case of PSE, the high rate of post-mortem glycolysis, induced by acute ante-mortem stress and leading to a rapid fall in tissue pH, is responsible for the meat quality problem (Ferket, 1995; van der Sluis, 1996; Barbut, 1996; McKee and Sams, 1997). It is not known if alterations in ante-mortem cell calcium homeostasis and sarcolemmal permeability predispose poultry to this condition as it does in pigs (Klont *et al.*, 1994).

The various mechanisms mediating cell damage or myopathy in mammals, however, have also been identified in muscles from poultry. Ionic imbalance leading to raised intracellular free calcium will induce altered sarcolemmal permeability, loss of intracellular components, cell dysfunction and necrosis. Myoplasmic calcium homeostasis is thus central to the aetiology of many muscle abnormalities in chickens, turkeys and other birds. Genetic and nutritional factors influencing this system should be fully characterized in order to develop appropriate strategies for reduction of the incidence of myopathies. All aspects of calcium regulation should be considered including channel-mediated release from the SR. There is some evidence that some disruption of calcium homeostasis leading to growth-associated muscle damage may be linked with artificial genetic selection for desirable production traits in poultry such as rapid growth rate, altered body conformation and improved feed conversion efficiency. Such lesions may render affected birds more susceptible to spontaneous and stress-induced muscle damage. It is not clear if the ante-mortem pathophysiological changes in muscle are directly responsible for post-mortem characteristics giving rise to meat quality problems such as PSE. Certainly mechanisms and lesions appear to be present in the skeletal muscle of rapidly growing modern poultry which would lead to tissue dysfunction and major derangements of metabolism prior to slaughter particularly in response to stress. It is essential that future studies address the issues of the basic physiology and biochemistry of skeletal muscle in poultry in order to provide a sound scientific foundation for reductions in muscle abnormalities and concomitant increased understanding of the biological basis of poultry meat quality.

ACKNOWLEDGEMENTS

The authors wish to thank Ailsa Carlisle, Dale Sandercock, Jo Mills and Richard Hunter for their assistance in the preparation of this manuscript and for their valuable contributions to the research programme which forms part of the body of work reviewed. We are also grateful to the Ministry of Agriculture, Fisheries and Food, Ross Breeders (UK) and the British Turkey Federation for providing the funding and support which allowed this research programme to be undertaken.

REFERENCES

Airey, J.A., Grinsell, M.M., Jones L.R., Sutko, J.L.. and Witcher, D. (1993a) Three ryanodine receptor isoforms exist in avian striated muscles. *Biochemistry* 32, 5739–5745.

Airey, J.A., Baring, M.D., Beck, C.F., Chelliah, Y., Deerinck, T.J., Ellisman, M.H., Houenou, L.J., McKemy, D.D., Sutko, J.L. and Talvenheimo, J. (1993b) Failure to make normal alpha ryanodine receptor is an early event associated with the crooked neck dwarf (cn) mutation in chicken. *Developmental Dynamics* 197, 169–188.

Airey, J.A., Deerinck, T.J., Ellisman, M.H., Houenou, L.J., Ivanenko, A., Kenyon, J.L., McKemy, D.D. and Sutko, J.L. (1993c) Crooked neck dwarf (cn) mutant chicken skeletal muscle cells in low density primary cultures fail to express normal alpha ryanodine receptor and exhibit a partial mutant phenotype. *Developmental Dynamics* 197, 189–202.

Armstrong, R.B. (1990) Initial events in exercise-induced muscular injury. *Medicine and Science in Sports and Exercise* 22, 429–435.

Ashley, R.H. (1995) Intracellular calcium channels. *Essays in Biochemistry* 30, 97–117.

Backstrom, L. and Kauffman, R. (1995) The porcine stress syndrome, a review of genetics, environmental factors and animal well-being implications. *Agricultural Practice* 16, 24–30.

Barbut, S. (1996) Occurrence of pale soft exudative meat in mature turkey hens. *British Poultry Science* 38, 74–77.

Barnard, E.A., Lyles, J.M. and Pizzey, J.A. (1982) Fibre types in chicken skeletal muscles and their changes in muscular dystrophy. *Journal of Physiology* 331, 333–354.

Barragry, T.B. (1994) Growth promoting agents. In: Barragry, T.B. (ed.) *Veterinary Drug Therapy*, Lea and Febiger, Philadelphia, pp. 597–621.

Bean, B.P. (1989) Classes of calcium channels in vertebrate cells. *Annual Review of Physiology* 51, 367–384.

Berridge, M.J. (1994) The biology and medicine of calcium signalling. *Molecular and Cellular Endocrinology* 98, 119–124.

Berridge, M.J. (1995) Capacitative calcium entry. *Biochemical Journal* 312, 1–11.

Berridge, M.J. (1997) Elementary and global aspects of calcium signalling. *Journal of Physiology* 499, 291–306.

Best, C.H. and Taylor, N.B.(1965) The physiology of nerve and muscle. In: *The Living Body*, 4th edn. Chapman and Hall, London, pp. 459–505.

Block, B.A. (1994) Thermogenesis in muscle. *Annual Review of Physiology* 56, 535–577.

Bodenstein, J.B. and Engel, A.G. (1978) Intracellular calcium accumulation in Duchenne dystrophy and other myopathies: a study of 567000 muscle fibres in 114 biopsies. *Neurology* 28, 439–446.

Bowman, W.C. and Marshall, I.G. (1971) Muscle. In: Bell, D.J. and Freeman, B.M. (eds) *Physiology and Biochemistry of the Domestic Fowl*, Volume 2. Academic Press, London, pp. 707–737.

Britt, B.A. (1977) The clinical and laboratory features of malignant hyperthermia management. In: Hensckel, E.O. (ed.) *Malignant Hyperthermia: Current Concepts*. Appleton-Century-Crofts, New York, pp. 9–45.

Bull, R. and Marengo, J.J. (1994) Calcium-dependent halothane activation of sarcoplasmic reticulum calcium channels from frog skeletal muscle. *American Journal of Physiology* 266, C391–C396.

Cappochi, G., Tassi, C., Ricci, S., Zampolini, M., Fausti, R. and Rossi, A. (1987) Creatine kinase BB activity in serum of patients with acute stroke: correlation with severity of brain damage. *Italian Journal of Neurological Science* 8, 567–570.

Carafoli, E. (1987) Intracellular Ca^{2+} homeostasis. *Annual Review of Biochemistry* 56, 395–433.

Carafoli, E. (1991) Calcium pump of the plasma membrane. *Physiological Reviews* 71, 129–153.

Cardona, C.J., Bickford, A.A., Galey, F.D., Charlton, B.R. and Cooper, G. (1992) A syndrome in commercial turkeys in California and Oregon characterized by a rear-limb necrotizing skeletal myopathy. *Avian Diseases* 36, 1092–1101.

Carlisle, A.J., Mitchell, M.A. and Tritten, C. (1997) Possible myoprotective effects of estradiol-17beta in the immature broiler chicken, effects of the anti-oestrogen tamoxifen. *British Poultry Science* 38, Suppl., S46–S48.

Cavaliere, M.J., Calore, E.E., Haraguchi, M., Gorniak, S.L., Dagli, M.L.Z., Raspantini, P.C., Calore, N.M.P. and Weg, R. (1997) Mitochondrial myopathy in *Senna occidentalis* seed fed chicken. *Ecotoxicology and Environmental Safety* 37, 181–185.

Cherel, Y., Wyers, M. and Dupas, M. (1995) Histopathological alterations of turkey skeletal muscle observed at the slaughterhouse. *British Poultry Science* 36, 443–453.

Cheville, N.F. (1966) The pathology of vitamin E deficiency in the chick. *Pathologica Veterinaria* 3, 208–225.

Christensen, N.H. (1986) Sub-gastrocnemial ischemic myopathy in broiler breeders. *Avian Diseases* 31, 910–912.

Claremont, D., Jackson, M.J. and Jones, D.A. (1984) Accumulation of calcium in experimentally damaged mouse muscles *in vitro. Journal of Physiology* 353, 57P.

Coronado, R., Morrissette, J., Sukhareva, M. and Vaughan, D.M. (1994) Structure and function of ryanodine receptors. *American Journal of Physiology* 266, C1485–C1504.

Damiani, E., Tarugi, P., Calandra, S. and Magreth, A. (1992) Sequential expression during postnatal development of specific markers of junctional and free sarcoplasmic reticulum in chicken pectoralis muscle. *Developmental Biology* 153, 102–114.

Dawson, D.M. and Boston, M.D. (1966) Leakage of enzymes from denervated and dystrophic chicken muscle. *Archives of Neurology* 14, 321–325.

Decanniere, C.P., Van Hecke, P., Vanstapel, F., Ville, H. and Geers, R. (1993) Metabolic responses to halothane in piglets susceptible to malignant hyperthermia: an *in vivo* ^{31}P-NMR study. *Journal of Applied Physiology* 75, 955–962.

Deluca, M., Hall, N., Rice, R. and Kaplan, M.O. (1981) Creatine kinase isoenzymes in human tumours. *Biochemical and Biophysical Research Communications* 99, 189–195.

Dowling, L. (1992) Ionophore toxicity in chickens: a review of pathology and diagnosis. *Avian Pathology* 21, 355–368.

Drittanti, L., Zanello, S. and Boland, R. (1994) Induction of a calbindin-D_{9k}-like protein in avian muscle cells by 1,25-dihydroxy-vitamin D_3. *Biochemistry and Molecular Biology International* 32, 859–867.

Dulhunty, A.F., Junankar, P.R., Eager, K.R., Ahern, G.P. and Laver, D.R. (1996) Ion channels in the sarcoplasmic-reticulum of striated muscle. *Acta Physiologica Scandinavica* 156, 375–385.

Duncan, C.J. (1978) Role of intracellular calcium in promoting muscle damage: a strategy for controlling the dystrophic condition. *Experientia* 34, 1531–1535.

Duncan, C.J. and Jackson, M.J. (1987) Different mechanisms mediate structural changes and intracellular enzyme efflux following damage to skeletal muscle. *Journal of Cell Science* 87, 183–188.

Eisner, D.A. and Lederer, W.J. (1985) Na–Ca exchange: stoichiometry and electrogenicity. *American Journal of Physiology* 248, C189–C202.

Eisner, D.A. and Trafford, A.W. (1996) A sideways look at sparks, quarks, puffs and blips. *Journal of Physiology* 497, 1.

el Mallakh, R.S., Egan, M. and Wyatt, R.J. (1992) Creatine kinase and enolase: intracellular enzymes serving as markers of central nervous system damage in neuropsychiatric disorder. *Psychiatry* 55, 392–402.

Eppenburger, H.M., Eppenburger, M., Richerich, R. and Aelu, H. (1967) The ontogeny of creatine kinase isoenzymes. *Developmental Biology* 10, 1–9.

Fabbrizio, E., Harricane, M.C., Pons, F., Leger, J. and Mornet, D. (1992) Properties of chicken cardiac dystrophin. *Biology of the Cell* 76, 167–174.

Farah, C.S. and Reinach, F.C. (1995) The troponin complex and regulation of muscle-contraction. *Faseb Journal* 9, 755–767.

Fay, R.S. and Gallant, E.M. (1990) Halothane sensitivity of young pigs *in vivo* and *in vitro*. *American Journal of Physiology* 259, R133–R138.

Ferket, P.R. (1995) Pale, soft, and exudative breast meat in turkeys. *Turkeys* 43(4), 19–21.

Ficken, M.D., Wages, D.P. and Gonder, E. (1989) Monensin toxicity in turkey breeder hens. *Avian Diseases* 33, 186–190.

Filipek, A. and Wojda, U. (1996) Chicken gizzard calcyclin – Distribution and potential target proteins. *Biochemical and Biophysical Research Communications* 225, 151–154.

Fletcher, J.E., Tripolitis, L., Rosenberg, H. and Beech, J. (1993) Malignant hyperthermia halothane- and calcium-induced calcium release in skeletal muscle. *Biochemistry and Molecular Biology International* 29, 763–772.

Franzini-Armstrong, C. (1995) Disposition of ryanodine and dihydropyridine receptors in striated muscle. Comparative and developmental clues to E-C coupling. *Journal of Physiology* 487, 2S.

Franzini-Armstrong, C. and Jorgensen, A.O. (1994) Structure and development of E-C coupling units in skeletal muscle. *Annual Reviews of Physiology* 56, 509–534.

Fujii, J., Otsu, K., Zorato, F., De Leon, S., Khanna, V.J., Weiler, J.E., O' Brien, P.J. and Maclennan, D.H. (1991) Identification of a mutation in the porcine ryanodine receptor associated with malignant hyperthermia. *Science* 253, 448–451.

Gagne, S.M., Li, M.X. and Sykes, B.D. (1997) Mechanism of direct coupling between binding and induced structural change in regulatory calcium binding proteins. *Biochemistry* 36, 4386–4392.

Gallant, E.M. and Goettl, V.M. (1989) Porcine malignant hyperthermia: halothane effects on force generation in skeletal muscles. *Muscle and Nerve* 12, 56–63.

Hamburg, R.J., Friedman, D.L. and Perrymen, M.B. (1991) Metabolic and diagnostic significance of creatine kinase isoenzymes. *Trends in Cardiovascular Medicine* 1, 195–200.

Hanrahan, L.A., Corrier, D.E. and Naqi, S.A. (1981) Monensin toxicosis in broiler chickens. *Veterinary Pathology* 18, 665–671.

Harper, J.A., Bernier, P.E. and Thompson-Cowley, L.L. (1983) Early expression of hereditary deep pectoral myopathy in turkeys due to forced wing exercise. *Poultry Science* 62, 2303–2308.

Harvey, A.L. and Marshall, I.G. (1983) Muscle. In: Freeman, B.M. (ed.) *Physiology and Biochemistry of the Domestic Fowl*, Volume 4. Academic Press, London, pp. 219–233.

Harvey, A.L. and Marshall, I.G. (1986) Muscle. In: Sturkie, P.D. (ed.) *Avian Physiology*, 4th edn. Springer-Verlag, Berlin, pp. 74–86.

Hassan, S., Hakkarainen, J., Jonsson, L. and Tyopponen, J. (1990) Histopathological and biochemical changes associated with selenium and vitamin E deficiency in chicks. *Journal of Veterinary Medicine* 37, 708–720.

Henckel, P. (1996) Physiology and biochemistry of muscle fibres in poultry. *Proceedings of the 2nd European Poultry Breeders Roundtable* 73, 79–89.

Hocking, P.M., Mitchell, M.A., Bernard, R. and Sandercock, D.A. (1997) Interactions of age, strain, sex and food restriction on plasma creatine kinase activity in turkeys. *British Poultry Science* 39, 360–361.

Hollands, K.G., Grunder, A.A., Williams, C.J. and Gavora, J.S. (1980) Plasma creatine kinase as an indicator of degenerative myopathy in live turkeys. *British Poultry Science* 21, 161–169.

Hollands, K.G., Grunder, A.A. and Gavora, J.S. (1986) Divergent selection for incidence of degenerative myopathy of the musculus supracoracoideus of meat-type chickens. *Poultry Science* 65, 417–425.

Holm, C.G.P. and Fletcher, D.L. (1997) Antemortem holding temperatures and broiler breast meat quality. *Journal of Applied Poultry Research* 6, 180–184.

Hoya, A. and Venosa, R.A. (1992) Ionic movements mediated by monensin in frog skeletal muscle. *Biochimica et Biophysica Acta* 1101, 123–131.

Hoya, A. and Venosa, R.A. (1995) Characteristics of Na^+/Ca^{2+} exchange in frog skeletal muscle. *Journal of Physiology* 486, 615–627.

Hudecki, M.S., Povoski, S.P., Gregorio, C.C., Granchelli, J.A. and Pollina, C.M. (1995) Efficacy of drug regimen exceeds electrostimulation in treatment of avian muscular dystrophy. *Journal of Applied Physiology* 78, 2014–2019.

Hughes, G., Starling, A.P., Sharma, R.P., East, J.M. and Lee, A.G (1996) An investigation of the mechanism of inhibition of the calcium ATPase by phospholamban. *Biochemistry Journal* 318, 973–979.

Ikura, M. (1996) Calcium-binding and conformational response in EF-hand proteins. *Trends in Biochemical Sciences* 21, 14–17.

Itoh, N. (1993) Serum enzyme activity evaluated in budgerigars (*Melopsittacus undulatus*) inflicted with muscle injury. *Research in Veterinary Science* 55, 275–280.

Ivanenko, A., McKemy, D.D., Kenyon, J.L., Airey, J.A. and Sutko, J.L. (1995) Embryonic chicken muscle cells fail to develop normal excitation–contraction coupling in the absence of the alpha ryanodine receptor – implications for a two ryanodine receptor system. *Journal of Biological Chemistry* 270, 4220–4223.

Jackson, M.J. (1993) Molecular mechanisms of muscle damage. In: Partridge, T. (ed.) *Molecular and Cell Biology of Muscular Dystrophy.* Chapman and Hall, London, pp. 257–282.

Jackson, M.J., Jones, D.A. and Edwards, R.H.T. (1984) Experimental skeletal muscle damage: the nature of the calcium-activated degenerative processes. *European Journal of Clinical Investigation* 14, 369–367.

Jackson, M.J., Jones, D.A. and Edwards, R.H.T. (1985) Measurements of calcium and other elements in muscle biopsy samples from patients with Duchenne muscular dystrophy. *Clinica Chimica Acta* 147, 215–221.

Jackson, M.J., Page, S. and Edwards, R.H.T. (1991) The nature of the proteins lost from isolated rat skeletal muscle during experimental damage. *Clinica Chimica Acta* 197, 108–112.

Jenkins, K.J., Collins, F.W. and Hidiroglou, M. (1992) Efficacy of various flavonoids and simple phenolics in prevention of nutritional myopathy in the chick. *Poultry Science* 71, 1577–1580.

Jones, D.A., Jackson, M.J. and Edwards R.H.T. (1983) Release of intracellular enzymes from an isolated mammalian skeletal muscle preparation. *Clinical Science* 65, 193–201.

Jones, D.A., Jackson, M.J., McPhail, G. and Edwards, R.H.T. (1984) Experimental mouse muscle damage. The importance of external calcium. *Clinical Science* 66, 317–322.

Jones, D.A., Newham, D.J., Round, J.M. and Tolfree, S.E.J. (1986) Experimental human muscle damage, morphological changes in relation to other indices of damage. *Journal of Physiology* 375, 435–448.

Julian, R.J. (1991) Poisons and toxins. In: Calnek, B.W. (ed.) *Diseases of Poultry,* 9th edn. Wolfe, London, pp. 863–884.

Kannan, G., Heath, C.J., Wabeck, C.J., Souza, M.C.P., Howe, J.C. and Mench, J.A. (1997) Effects of crating and transport on stress and meat quality characteristics in broilers. *Poultry Science* 76, 523–529.

Karkela, J., Bock, E. and Kaukinen, S. (1993) CSF and serum brain specific creatine kinase isoenzyme (CK-BB), neuron-specific enolase (NSE) and neural cell adhesion molecule (NCAM) as prognostic markers for hypoxic brain injury after cardiac arrest in man. *Journal of Neurological Science* 116, 100–109.

Kawasaki, H. and Kretsinger, R.H. (1995) Calcium binding proteins 1. EF-Hands. *Protein Profile* 2(4), 305–490.

Kenyon, G.L. and Reed, G.H. (1983) Creatine kinase: structure-activity relationships. *Advances in Enzymology* 54, 367–426.

Klein, M.G., Cheng, H., Santana, L.F., Jiang, Y.H., Lederer, W.J. and Schneider, M.F. (1996) Two mechanisms of quantized calcium-release in skeletal muscle. *Nature* 379, 455–458.

Klont, R.E., Lambooy, E. and Van Logtestijn, J.G. (1994) Effect of dantrolene treatment on muscle metabolism and meat quality of anesthetized pigs of different halothane genotypes. *Journal of Animal Science* 72, 2008–2016.

Konishi, M., Hollingworth, S., Harkins, A.B. and Baylor, S.M. (1991) Myoplasmic calcium transients in intact frog skeletal muscle fibres monitored with the fluorescent indicator furaptra. *Journal of General Physiology* 97, 271–301.

Kunst, U., Pingel, H. and V. Lengerken, G. (1996) The effects of high temperatures on carcass composition and meat quality of ducks. *World Poultry* 12, 27–28.

Lumeij, J.T., De Bruijne, J.J., Slob, A., Wolfswinkel, J. and Rothuizen, J. (1988a) Enzyme activities and elimination half-lives of homologous muscle and liver enzymes in the racing pigeon (*Columba livia domestica*). *Avian Pathology* 17, 851–864.

Lumeij, J.T., Meidam, M, Wolfswinkel, J., van der Hage, M.H. and Dorrenstein, G.M. (1988b). Changes in plasma chemistry after drug-induced liver disease or muscle necrosis in racing pigeons (*Columba livia domestica*). *Avian Pathology* 17, 865–874.

McDowell, L.R. (1989) Vitamin E. In: *Vitamins in Animal Nutrition – Comparative Aspects to Human Nutrition.* Academic Press Harcourt Brace Jovanovich, London, pp. 93–131.

McKee, S.R. and Sams, A.R. (1997) The effect of seasonal heat stress on rigor development and the incidence of pale, exudative turkey meat. *Poultry Science* 76, 1616–1620.

MacLennan, D.H. (1992) The genetic basis of malignant hyperthermia. *Trends in Physiological Sciences* 13, 330–334.

MacLennan, D.H., Duff, C., Zorzato, F., Fujii, J., Phillips, M.S., O'Brien, P.J., Korneluk, R.G. Frodis, W., Britt, B.A. and Worton, R.G. (1990) Ryanodine receptor gene. *Nature* 343, 559–561.

MacLennan, D.H. and Phillips, M.S. (1992) Malignant hyperthermia. *Science* 256, 789–794.

Martindale, L., Siller, W.G. and Wight, P.A.L. (1979) Effects of subfascial pressure in experimental deep pectoral myopathy of the fowl, an angiographic study. *Avian Pathology* 8, 425–436.

Martonosi, A.N. (1984) Mechanisms of Ca^{2+} release from sarcoplasmic reticulum of skeletal muscle. *Physiological Reviews* 64, 1240–1319.

Meissner, G. (1986) Ryanodine activation and inhibition of the calcium release channel of sarcoplasmic reticulum. *Journal of Biological Chemistry* 261, 6300–6306.

Meissner, G. (1994) Ryanodine receptor/Ca^{2+} release channels and their regulation by endogenous effectors. *Annual Review of Physiology* 56, 485–508.

Meissner, G. and Lu, X.Y. (1995) Dihydropyridine receptor–ryanodine receptor inter-actions in skeletal muscle excitation contraction coupling. *Bioscience Reports* 15, 399–408.

Michalak, M., Milner, R.E., Burns, K. and Opas, M. (1992) Calreticulin. *Biochemical Journal* 285, 681–692.

Mickelson, J.R. and Louis, C.F. (1996) Malignant hyperthermia – excitation–contraction coupling, Ca^{2+} release channel and cell Ca^{2+} regulation defects. *Physiological Reviews* 76, 537–592.

Miller, E.K., Word, R.A., Goodall, C.A. and Iacopino, A.M. (1994) Calbindin-D-9k gene expression in human myometrium during pregnancy and labour. *Journal of Clinical Endocrinology and Metabolism* 79, 609–615.

Ming-Tsao, C., Lin, S.S. and Lin, L.C. (1991) Effect of stresses before slaughter on changes to the physiological, biochemical and physical characteristics of duck muscle. *British Poultry Science* 3, 997–1004.

Mitchell, M.A. and Sandercock, D.A. (1994a) Age dependent changes in plasma creatine kinase activity in broiler chickens. In: *Proceedings 9th European Poultry Conference,* United Kingdom Branch of the World's Poultry Science Association, pp. 266–267.

Mitchell, M.A. and Sandercock, D.A. (1994b) Mechanism of monensin myotoxicity in the broiler chicken — an *in vitro* model. *British Poultry Science* 35, 824.

Mitchell, M.A. and Sandercock, D.A. (1995a) Creatine kinase isoenzyme profiles in the plasma of the domestic fowl (*Gallus domesticus*): effects of acute heat stress. *Research in Veterinary Science* 59, 30–34.

Mitchell, M.A. and Sandercock, D.A. (1995b) Increased hyperthermia induced skeletal muscle damage in fast growing broilerchickens? *Poultry Science* 74, Suppl. 1, 74.

Mitchell, M.A. and Sandercock, D.A. (1995c) Mechanisms of monensin induced myotoxicity: the basis for therapeutic strategies. In: *European Society of Veterinary Pathology, 13th European Congress for Veterinary Pathology, Edinburgh, 27th–30th September 1995.* UnivEd Technologies, Edinburgh, Abstract 4B–4.

Mitchell, M.A. and Sandercock, D.A. (1996) An estrogen induced amelioration of growth associated myopathy in female broiler chickens?*Poultry Science,* 75, Suppl. 1, 20.

Mitchell, M.A. and Sandercock, D.A. (1997) Possible mechanisms of heat stress induced myopathy in the domestic fowl. *Journal of Physiology and Biochemistry* 53, 75.

Mitchell, M.A. and Sandercock, D.A. (1998) Monensin induced myopathy in broilers: the effects of dose and acute heat stress. *Poultry Science*, Suppl. 1 (in press).

Mitchell, M.A., Kettlewell, P.J. and Maxwell, M.H. (1992) Indicators of physiological stress in broiler chickens during road transportation. *Animal Welfare* 2, 91–103.

Mitchell, M.A., Sandercock, D.A. and Whitehead, C.C. (1994) Mechanism of stress induced efflux of intracellular muscle enzymes in broiler chickens – effects of alpha-tocopherol. *British Poultry Science* 35, 186.

Mitchell, M.A., Hocking, P.M., Hunter, R.R. and Sandercock, D.A. (1996) A relationship between growth and plasma creatine kinase activity in sire line and traditional turkeys. *British Poultry Science* 37, Suppl. S86–S87.

Moran, E.T. and Bilgili, S.F. (1995) Influence of broiler livehaul on carcass quality and further-processing yields. *Journal of Applied Poultry Science* 4, 13–22.

Moro, G., Saborido, A., Delgado, J., Molano, F. and Megias, A. (1995) Dihydropyridine receptors in transverse tubules from normal and dystrophic chicken skeletal muscle. *Journal of Muscle Research and Cell Motility* 16, 529–542.

Ngoka, D.A., Froning, G.W., Lowry, S.R. and Babji, A.S. (1982) Effects of sex, age preslaughter factors and holding conditions on the quality characteristics and chemical composition of turkey breast meat. *Poultry Science* 61, 1996–2003.

Nicotera, P., Bellomo, G. and Orrenius, S. (1990) The role of Ca^{2+} in cell killing. *Chemical Research and Toxicology* 3, 484–494.

Nicotera, P., Bellomo, G. and Orrenius, S. (1992) Calcium-mediated mechanisms in chemically induced cell death. *Annual Review of Pharmacology and Toxicology* 32, 449–470.

Niki, I., Yokokura, H., Sudo, T., Kato, M. and Hidaka, H. (1996) Calcium signalling and intracellular calcium binding-proteins. *Journal of Biochemistry* 120, 685–698.

Obinata, T. (1993) Contractile proteins and myofibrillogenesis. *International Review of Cytology – A Survey of Cell Biology* 143, 153–189.

O'Brien, P.J. (1987) Etiopathogenetic defect of malignant hyperthermia: hypersensitive calcium-release channel of skeletal muscle sarcoplasmic reticulum. *Veterinary Research Communications* 11, 529–559.

O'Brien, P.J., Pook, H.A., Klip, A., Britt, B.A., Kalow, B.I., Mclaughlin, R.N., Scott, E. and Elliot, M.E. (1990a) Canine stress syndrome/malignant hyperthermia susceptibility: calcium-homeostasis defect in muscle and lymphocytes. *Research in Veterinary Science* 48, 124–128.

O'Brien, P.J., Klip, A., Britt, B.A. and Kalow, B.I. (1990b) Malignant hyperthermia susceptibility: basis for pathogenesis and diagnosis. *Canadian Journal of Veterinary Research* 54, 83–92.

Ogawa, Y. (1994) Role of ryanodine receptors. *Critical Reviews in Biochemistry and Molecular Biology* 29, 229–274.

Oguni, M., Setogawa, T., Tanaka, Shinoara, H. and Kato, K. (1992) Immunohistochemical study on the distribution of creatine kinase sub-units in early human embryos. *Acta Histochemica and Cytochemica* 25, 483–489.

Ostrowski-Meissner, H.T. (1981) The physiological responses of broilers exposed to short-term thermal stress. *Comparative Biochemistry and Physiology* 70A, 1–8.

Ottini, L., Marziali, G., Conti, A., Charlesworth, A. and Sorrentino, V. (1996) Alpha-isoforms and beta-isoforms of ryanodine receptor from chicken skeletal muscle are the homologs of mammalian RYR1 and RYR3. *Biochemical Journal* 315, 207–216.

Parker, I., Zang, W.-J. and Wier, W.G. (1996) Calcium sparks involving multiple calcium release sites along Z-lines in rat heart cells. *Journal of Physiology* 497, 31–38.

Percival, A.L., Williams, A.J., Kenyon, J.L., Grinsell, M.M. and Airey, J.A. (1994) Chicken skeletal muscle ryanodine receptor isoforms – ion channel properties. *Biophysical Journal* 67, 1834–1850.

Perelman, B. and Avidar, Y. (1994) Trembling syndrome (metabolic myopathy) in broiler breeder pullets. *Israel Journal of Veterinary Medicine* 49, 73–76.

Phoenix, J., Edwards, R.H.T. and Jackson, M.J. (1989) Inhibition of calcium induced cytosolic enzyme efflux from skeletal muscle by vitamin E and related compounds. *Biochemical Journal* 287, 207–213.

Piper, H.M. (1989) Energy deficiency, calcium overload or oxidative stress, possible causes of irreversible ischemic myocardial injury. *Klinische Wochenschrift* 67, 465–476.

Pozzan, T., Rizzuto, R., Volpe, P. and Meldolesi, J. (1994) Molecular and cellular physiology of intracellular calcium stores. *Physiological Reviews* 74, 596–636.

Quest, A.F.G., Eppenburger, H.M. and Wallimann, T. (1990) Two different B-type creatine kinase subunits dimerize in a tissue-specific manner. *FEBS Letters* 262, 299–304.

Rall, J.A. (1996) Role of parvalbumin in skeletal muscle relaxation. *News in Physiological Science* 11, 249–255.

Randall, C.J. (1981) Acute pectoral myopathy in broiler breeders. *Avian Pathology* 11, 245–252.

Reiner, G., Hartmann, J. and Dzapo, V. (1995) Skeletal muscle sarcoplasmic calcium regulation and Sudden Death Syndrome in chickens. *British Poultry Science* 36, 667–675.

Rémignon, H., Desrosiers, V. and Marche, G. (1996) Influence of increasing breast meat yield on muscle histology and meat quality in the chicken. *Reproduction, Nutrition and Development* 36, 523–530.

Rempel, W.E., Lu, Ming-Yu, Kandelgy, S.E., Kennedy, C.F.H., Irvin, L.R., Mickelson, J.R. and Louis, C.F. (1993) Relative accuracy of the halothane challenge test and a molecular genetic test in detecting the gene for porcine stress syndrome. *Journal of Animal Science* 71, 1395–1399.

Rios, E. and Pizarro, G. (1988) Voltage sensors and calcium channels of excitation–contraction coupling. *News in Physiological Sciences* 3, 223–227.

Rios, E. and Pizarro, G. (1991) Voltage Sensor of excitation-contraction coupling in skeletal muscle. *Physiological Reviews* 71, 849–908.

Rios, E., Pizarro, G. and Stefani, E. (1992) Charge movement and the nature of signal transduction in skeletal muscle excitation–contraction coupling. *Annual Review of Physiology* 54, 109–133.

Rosenberg, H., Fletcher, J.E and Seitman, D. (1992) Pharmacogenetics. In: Barash, P.G. and Cullen, B.F. (eds) *Clinical Anaesthesia*. J.B. Lippincott, Philadelphia, pp. 589–613.

Sandercock, D.A. and Mitchell, M.A. (1995) The possible roles of Na⁺ and Ca²⁺ overload in the mechanism of monensin-induced myotoxicity in isolated avian (*Gallus domesticus*) skeletal muscle. *Journal of Physiology* 485, 41P–42P.

Sandercock, D.A. and Mitchell, M.A. (1996) Dose dependent myopathy in monensin supplemented broiler chickens: effects of acute heat stress. *British Poultry Science*, 37, Suppl., S92–S94.

Sandercock, D.A., Mitchell, M.A. and Macleod, M.G. (1995) Metabolic heat production in fast and slow growing broiler chickens during acute heat stress. *British Poultry Science* 36, 868.

Sandercock, D.A., Mitchell, M.A. and Whitehead, C.C. (1996) The possible roles of Na⁺ and Ca²⁺ overload in the mechanism of monensin induced myotoxicity in isolated avian skeletal muscle. *Poultry Science*, 75 Suppl. 1, 50.

Satyshur, K.A., Pyzalska, D., Greaser, M., Rao, S.T. and Sundaralingam, M. (1994) Structure of chicken skeletal muscle-troponin-C at 1.78 angstrom resolution. *Acta Crystallographica (Section D-Biological Crystallography)* 50, 40–49.

Schafer, B.W. and Perriard, J.-C. (1988) Intracellular targeting of isoproteins in muscle cytoarchitecture. *Journal of Cell Biology* 106, 1161–1170.

Schanne, F., Kane, A.B., Young, E.E. and Farber, J.L. (1979) Calcium dependence of toxic cell death: a final common pathway. *Science* 206, 700–702.

Schatzmann, H.J. (1989) The calcium pump of the surface membrane and of the sarcoplasmic reticulum. *Annual Review of Physiology* 51, 473–485.

Schmoelzl, S., Leeb, T., Brinkmeier, H., Brem, G. and Brenig, B. (1996) Regulation of tissue-specific expression of the skeletal muscle ryanodine receptor gene. *Journal of Biological Chemistry* 271, 4763–4769.

Schneider, M.F. (1994) Control of calcium release in functioning skeletal muscle fibres. *Annual Review of Physiology* 56, 463–484.

Schneider, M.F. and Chandler, W.K. (1973) Voltage dependent charge movement in skeletal muscle. *Nature* 242, 244–246.

Schneider, M.F., Simon, B.J. and Szucs, G. (1987) Depletion of calcium from the sarcoplasmic reticulum during calcium release in frog skeletal muscle. *Journal of Physiology* 392, 167–192.

Shibata, T. (1996) The causal mutation for malignant hyperthermia in commercial pigs and pale, soft and exudative meats. *Animal Science and Technology* 5, 476–481.

Siller, W.G. (1980) Recent developments concerning Oregon disease. *Turkeys* (Jan/Feb), 47–52.

Siller, W.G. (1985) Deep pectoral myopathy: a penalty of successful selection for muscle growth. *Poultry Science* 64, 1591–1595.

Siller, W.G. and Wight, P.A.L. (1978) The pathology of deep pectoral myopathy of turkeys. *Avian Pathology* 7, 583–617.

Siller, W.G., Wight, P.A.L., Martindale, L. and Bannister, D.W. (1978) Deep pectoral myopathy: an experimental simulation in the fowl. *Research in Veterinary Science* 24, 267–268.

Siller, W.G., Martindale, L. and Wight, P.A.L. (1979a) The prevention of experimental deep pectoral myopathy of the fowl by fasciotomy. *Avian Pathology* 8, 301–307.

Siller, W.G., Wight, P.A.L. and Martindale, L. (1979b) Exercise-induced deep pectoral myopathy in broiler fowls and turkeys. *Veterinary Science Communications* 2, 331–336.

Slack, J.P., Grupp, I.L., Luo, W. and Kranias, E.G. (1997) Phospholamban ablation enhances relaxation in the murine soleus. *American Journal of Physiology* 273, C1–C6.

Soike D. (1995) Versleichende histopathologische, elektronenmikroskopische, histo-chemische und morphometrische untersuchungen an ausgwahlten muskeln von huhnern der lege- und mastrichtung. Dissertation (Dr. Vet. Med.) Berlin 1995.

Sosnicki, A.A. and Wilson, B.W. (1991) Pathology of turkey skeletal muscle: implications for the poultry industry. *Food Structure* 10, 317–326.

Sosnicki, A., Cassens, R.G., McIntyre, D.R., Vimini, R.J. and Greaser, M.L. (1989) Incidence of microscopically detectable degenerative characteristics in skeletal muscle of turkey. *British Poultry Science* 30, 69–80.

Sosnicki, A.A., Cassens, R.G., Vimini, R.J. and Greaser, M.L. (1991a) Histopathological and ultrastructural alterations of turkey skeletal muscle. *Poultry Science* 70, 349–357.

Sosnicki, A.A., Cassens, R.G., Vimini, R.J. and Greaser, M.L. (1991b) Distribution of capillaries in normal and ischemic turkey skeletal muscle. *Poultry Science* 70, 343–348.

Suarez-Kurtz, G. and Eastwood, A.B. (1981) Release of sarcoplasmic enzymes from frog skeletal muscle. *American Journal of Physiology* 241, C98–C105.

Sulieman, M.S., Minezaki, K.K. and Chapman, R.A. (1992) A phospholipase A2 inhibitor (Ro 31-4493) prevents the protein loss associated with the Ca-paradox in isolated guinea-pig hearts and is without effect on L-type channels of isolated myocytes. *Journal of Physiology* 446, 439P.

Sutko, J.L. and Airey, J.A. (1996) Ryanodine receptor Ca^{2+} release channels: does diversity in form equal diversity in function? *Physiological Reviews* 76, 1027–1069.

Sutko, J.L., Airey, J.A., Murakami, K., Takeda, M. and Beck, C. (1991) Foot protein isoforms are expressed at different times during embryonic chick skeletal muscle development. *Journal of Cell Biology* 113, 793–803.

Szczesna, D., Guzman, G., Miller, T., Zhao, J.J., Farokhi, K., Ellemberger, H. and Potter, J.D. (1996) The role of the 4 calcium binding sites of troponin-C in the regulation of skeletal-muscle contraction. *Journal of Biological Chemistry* 271, 8381–8386.

Tani, M. (1990) Mechanisms of Ca^{2+} overload in reperfused ischemic myocardium. *Annual Review of Physiology* 52, 543–559.

Tharin, S., Hamel, P.A., Conway, E.M., Michalak, M. and Opas, M. (1996) Regulation of calcium-binding proteins calreticulin and calsequestrin during differentiation in the myogenic cell-line L6. *Journal of Cellular Physiology* 166, 547–560.

Toury, R., Stelly, N., Boisonneau, E., Convert, M. and Dupuis, Y. (1990) Relationship between vitamin D status and deposition of bound calcium in the skeletal muscle of the rat. *Biology of the Cell* 69, 179–189.

Toury, R., Dupuis, Y., Balmain, N. and Mathieu, H. (1994) The effects of vitamin D deficiency on rat skeletal muscle ultrastructure and calbindin-D-9k and calbindin-D-28k. *Cells and Materials* 4, 165–177.

Tripp, M.J. and Schmitz, J.A. (1982) Influence of physical exercise on plasma creatine kinase activity in healthy and dystrophic turkeys and sheep. *American Journal of Veterinary Research* 43, 2220–2223.

Trump, B.F., Berezesky, I.K., Smith, M.W., Phelps, P.C. and Elliget, K.A. (1989) The relationship between cellular ion deregulation and acute and chronic toxicity. *Toxicology and Applied Pharmacology* 97, 6–22.

Tsien, R.W. and Tsien, R.Y. (1990) Calcium channels, stores and oscillations. *Annual Review of Cell Biology* 6, 715–760.

Tsugorka, A., Rios, E. and Blatter, L.A. (1995) Imaging elementary events of calcium release in skeletal muscle cells. *Science* 269, 1723–1726.

van der Sluis, W. (1996) PSE a new problem in turkey breast meat. *World Poultry* 12, 24–25.

Vergara, J., Difranco, M., Compagnon, D. and Suarez-Isla, A. (1991) Imaging of calcium transients in skeletal muscle fibers. *Biophysical Society* 59, 12–24.

Vretou-Jockers, E. and Vassilopoulos, D. (1989) Skeletal muscle CK-B activity in neurogenic muscular atrophies. *Journal of Neurology* 236, 284–287.

Wages, D.P. and Ficken, M.D. (1988) Skeletal muscle lesions in turkeys associated with the feeding of monensin. *Avian Diseases* 32, 583–586.

Watanabe, T., Takemasa, T., Yonemura, I. and Hirabayashi, T. (1997) Regulation of troponin T gene expression in chicken fast skeletal muscle: involvement of an M-CAT-like element distinct from the standard M-CAT. *Journal of Biochemistry* 121, 212–218.

Weisman, Y., Wax, E. and Bartov, I. (1994) Monensin toxicity in two breeds of laying hens. *Avian Pathology* 23, 575–578.

Wight, P.A.L., Siller, W.G., Martindale, L. and Filshie, J.H. (1979) The induction by muscle stimulation of a deep pectoral myopathy in the fowl. *Avian Pathology* 8, 115–121.

Williamson, J.R. and Monck, J.R. (1989) Hormone effects on cellular calcium fluxes. *Annual Review of Physiology* 51, 107–124.

Wilson, B.W. (1990) Developmental and maturational aspects of inherited avian myopathies. *Proceedings of the Society of Experimental Biology and Medicine* 194, 87–96.

Wilson, B.W., Nieberg, P.S. and Buhr, R.J. (1990) Turkey muscle growth and focal myopathy. *Poultry Science* 69, 1553–1562.

Wrogemann, K. and Pena, S.J.G. (1976) Mitochondrial overload: a general mechanism for cell necrosis in muscle diseases. *Lancet* ii, 672–674.

Yano, K. and Zarainherzberg, A. (1994) Sarcoplasmic-reticulum calsequestrins – structural and functional properties. *Molecular and Cellular Biochemistry* 135, 61–70.

Yao, Y., Kirinoki, M. and Hirabayashi, T. (1994a) Persistent expression of tissue-specific troponin-T isoforms in transplanted chicken skeletal muscle. *Journal of Muscle Research and Cell Motility* 15, 21–28.

Yao, Y., Miyazaki, J.I. and Hirabayashi, T. (1994b) Coexistence of fast-muscle type and slow-muscle type troponin-T isoforms in single chimeric muscle-fibers induced by muscle transplantation. *Experimental Cell Research* 214, 400–407.

Zimmer, D.B., Cornwall, E.H., Landar, A. and Song, W. (1995) The S100 protein family – history, function, and expression. *Brain Research Bulletin* 37, 417–429.

CHAPTER 4
Biochemical basis of meat texture

C.E. Lyon and R.J. Buhr

Poultry Processing and Meat Quality Research Unit, United States Department of Agriculture, Agricultural Research Service, Russell Research Center, Athens, GA 30604, USA

INTRODUCTION

The preceding chapter dealt with the development and structure of muscle tissue. In this chapter, the conversion of muscle (a living organ) to meat (an edible tissue) is discussed. Muscles vary in function, and therefore they vary in composition to provide contraction for movement and/or tension. Meat is composed of all of the support tissues (nervous, vascular, adipose and connective) that comprise a muscle and the quantity of support tissue varies by location within and among muscles. The post-mortem (PM) depletion of energy reserves within the muscle initiates the onset of rigor and the demarcation between muscle and meat. The degree of muscle contraction at the onset of rigor is variable, can be influenced by several physiological pathways and processing procedures, and is the main factor determining meat tenderness (Locker, 1960). It is important to remember that all the genetic improvements, live bird management practices and nutritional expertise used to enhance optimum broiler muscle growth and yield can be lost to the consumer if processing mistakes are made during the conversion of muscle to meat.

Historically, commercial poultry meat has been associated with the term 'tender'. When consumers purchase whole carcasses, there are few complaints of tough breast meat, because the muscles complete the rigor process while attached to the skeleton. Increasing demand for further-processed poultry products, especially those containing breast meat, propelled the rapid expansion of the industry, but earlier boning time ended the era when tender breast meat was guaranteed. In the United States, this association began to change when the volume of breast meat used for further-processed items steadily increased in the 1970s and 1980s. The changing market shifted the product mix from whole carcasses to cut-up and deboned breast meat.

In this chapter, the following topics are summarized: post-mortem muscle biochemistry and meat texture, methods for measuring meat texture and processing procedures that directly affect the texture of cooked poultry meat. The emphasis will be on meat from the breast muscles (the fillet, pectoralis and the tender, supracoracoideus) because of their economic importance to the poultry industry and the subsequent volume of research conducted using these muscles. The core of this review deals with poultry, broilers and turkeys, but, important contrasts between poultry and red meat are included. When evaluating experimental results, it is important to be cognizant that tenderness is a property of cooked meat and not raw meat.

POST-MORTEM MUSCLE BIOCHEMISTRY AND MEAT TEXTURE

The myofibrillar proteins actin and myosin comprise over half of the protein of skeletal muscle and are major factors in PM onset and resolution of rigor, tenderness, water holding capacity, emulsification and binding properties of meat. As noted in Chapter 3, muscles store chemical energy which can be utilized to produce mechanical contraction (shortening) resulting in skeletal movement for purposes such as locomotion. This renewable energy conversion from chemical into mechanical is interrupted by the cessation of blood flow at the time of death. Termination of vascular–cellular respiration results in the depletion of intracellular oxygen and initiates the consumption of all cellular energy reservoirs. The quantity of adenosine triphosphate (ATP) and creatine phosphate (CP) stored in the muscle are small and cannot be maintained in the PM muscle cell (fibre) for longer than a few minutes without regeneration. PM regeneration of ATP requires cellular metabolism to change from aerobic to anaerobic pathways. Anaerobic glycolysis causes the rapid utilization of muscle glycogen and results in the accumulation of lactic acid as a waste product.

As lactic acid accumulates, muscle pH declines from > 7.1 (de Fremery and Lineweaver, 1962; Stewart *et al.*, 1984; McGinnis *et al.*, 1989) to a metabolic ultimate of pH 5.4, below which glycolysis is inhibited. Consequently, the magnitude of the pH decline and the quantity of lactic acid accumulated PM depend on the amount of glycogen present in tissue at the time of death. Because of this relationship, meat quality is influenced by the circumstances of death, rate of PM glycolysis, concomitant falls of ATP and pH, time and temperature at onset of rigor and the resulting degree of muscle shortening (Lister *et al.*, 1970). The time PM to the onset of rigor is the delay phase and is characterized as muscle extensibility and minimal change in length. The duration of the delay phase is determined by ultimate pH and the elapsed time taken to reach ultimate pH (i.e. high ultimate pH reached rapidly corresponds to a short delay period). The onset of rigor is not triggered at a specific pH (above pH 6.0) but occurs irrespective of pH when > 60% of initial ATP is utilized (Khan, 1975). In the subsequent rapid phase of rigor, there is abrupt sarcomere shortening and decrease in extensibility. The pH at the onset of the rapid phase is linearly related to ultimate pH, which is determined by the initial glycogen reserves of the muscle at the time of slaughter (pH onset = 0.76 (ultimate pH + 2.2)) (Bate-Smith and Bendall, 1949). The rate of pH change at any pH (between 7.0 and 5.8) is remarkably consistent from animal to animal at a uniform temperature, with a minimal rate at pH 6.7. Minimal change in muscle tension also occurs within the pH range 6.7–6.4, and the sarcoplasmic reticulum continues to sequester calcium. Both PM muscle shortening and the development of tension occur rapidly as the pH drops below 6.3–6.2 with peak tension at pH 6.0 as the muscle reaches full rigor (Newbold, 1966). When a muscle is in full rigor, the shortest sarcomere lengths are attained (1.4–2.0 µm at 2–8 h PM) and the muscle becomes inextensible (Khan, 1974; Dunn *et al.*, 1993). Onset of rigor in breast fillets can occur within 15 min PM, whereas rigor onset for leg muscles may occur within 3 min PM. Full rigor for breast fillets occurs at 2–4 h PM and for leg muscles by 2 h (Kijowski *et al.*, 1982). Research on fillets boned immediately PM (aged at 8°C) revealed significant sarcomere shortening between 2 and 4 h PM. Sarcomere shortening and corresponding R values from 1.07 to 1.26 indicating the approximate time of rigor onset and full rigor (Papa and Fletcher, 1988b). The R value is calculated as the ratio of absorbance between adenine nucleotides (260 nm, ATP + ADP + AMP) and inosine (250 nm, inosine + inosine monophosphate + hypoxanthine metabolites of AMP), and thus is an indicator of ATP depletion within a muscle (Khan and Frey, 1971; Honikel and Fischer, 1977). The last phase of rigor is resolution or postrigor when a muscle is again extensible, but in contrast to the onset of rigor, muscle in this phase remains extended after loading.

The onset of rigor is related to the rate of intramuscle pH decline, occurring in broilers and turkeys at 2–4 h PM as compared to 10 h PM for beef. In poultry muscles, the ultimate (terminal) pH for predominantly white or predominantly red fibre type muscles differs. Red leg muscle reaches ultimate pH within 2–3 h PM (pH 6.0–5.9), whereas white breast muscle pH may continue to decline beyond 24 h (pH 5.6–5.4) when carcasses are rapidly chilled PM. Ultimate pH for broiler fillets (a white muscle) may be attained by 8 h PM (de Fremery and Pool, 1960; Khan, 1974; Stewart *et al.*, 1984). The longer period for rigor onset and the longer pH decline in white fibre type muscles is due to greater initial energy reserves, mainly in the form of glycogen (Hay *et al.*, 1973). Initial ATP levels are also higher in chicken fillets (4.8 mg g^{-1}) than beef muscles (3.1 mg g^{-1}). Rigor mortis not only develops, but resolves earlier PM in leg muscles than in breast muscles (Kijowski *et al.*, 1982). This observation was confirmed by evaluating muscles composed entirely of red-aerobic fibres (anterior latisimus dorsi) or white-anaerobic fibres (pectoralis). Aerobic muscle had completed metabolic activity after 2 h PM, but anaerobic muscle was still metabolically active at 8 h PM (Sams and Janky, 1991).

When glycolysis is prevented by iodoacetate injection, or when energy is depleted ante-mortem by adrenaline injection, there is no PM pH drop, sarcomeres do not shorten, and meat remains tender as muscles enter rigor immediately PM without shortening (de Fremery, 1966; Khan and Nakamura, 1970; Sayre, 1970). The most closely related biochemical event to the onset of rigor mortis is the depletion of ATP to less than 30–40% of initial levels (Erdos, 1943; de Fremery and Pool, 1960; Khan, 1975; Kijowski, *et al.*, 1982). The depletion of ATP is indicated by an R value near 1.0 at the onset of rigor and near 1.3 at full rigor (Khan and Frey, 1971; Davidek and Velisek, 1973; Papinaho and Fletcher, 1996).

The degree of struggling at death accelerates the rate of PM glycolysis due to elevation of muscle temperature (Dodge and Peters, 1960), resulting in more rapid consumption of glycogen, lower initial pH, and an earlier onset of rigor (de Fremery, 1966). However, minimal differences in fillet tenderness were detected among shear force values for anaesthetized (3.3 kg), electrically stunned (4.0 kg), and non-stunned (4.1 kg) broilers, after ageing carcasses at 2°C for 24 h (de Fremery, 1966). The rate of PM glycolysis is determined by muscle ATP utilization, pH and temperature. The muscles of stress susceptible pigs (pale, soft, exudative, PSE) become anoxic by reduced blood flow before stunning for slaughter, and not by struggling during slaughter (initial pH 6.25, Bate-Smith and Bendall, 1949; Kastenschmidt, 1970). In addition, electromyograph recordings revealed greater post-stun muscle activity for stress-resistant than stress-susceptible pigs (Kastenschmidt, 1970). However, prolonged feed withdrawal and ante-mortem physical exhaustion will lower initial glycogen content, thereby shortening the time to onset of rigor. This results in a higher ultimate pH because ante-mortem lactic acid was removed from the muscle by the vascular system (de Fremery and Lineweaver, 1962). Lyon *et al.* (1991) subjected broilers to feed withdrawal periods of 0, 8, 16 or 24 h and detected small differences in pH for fillets boned at 2 and 4 h PM, but lower shear values for all feed-withdrawal periods (5.84–6.01 kg) compared to values for full feed broilers (7.09 kg). The lower shear values can be explained by an earlier onset of rigor with reduced initial muscle glycogen and therefore less potential for shortening of the fillet after boning at 2 and 4 h.

The PM relationship between the onset and resolution phases of rigor and subsequent meat tenderness is fundamental to understanding present limitations to early boning of breast meat. Rigidity in rigor is a direct result of PM muscle shortening and loss of muscle extensibility. Full rigor can occur between 1 and 2 h PM in the chicken fillet chilled at 15°C (Sayre, 1970). Inextensibility must occur or the muscle would return to resting length immediately after depletion of ATP. The process of muscle fibre contraction or relaxation requires actin–myosin filaments to uncouple, and consume ATP. Loss of muscle extensibility is related to ATP depletion to less than 20% of initial levels. Inextensibility occurs with nearly 100% of overlapped actin–myosin filaments cross-linked compared to only 20% during typical ante-mortem muscle contractions (Huxley and Brown, 1967). Loss of elasticity, increased inextensibility and tension development all accompany sarcomere shortening and the onset of rigor. Therefore, rigor shortening must precede loss of extensibility.

The mechanics for PM rigor shortening are attributed to the pH decline and the optimal pH range (7–6) for the sarcoplasmic reticulum to sequester calcium and maintain an electrochemical gradient (from 10^{-4} to 10^{-7}M). As the pH drops below 6.0 PM, calcium diffusion from the sarcoplasmic reticulum exceeds the rate of calcium accumulation. When sarcoplasmic calcium concentration reaches 10^{-6}M and ATP is available, muscle contraction occurs. PM fibre shortening and ante-mortem muscle contraction also differ in that there is no neural stimulation necessary for PM shortening. Within 5 min PM, all electrical activity ceases in terms of action potentials from the nervous system as well as spontaneous propagation along the muscle sarcolemma (Kastenschmidt, 1970). In rare cases (excluding physical exhaustion) the earliest onset of rigor occurs within 15 min PM, well after the 5 min electrical conduction potential of nervous or muscle tissue.

Not all fibres within a muscle shorten uniformly PM. Variation in muscle composition (fibre type) and innervation (motor units) provides gradation in muscle contraction ante-mortem and ensures diverse PM energy reserves, onset of rigor, and degree of fibre shortening. Passive fibre shortening occurs due to connective tissue structural attachment of adjacent fibres, resulting in many wavy or kinky fibres (up to 80%; Cooper *et al.*, 1969). Furthermore, even if a muscle is composed entirely of a single fibre type, the degree of shortening throughout the muscle at any time PM will not be uniform (Smith and Fletcher, 1988) due to variable energy reserves and their utilization. Therefore, toughness of meat may not correlate directly to a decrease in mean sarcomere length. Instead, toughness may correlate to an increased incidence of highly shortened (< 1.5 μm) sarcomeres in which both ends of the myosin filaments interdigitate adjacent Z-discs, resulting in a ridged continuum. In general, sarcomere length prerigor and during rigor has been positively correlated ($r = 0.80$) with tenderness, whereas fibre diameter was negatively correlated ($r = -0.73$) with tenderness (Herring *et al.*, 1965). These opposite correlations with tenderness are expected since the degree of sarcomere shortening is directly related to the cross-sectional area of muscle fibres. Herring *et al.* (1965) reported that tenderness of beef was linearly related to fibre diameter and curvilinearly with sarcomere length.

Resolution of rigor is due to degradation of muscle ultrastructure, specifically the rupture of the actin–Z-disc connection. Some evidence has been reported for weakening of the actin–myosin interaction by proteolysis (Goll, 1968), but there is no evidence for uncoupling of actin–myosin cross-links (in the absence of ATP) or the sliding of thick and thin filaments to lengthen sarcomeres. Resolution of rigor is the gradual loss of ability to maintain isometric tension due to loss of Z-disc integrity within the muscle fibre, and it is associated with increased tenderness. Loss of calcium accumulating ability by the sarcoplasmic reticulum and mitochondria is thought to raise calcium levels high enough to induce cleavage of the actin–Z-disc complex (Greaser, 1968; Greaser *et al.*, 1969). Support for the role of calcium is provided by the fact that Z-discs remain intact PM when muscles are treated with the calcium chelators EDTA or EGTA (Goll *et al.*, 1970, 1983). Additional evidence that the actin–Z-disc region is a weak point of the sarcomere is that kinking, buckling and transverse splitting of myofibrils almost exclusively occurs within the I-zone and rarely across the A-zone (Takahashi *et al.*, 1967; MacNaughtan, 1978). Fibres that have lost their Z-disc integrity are also easier to tease into individual fibres, therefore interfibrillar attachment, as well as intrafibrillar Z-discs, have deteriorated. Z-disc degradation can occur within 24 h if meat is held at 37°C, but will require 3–5 days when meat is held at 2°C. Z-discs of red fibres are more stable PM than Z-discs of white fibres (Goll *et al.*, 1970; Abbott *et al.*, 1977), and Z-discs in older animals are more resistant to degradation than in younger animals. Myofibrils of chickens are fragmented into progressively smaller sarcomere segments when homogenized after increasing periods of PM storage (Takahashi *et al.*, 1967). The most rapid change in fragmentation and tenderization occurs during the initial 8 h PM (Pool *et al.*, 1959). Ageing results in increased fibre extension to twice equilibrium length, loss of intermyofibrillar adhesion, dissolution of the Z-discs, loss of gap filaments and has been attributed to endogenous proteolytic enzymes (Davey and Dickson, 1970; Davey, 1984).

Postmortem Muscle pH Drop

The rate of pH decline in the muscle plays a significant role in cooked meat texture and the appropriate timing for product fabrication. Tenderness can be affected by both very slow and very fast rates of early PM glycolysis. Muscle pH is also critical to binding properties and moisture characteristics of the cooked meat. Many poultry products incorporate polyphosphates to enhance water-holding capacity. This increase in functional property is due to maintaining higher pH PM (Hamm, 1960, 1970). Protein extraction is also greater in muscle with a high pH, and this enhances binding ability in a formed product (Solomon and Schmidt, 1980).

The relationship between the rate of pH change and the resulting meat quality (as water-holding capacity, colour and toughness) is a function of the temperature of the muscle when pH 6.0 is attained. A rapid pH drop will occur at higher muscle temperature, resulting in earlier onset of rigor and greater degree of rigor shortening (Khan, 1974). Muscle shortening and the degree of sarcomere contraction at rigor are negatively correlated with meat tenderness (Lowe, 1948; Herring *et al.*, 1965; Welbourn *et al.*, 1968; Bilgili *et al.*, 1989). Temperature has a marked influence on the rate of pH decline. High temperatures accelerate pH decline, whereas low temperatures retard rates of glycolysis and lactic acid production (Marsh, 1954). Prerigor beef is tender when cooked immediately and toughens as rigor progresses to completeness. Cooking prerigor broiler fillets immediately after boning (2 min PM) resulted in greater tenderness, measured by lower W-B shear values (5.6 kg), than for fillets cooked after 1 h ageing at 21°C (7.8 kg). With the resolution of rigor, there is an increase in tenderness with ageing (Ramsbottom and Strandine, 1949; Paul *et al.*, 1952; de Fremery, 1966). At the isoelectric point of muscle (pH < 5.4), water-binding ability of muscle proteins is at a minimum, proteins become denatured, and can precipitate. In addition, glycolysis is inhibited and there is an equalization of intra- and intercellular pH and ion concentrations. A rapid pH drop while muscle temperature is high, is responsible for PSE pork meat which is characterized by low water-holding capacity, loose muscle structure (soft texture) and physically disrupted fibres.

Rigor Onset

An earlier onset of rigor can occur when the carcass is maintained at a high temperature PM (> 19°C), resulting in the more rapid utilization of ATP and attaining a high ultimate pH, and is termed 'heat' or 'alkaline' rigor. Dark cutting beef (dark, firm and dry) results from pre-slaughter glycogen depletion, causing an early onset of rigor at a higher muscle temperature with minimal shortening. This meat has a high pH, greater water-binding capacity, dark colour, stickiness and increased tenderness. Rigor onset at a high pH (> 6.0) results in less sarcomere shortening due to limited calcium release from the sarcoplasmic reticulum. Grinding prerigor meat results in a high ultimate pH due to increased oxygen availability for ATP regeneration, and the addition of salt inhibits glycolysis. Similarly, administering oxygen immediately ante-mortem, injection of magnesium sulphate (anaesthetic and vasodilator properties) or exposing excised muscle strips to oxygen during PM glycolysis delays the onset of rigor mortis by maintaining higher levels of ATP and CP, resulting in lower lactic acid production and a higher pH (Lister *et al.*, 1970; Sair *et al.*, 1970; Buege and Marsh, 1975).

Cold shortening occurs when the rate of the PM pH decline is slow (pH > 6.7) and muscles are rapidly cooled below 14°C. Cold shortening results in the disappearance of the I-zone due to sarcomere shortening (> 40%) caused by excessive release of calcium (sarcotubular and mitochondrial) in the presence of ATP (Locker and Hagyard, 1963; Buege and Marsh, 1975; Jeacocke, 1984). Calcium diffuses into the sarcoplasm, induced by the electrochemical gradient, exceeding the temperature-reduced ability of the sarcoplasmic reticulum to sequester calcium. Cold shortening has been reported only in red muscles during whole carcass chilling. This may occur since red muscles have less developed sarcoplasmic reticulum systems and more numerous mitochondria than white muscles (Welbourn *et al.*, 1968). This less developed sarcoplasmic reticulum system results in sufficient concentrations of sarcoplasmic calcium (10^{-6}M) to induce contraction when red meat is subjected to cold temperatures (14°C). Cold shortening occurs primarily in superficial muscles or the musculature of smaller animals, and occurs in less than half the fibres of a red muscle (Voyle, 1969). The rapid pH decline in the white breast fillets of poultry PM, reduces the potential for cold shortening due to improbability of attaining muscle temperatures below 14°C before the pH drops below 6.7.

Thaw rigor occurs when meat frozen prerigor is thawed, and muscle shortening occurs in the presence of sufficient quantities of both ATP and calcium. Freezing ruptures the sarcoplasmic reticulum membrane, and calcium is released during defrosting. Within 30 min of thawing, there is rapid depletion of ATP and glycogen, resulting in the rapid onset of rigor shortening (> 40%) and severe toughening (de Fremery, 1966). Cooking frozen prerigor meat intensifies thaw rigor and toughness since the transformation from frozen to cooked is not instantaneous. However, if prerigor meat is frozen and held at −3 to −5°C for 48 h during thaw, insufficient quantities of ATP will remain and thaw rigor can be prevented. This was demonstrated by Lyon *et al.*

(1992a) when fillets boned at 0, 1 or 24 h after chilling were frozen (–32°C) immediately or after an additional 12 or 24 h of refrigeration (2°C). Shear values where higher for fillets boned at 0 or 1 h postchill compared to 24 h, but immediately freezing and defrosting (2°C for 20 h), or an additional 12 or 24 h of refrigeration after boning did not alter shear values.

Postmortem Proteolysis

Endogenous PM proteolysis by the calcium-dependent, neutral proteolytic system calpain–calpastatin (μ-calpain and m-calpain), has been suggested to be responsible for Z-disc degradation, as well as degradation of other cytoskeletal proteins (desmin, connectin, and nebulin). Calpain is most active at neutral pH, and the two isoforms differ in their calcium requirement for activity (Dayton *et al.*, 1981; Murachi, 1983). The activity of the calpain–calpastatin system is severely restricted *in vitro* as PM pH drops below 6.0. This limitation brings into question the role of the neutral proteolytic system in the later stages of ageing-induced tenderization. However, ageing-induced tenderness is associated with decreases in calpain but not catheptic enzyme levels (Koohmaraie, 1988, 1992). Lysosomal acid proteinases (cathepsins D, B, L and H) and their inhibitors (cystatins) regulate the degradation of actin and myosin *in situ*. These lysosomal enzymes are active at pH as low as 2.5 and may complete tenderization initiated by the calpain–calpastatin system PM (Matsukura *et al.*, 1981). A third set of longitudinal myofilaments that are related to meat tenderness, called gap filaments, were described by Locker *et al.* (1977) and Locker and Wild (1982). Gap filaments disappear with ageing and after certain cooking conditions. Gap filaments are composed of the protein connectin, and are present in M-lines, Z-discs the A-I junction, and through the entire A-band (Maruyama *et al.*, 1981). An additional myofibular protein, nebulin, is found within the N₂-line, and provides a cytoskeletal role in the myofibril (Wang, 1981). Apparently, connectin and nebulin are susceptible to proteolytic degradation during ageing, especially by calcium-activated enzymes, and their degradation during ageing is associated with tenderness.

METHODS FOR MEASURING MEAT TEXTURE

Cooking generally results in increased tenderness of poultry muscles, but the method of cooking can affect tenderness. Paradoxically, cooking induces fibre shrinkage as measured by shorter sarcomeres, and it increases meat tenderness (Williams *et al.*, 1986). Shear resistance of cooked meat appears to behave as a three component system: connective tissue orientation, actin–myosin overlap and water content (Currie and Wolfe, 1980). Collagen shrinks at temperatures of 60–70°C pulling myofibres passively together into a wavy appearance during cooking. At temperature > 80°C, collagen is solubilized, or converted into gelatin, resulting in progressive tenderization, dependent on the rate of heating and length of time above 80°C (Voyle, 1979).

Objective Instrumental Measurements

Instrumental measures of meat tenderness have been determined by shear, tensile or compression tests done unidirectionally across the fibre orientation of the meat samples. Variation within a muscle can exceed 20% (Chrystall, 1994). Shear measures the force required to cleave samples under a set of standard conditions. Several instruments are available to evaluate the force required to shear and/or compress meat samples. The Warner-Bratzler (W-B) shear method (Bratzler, 1932) uses a single blade to shear a meat sample, and the maximum force is usually recorded in kilograms. The Allo-Kramer (A-K) shear method (Kramer *et al.*, 1951) uses multiple blades that first compress and then shear a sample through the bottom of a slotted cell. The force to shear is usually recorded in kg g^{-1} of sample weight. Both the W-B and A-K shear tests are empirical methods. Texture profile analysis (TPA) with an Instron Universal Testing Machine uses a dual compression of a sample to simulate mastication. The results of TPA for meat samples include values for the attributes of hardness, springiness, cohesiveness, guminess and chewiness. Definitions of the TPA terms and their relationship to sensory evaluation of food samples were recently documented (Meullenet *et al.*, 1997). The TPA test is an example of an imitative method that yields multiple attributes and may be related to the consumer acceptability of a meat product.

Sample dimensions also play a major role in results, and should be described in detail or referenced. Physical characteristics of the product as used by the consumer should be taken into account when evaluating the meat sample. If the treatment imposed has a direct effect on meat thickness due to muscle contraction, then the difference in sample thickness at the point of evaluation should be part of the test. However, if the research goal is to evaluate the sensitivity of instrumental procedures, then uniform thickness of the samples would be required. For example, increasing sample surface area from 4 to 16 cm^2 (both 3 mm thick) resulted in a 36% lower A-K peak shear force per gram of sample. Dividing peak force by sample weight did not proportionally correct for sample surface area (Heath and Owens, 1997). Smith and Fletcher (1990) reported similar differences between intact broiler fillet samples (3 cm^2) and diced samples (1 cm^3) using the A-K shear device. Four PM boning times were used to assure a wide range of texture (0.5, 1, 4 or 24 h). Dicing resulted in 30% lower force to shear values per weight of sample compared to the larger sample. Smith and Fletcher (1990) suggested that greater differences between shear methods for the earlier boning times indicated that dicing samples may result in less sensitivity when evaluating relatively tough fillets.

Subjective Panel Evaluation

An accurate description of meat tenderness involves more than a single instrumental value such as force to shear, especially for treatments that may alter PM biochemical events and affect not only tenderness, but also moisture binding characteristics. Sensory evaluation is more complicated, but yields significantly more detail on changes that occur before, during and after mastication. It is essential that the validity of the instrumental values be documented with sensory information. Lyon and Lyon (1990a, b, 1991) established the relationships between four objective shear procedures (A-K, table-top W-B, Instron W-B, and single blade A-K) and sensory responses to tenderness for broiler breast fillets. A spectrum of PM boning times from immediately after picking to 24 h were used to provide a range of texture. A 24 member untrained panel evaluated the cooked meat using 5–6-item categorical intensity scales for tenderness, juiciness and overall texture acceptability. Instrumental shear values were significantly affected by early PM boning time. The data provide ranges of the sensory perception of tenderness from very tough to very tender and the appropriate range of shear values for each instrument that corresponds to the sensory scale. For example, W-B shear values between 6.6 and 3.6 kg correspond to the slightly to the moderately tender portion of the sensory scale, whereas at the extremes of the scale, W-B shear values greater than 12.6 kg correspond to very tough and W-B values less than 3.6 kg correspond to very tender. Another approach was used to test the relationships between instrumental (W-B, A-K shear) and sensory tenderness by using broiler fillets boned at 2, 6 and 24 h PM. The 11-member trained panel developed 20 sensory descriptive texture attributes which were separated by variable cluster analysis into five groups representing mechanical, moisture and chewdown characteristics. Both instrumental methods indicated differences due to boning time and correlated highly ($r > 0.90$) with mechanical and chewdown sensory characteristics (Lyon and Lyon, 1997).

Sarcomere Length

Sarcomere length (distance between adjacent Z-discs) is used as a measure of muscle contraction and is highly correlated with tenderness of prerigor and rigor meat. Comparison of methods for sarcomere length determination by oil immersion phase-contrast light microscopy (single sarcomere within a myofibril) or laser diffraction (average of all illuminated sarcomeres within a muscle fibre) has resulted in high correlations ($r > 0.8$) for prerigor and rigor muscle (Ruddick and Richards, 1975) and for stretched and non-restrained prerigor muscle (Cross *et al.*, 1980). Postrigor comparisons were less well correlated ($r = 0.68$). Young *et al.* (1990) also reported good correlations between the laser and microscopic methods for sarcomeres 1.60 μm or longer ($r = 0.75$; 24% shortening with myosin filaments reaching adjacent Z-discs), but the laser overestimated sarcomere length for shorter sarcomeres and the correlation coefficient was lower ($r = 0.37$). These studies agree with the peak in resistance for shear data at 35–40% sarcomere shortening (1.4 μm) when actin filaments touch opposite Z-discs and myosin filaments penetrate Z-discs (Marsh and Carse, 1974). Lower resistance to shearing and greater tenderization are associated with longer and shorter sarcomeres.

PROCESSING PROCEDURES THAT DIRECTLY AFFECT TEXTURE OF COOKED POULTRY MEAT

The incorporation of chicken items into fast-food menus has dramatically increased the consumption of broiler meat. Breast meat is the driving force for the increase in demand and consumption. Product form ranges from intact breast fillets to nuggets, strips and popcorn pieces, and the demand continues to increase every year for further-processed items. The demand for more meat in diverse forms has resulted in more broilers being processed, with most plants operating two shifts per day. For example, in the US approximately 5.24 billion broilers were slaughtered in 1988, compared to 7.69 billion in 1996.

To ensure optimum tenderness in cooked breast meat, a minimum post-chill ageing time of 4 h prior to boning is required (Lyon *et al.*, 1985). From the plant standpoint, keeping the processing lines and product moving through the chiller to the loading dock in an orderly fashion is desirable. This optimum plant schedule would result in removal of the fillet from carcasses immediately after ice–water immersion chilling for times ranging from 45 min to 1 h. Filleting after chilling for 1 h would eliminate the need to provide refrigerated cooler space and labour to put the carcasses into meat lugs, move them into the coolers and then remove them and hang back on the line 4–24 h later. Many US processors consider the time and money involved in holding carcasses or front halves prior to boning to be their biggest economic barrier. The costs associated with holding broiler front-halves, including cost of purchasing and cleaning containers, labour, refrigeration, space and loss in yield totalled over $5 million per year for one US company (Sams, 1997). This desire to save on equipment, space and labour has been the impetus for researchers to evaluate various treatments to minimize PM ageing while striving to optimize tenderness in the finished meat products.

Over the last 10 years, numerous treatments have been evaluated with the goal of reducing or eliminating ageing of carcasses postchill while optimizing cooked meat texture. Generally, treatments that accelerate PM glycolysis cause a sharp pH drop that hastens the onset of rigor at a higher temperature, resulting in greater fibre shortening and increased toughness of meat aged on-the-frame (de Fremery and Lineweaver, 1962; Khan, 1975). Alternatively, factors that maintain PM resynthesis of ATP and inhibit ATP breakdown delay the onset of rigor until after chilling. Lowering carcass temperature resists fibre shortening resulting in increased tenderness of meat aged on-the-frame. A variety of treatments has been applied to alter ATP breakdown to enhance tenderness with variable results: gas stunning, electrical stimulation, muscle tensioning, belt flattening, high temperature conditioning, extended chilling, incorporation of additives and combinations of the above treatments. All of these treatments affect the rate of PM biochemical reactions and/or the physical integrity of the muscle fibres. The following section details some of the research in these areas.

On-Frame Ageing and Boning Time

There are numerous reports documenting the need for on-the-frame ageing of fillets to ensure adequate tenderness after cooking (Pool *et al.*, 1959; Stewart *et al.*, 1984; Lyon *et al.*, 1985; Dawson *et al.*, 1987). Lyon *et al.* (1985) conducted a study under commercial conditions to determine the postchill whole carcass ageing time (0, 1, 2, 4, 6, 8 or 24 h) necessary to ensure tenderness in boned broiler fillets. Fillets boned immediately after ice–water immersion chilling for 45 min exhibited significantly higher pH values (6.22) than any of the later postchill samples, which varied little. The high pH for the 0 h postchill muscle indicates that little lactic acid had accumulated, and indirectly indicates that more ATP was present in the muscle. This 0 h postchill boned group (after fillet ageing for 24 h) exhibited significantly higher W-B shear values than any later boned group (15.19 kg). The force required to shear the meat boned at 1 and 2 h postchill was statistically lower than for those boned immediately after chilling (10.61 and 10.85 kg, respectively). Shear values for muscles boned 4, 6, 8 or 24 h postchill were not significantly different and ranged from 5.23 to 7.73 kg. These results illustrate the importance of on-the-frame postchill ageing times to ensure adequate tenderness in broiler fillets. The larger carcass size of turkeys requires additional ageing time before boning. Boning turkey fillets after 3 or 24 h of ageing resulted in no detectable difference in tenderness (Raj and Nute, 1995). The lack of difference between 3 and 24 h indicates that turkey fillets had entered rigor by 3 h PM and boning did not induce significant shortening or detectable differences in shear force.

Boning prior to chilling (hot boning) dramatically increases fillet toughness (Lowe, 1948; Pool *et al.*, 1959; Lyon *et al.*, 1973, Stewart *et al.*, 1984; Dawson *et al.*, 1987). High temperature accelerates the onset of rigor in hot boned fillets and muscle fibres shorten significantly in the absence of restraint, resulting in toughening compared to cold boned fillets. Skeletal restraint is removed during boning and hot boned prerigor meat will shorten and toughen (Papa *et al.*, 1989). Similarly, carcass portioning that requires transverse cuts across the breast will result in significantly higher shear values when cuts are made at 2 h PM compared to 48 h PM (Lyon *et al.*, 1973). Ultimate pH is not affected by ageing-boning time (Stewart *et al.*, 1984; Sams *et al.*, 1990), although early boning results in consistently shorter sarcomere lengths even after additional ageing.

Breast Muscle Tensioning

Locker (1960) noted that beef tenderness is affected by the degree of muscular contraction during the early PM period and that muscles not allowed to contract during rigor are more tender than muscles that are allowed to contract. He suggested that contracted muscle is less tender than relaxed muscle since there are more myofilaments per unit of muscle cross-section and greater density of actin–myosin binding. The importance of skeletal restraint in broilers was demonstrated by Cason *et al.* (1997) who showed that severing the tendon of insertion for the supracoracoideus muscle postevisceration resulted in greater shear of both antagonistic muscles, the pectoralis (fillet) and supracoracoideus (tender) at 2 and at 24 h PM.

Several attempts to achieve tension induced tenderization with various methods of binding the wings to apply tension to the breast muscles have produced small improvements in tenderness although all early boned fillets were considered tough (Janky *et al.*, 1992). Experiments with binding the elbows above the back after bleeding have had limited impact on fillet tenderness or sarcomere length (Birkhold *et al.*, 1992). Wing restraint during evisceration and chilling, and boning at 24 h also produced minimal changes in sarcomere length and all shear values were considered tender (Papa and Fletcher, 1988a). Restraining the wings in combination with other treatments has been shown to increase breast meat tenderness. Lyon *et al.* (1992b) combined wing restraints with an additional 1 h ageing after ice–water immersion chilling for 1 h. Cooked fillets from carcasses subjected to this treatment combination required 53% less force to shear (W-B) than fillets from a control group (no restraints, 1 h chill). Birkhold and Sams (1993) combined wing restraints and electrical stimulation to significantly reduce A-K shear values by 39% and measured longer sarcomeres compared to a control group. A later study (Lyon and Lyon, 1994) combined electrical stimulation during bleeding with wing restraints in two locations on the wings to evaluate the incidence of residual blood adjacent to the shoulder joints as well as sarcomere length and shear values for fillets boned at 75 min PM. Placing restraints as proximal to the shoulder as possible resulted in a significant increase in residual blood adjacent to the shoulder joints. Regardless of location, sarcomeres were longer and W-B shear values lower for carcasses with restraints. The increased incidence of a quality defect like accumulated blood adjacent to the shoulder joints poses a serious problem which other researchers have also noted (Raj *et al.*, 1990).

Chilling and Ageing Temperature

Poultry carcasses are chilled after evisceration to lower carcass temperature to 4.4°C within 4 h PM to minimize rigor shortening and toughness. High temperature ageing (> 16°C) results in more rapid pH decline and Z-disc degradation (Goll *et al.*, 1970). In a study evaluating both high temperature conditioning and electrical stimulation, Sams (1990) noted that high temperature conditioning did not affect ultimate R value or shear unless accompanied by electrical stimulation. In combination, the treatments resulted in a moderate increase in tenderness for fillets boned 1 h PM. This difference is attributed to a greater degree of shortening and toughening after boning (at 1 h PM) for the chilled non-stimulated fillets. High temperature ageing (41°C) resulted in longer sarcomeres from 1 to 4 h PM, but higher shear values (deboned 5 h PM) than those ageing at 0°C prior to boning (Bilgili *et al.*, 1989). Apparently, the accelerated onset of rigor associated with high temperature ageing improved tenderness only for fillets boned before 4 h PM.

Electrical Stunning

The main reason for stunning poultry is to achieve rapid immobilization and ensure an accurate neck cut resulting in a uniform rate of bleeding and assure death prior to scalding. From a welfare concern, stunned poultry should not experience any additional stressors associated with death. Use of electrical current for processing poultry goes back to 1749 and the British colonies in North America when Ben Franklin hosted a party for his friends who were interested in the use of electricity (Lopez and Herbert, 1975). The *pièce de resistance* was to be a turkey killed by electric shock. Franklin noted that killing turkeys electrically had the pleasant side-effect of making the meat uncommonly tender, reportedly the first practical application that had been found for electricity. An electrocuted turkey would have minimal struggling at death resulting in high initial glycogen levels and lower muscle temperature that would prolong ATP availability. Compared to the common practice of decapitation, the absence of clonic convulsions with electrocution would have resulted in a lower PM muscle temperature at the onset of rigor, and thus minimum muscle rigor shortening and improved tenderness. Franklin tried to perfect the technique and found he could easily put chicken hens to death using electricity, but that the larger turkeys had a tendency to faint and then recover consciousness a short time later unless a stronger dose was administered.

A more recent comparison between broilers electrically stunned or not stunned and processed under commercial conditions was reported by Lee *et al.* (1979). Muscle biochemical changes and ground cooked meat objective texture were determined after immersion chilling from carcasses aged at 2°C for either 4 or 24 h. Fillets from stunned carcasses exhibited higher levels of ATP, CP and pH values during the early processing steps (after bleeding, after picking, after chilling). It was concluded that electrical stunning delayed the onset of rigor by slowing the depletion of ATP until after chilling when the muscle temperature was around 4°C, thus resisting rigor shortening. After ageing for 24 h, ground meat from electrically stunned broilers required 28% less force to shear than the meat from non-stunned broilers (Lee *et al.*, 1979). These results are explained by the clonic convulsions during death of non-stunned broilers resulting in an increase in muscle temperature, rapid ATP utilization, and greater rigor shortening at the higher temperature. However, when the shear data were analysed from muscles boned immediately after chilling and then cooked, the trend was reversed with meat from electrically stunned broilers requiring 33% more force to shear than meat from non-stunned broilers. Lee *et al.* (1979) noted that all the meat cooked after chilling was tough (> 82 kg 20 g⁻¹). Fillets from stunned broilers had higher ATP (3.1 vs 0.2 µmol g⁻¹) and CP (0.02 µmol g⁻¹) than fillets from non-stunned broilers. The higher ATP and CP levels for the stunned broilers would have provided energy for greater rigor shortening after boning.

Extending stunning (100 V) duration for a total of 20 or 40 s appeared to accelerate ATP depletion, as indicated by elevated R values (0.92) measured immediately after stunning. These values were comparable to values for non-stunned broilers (0.91), but were higher than those for broilers stunned for 10 s (0.88). However, broilers stunned for 20 or 40 s had high initial pH values (6.38) that were not different from the pH values of those stunned for 10 s (6.42), but were higher than pH values for broiler that were not stunned (6.23; Fletcher, 1993). Ultimate pH, R value and A-K shear were similar for all treatments. In another study, extending carcass chilling for 1, 2 or 3 h did not affect the pH decline (remaining > 6.0), but fillets boned after 3 h revealed elevated R values and lower shear values compared to those boned after chilling for 1 or 2 h. These results indicate that extended ice chilling differentially inhibited glycolysis but not ATP utilization (Dickens and Lyon, 1995).

Thomson et al. (1986) examined the effects of electrical stunning and hot boning (after defeathering at 20 min PM) on pH and objective texture of broiler fillets. Stunned broilers received 55 V AC for 10 s, and both stunned and non-stunned broilers were bled in restraining cones for 120 s. One fillet was removed from each carcass after picking, the carcasses were then eviscerated, chilled for 30 min and stored at 2°C for 24 h at which time the remaining fillet was removed. Fillets from stunned broilers exhibited higher pH values at 20 min PM compared to fillets from non-stunned broilers. Both initial and ultimate pH varied significantly among replications, but ultimate pH was not affected by stunning. Fillets cooked at 20 min PM resulted in higher W-B shear values compared to fillets aged on the carcass for 24 h prior to boning and cooking. Thomson et al. (1986) noted that PM ageing prior to boning had a more pronounced effect on objective texture than electrical stunning.

Raising the stunning current from 0 to 50 or 100 mA resulted in higher pH and lower R value at boning times from 12 min to 4 h PM (Papinaho and Fletcher, 1996). After ageing fillets for 48 h, shear values were considered tough for all fillets boned at 8 h or less. In contrast, all shear values were considered tender, regardless of stunning amperage with on-the-frame ageing for 10–24 h. The duration of electrical stunning also influences tenderness of fillets boned at 1 h PM. Stunning durations of 6, 8 or 10 s at a constant potential of 50 V (30–32 mA) resulted in increased shear values compared to shorter durations of 2 or 4 s for fillets cooked after boning, at 1 h PM. Also as stunning duration increased, fillet pH values at 1 h PM were significantly higher (Young et al., 1996; Young and Buhr, 1997).

Electrical stunning treatments at currents that induce death have been applied to poultry. This concept of electrocution or irreversible stunning has been suggested by Heath et al. (1983) as a humane method of poultry slaughter that assures death prior to scalding. Heath noted that fillet pH values measured 2 h PM were not different for electrocuted or electrically stunned broilers. Lyon and Dickens (1993) reported on the effects of electrical stunning (50 V AC 34 mA, 10 s) and electrocution (200 V AC 132 mA, 10 s) treatments on the rate of PM pH and R value changes of broiler fillets and objective texture. After chilling for 75 min, fillets from broilers that had been electrocuted exhibited lower R values (1.02 vs 1.07) indicating higher levels of ATP. The W-B shear values were significantly higher for early boned fillets (75 min postchill) from broilers that had been electrocuted compared to broilers that had been stunned, 10.0 vs 7.3 kg, respectively. A later report (Dickens and Lyon, 1993) demonstrated that although shear values differed for stunned and electrocuted broilers boned at 2 h PM, boning at 4 h resulted in acceptable tenderness for both (4.5–4.9 kg). Therefore, the lower R value determined for electrocuted broilers than for stunned broilers appears to be an extension of the differences reported between stunned and non-stunned broilers for early boned fillets.

The results from these studies indicate that electric current may be a humane way to kill poultry, but it slows the rate of early PM biochemical reactions to the point that is not feasible to debone fillets prior to 4 h PM when electrocution or high voltage stunning is used (Kim *et al.*, 1988). Stunning minimizes peri-mortem struggling which results in utilizing 50% less glycogen and retaining a higher initial pH (de Fremery and Lineweaver, 1962). Papinaho *et al.* (1995) demonstrated that preventing struggling during slaughter by physical restraint or denervation, in combination with increasing stunning currents from 50 to 125 mA, had no affect on initial pH (15 min) or R value.

Gas Stunning

It was previously noted that electrical stunning is the most common method used in both the US and Europe, although several gas stunning systems are available. Over the past 5 years there has been a renewed interest in gas stunning. The basics of both gas and electrical stunning for poultry were recently summarized by Sams (1996). Gases such as carbon dioxide (CO_2), nitrogen (N_2) and argon (Ar) have been used for both chickens and turkeys. Extreme concentrations of any gas displaces oxygen and causes hypoxia which renders animals unconscious. Raj *et al.* (1990) measured pH (at 20 min and 24 h PM), texture and colour of cooked fillets, as well as carcass appearance (broken bones and haemorrhages) for broilers subjected to gas stunning. Broilers were exposed to Ar (98%) or CO_2 (45%) in crates (placed into a well containing the gas for 120 s) or shackled and electrically stunned using a water-bath for 4 s (107 mA). The fillets from electrically stunned broilers retained significantly higher pH at 20 min PM (pH 6.55) compared to muscles from carcasses stunned with CO_2 (pH 6.34) or Ar (pH 5.93). At 24 h PM, the ultimate fillet pH from carcasses subjected to these stunning treatments was not significantly different (pH 5.75, 5.84 or 5.79, respectively). This lack of an effect of gas stunning methods on ultimate pH is in agreement with results reported for electrical stunning and electrocution (Thomson *et al.*, 1986; Papinaho and Fletcher, 1996; Poole, 1997). Since ultimate pH was not affected by gas stunning, significant quantities of lactic acid were not removed from muscle tissue during the characteristic clonic convulsions that occur. Therefore, gas stunning and electrical stimulation have similar effects on PM muscle biochemistry (lower initial pH but unaffected ultimate pH). This differs from ante-mortem exhaustion or the occurrence of a death struggle of non-stunned broilers which both result in lower initial pH and higher ultimate pH.

Poole and Fletcher (1995) compared a flow-through gas killing system (2 min) for broilers subjected to Ar, CO_2 or N_2. Broilers reacted very quickly to CO_2 compared to Ar or N_2, although time from exposure to death, noted as cessation of respiratory ventilation, was essentially the same for CO_2, N_2 and Ar. Broilers subjected to Ar and N_2 exhibited more severe clonic convolutions with wing flapping and muscular contractions, and these physical observations were verified by lower 15 min PM fillet pH values for broilers subjected to Ar (pH 6.40) and N_2 (pH 6.44) than for CO_2 (pH 6.55). Ultimate pH after ageing for 24 h did not differ among gas stunning methods (pH 5.71).

Large turkeys stunned with CO_2 or Ar, and sampled at 2, 3, 5 and 18 h PM had lower pH (5.87 and 5.82) and lower fillet shear values (3.9 and 3.7 kg) than electrically stunned turkeys (pH 6.09 and shear 4.7 kg; Raj, 1994). Turkeys stunned with 40 or 60% CO_2 had lower pH (6.1, at 24 h ageing) than electrically (200 mA) stunned turkeys (pH 6.31; Fleming *et al.*, 1991). Fillet shear force was lowest for turkeys stunned with 40% CO_2 but higher for those stunned with 60% CO_2, and all were considered slightly to moderately tender (3.86–4.73 kg).

Raj *et al.* (1990) determined tenderness for fillets that were boned after ageing overnight (1°C) and cooked to an internal temperature of 90°C from electrically and gas stunned broilers. Fillets from electrically stunned broilers were 3.6% tougher than fillets from Ar stunned broilers and <1% tougher than fillets from CO_2 stunned broilers. All the meat would be considered very tender (2.15–2.23 kg shear). Raj *et al.* (1990) suggested that wing flapping induced by the Ar stunning treatment accelerated PM glycolysis resulting in an early onset of rigor, indicated by the lower 20 min PM pH value, and that this flapping was a 'natural flight movement'.

Raj and Nute (1995) determined the sensory profile and objective texture of turkey fillets boned 3 or 24 h PM from broilers stunned with Ar-induced anoxia and electrocution (150 mA). After cooking to 85°C, meat from anoxia stunned turkeys was rated less firm on cutting (9%), more tender (13%), and exhibited a more powdery residue (16%) upon mastication. Instrumental texture values (kg yield force) confirmed that the fillets from the anoxia stunned turkeys were more tender (by 15%, 3.09 kg) than fillets from electrically stunned (3.63 kg) turkeys, although correlation coefficients between instrumental and panel tenderness assessments were not significant. The sensory evaluation portion of the Raj and Nute (1995) study utilized ten experienced assessors to rate attributes grouped into four categories (texture characteristics on: cutting, initial mouthfeel, eating and residue). Principal component analysis was used to interpret the sensory data and create a sensory space. This type of analysis allowed for the separation of variation into components and revealed that the first two principal components (cutting and initial mouthfeel) accounted for 59% of the total variation. This type of sensory analysis is worthy of note because it again illustrates the complexity of mastication rated by the experienced panelists compared to a single force measurement for the instrumental procedure.

Raj *et al.* (1997) recently compared broiler carcass and meat quality after gaseous and electric stunning. A gas mixture of 30% CO_2, 60% Ar and 10% air was compared to electrical stunning at 80 mA, 50 Hz. Gas stunning in crates substantially reduced carcass and meat quality defects compared to electric stunning in shackles. Breast meat boned at 24 h PM from gas stunned broilers was more tender than meat from electrically stunned broilers (1.3 and 1.5 kg yield force, respectively). Meat from broilers that were gas stunned and boned 4 h PM and that from birds electrically stunned and boned 24 h PM were equivalent in tenderness (1.2 kg yield force).

Research indicates some benefits of gaseous stunning compared to electrical stunning in potentially hastening the onset of rigor (lower pH values 15 min PM) and reducing total carcass defects, but in the US electrical stunning continues to be used by the vast majority of broiler processors.

Electrical Stimulation

Electric current can also be used to hasten the onset of rigor in muscles and thus shorten PM ageing times prior to boning. Ashgar and Henrickson (1982) concluded that electrical stimulation accelerated the onset of rigor by depletion of ATP which resulted in rapid glycolysis, a pH drop, and an elevated R value. A biological and meat science review of electrical stimulation of beef and lamb carcasses was presented by Bendall (1980) and for poultry by Li *et al.* (1993). For beef carcasses, it was noted that ATP was fully depleted in less than 3 h after stimulation, whereas in non-stimulated carcasses the ATP level remained at 100%. Nichols and Cross (1980) reported that electrical stimulation caused a rapid pH decline up to 6 h PM in beef muscle, whereas non-stimulated muscles exhibited a gradual linear decline over time. The absence of any electrical stimulation effect on sarcomere length indicated that the prevention of cold shortening in excised muscles following electrical stimulation was not a concern (Will *et al.*, 1979; Nichols and Cross, 1980). Electrically stimulated beef sides exhibited lower W-B shear values and sustained greater cooking losses than did non-stimulated sides, indicating more tender meat due to the stimulation treatment (Savell *et al.*, 1978; Will *et al.*, 1979). Light micrographs revealed contraction bands and stretched areas on either side of the bands, whereas electron micrographs showed both contraction bands and physical disruption of the myofibrils on either side of the bands (Savell *et al.*, 1978). It was concluded that electrical stimulation improved tenderness by physical disruption and the formation of contraction bands, and not by prevention of cold shortening.

Bendall (1980) stated that stimulation had become one of the most useful tools in meat technology, particularly in view of the increasing tendency in commercial practice to cool carcasses as rapidly as possible after slaughter. In an earlier study, Bendall *et al.* (1976) reported that electrical stimulation was a very effective means to rapidly lower ATP levels and pH of major beef muscles. The greater pH decline for stimulated carcasses (nearly twice the normal rate) was attributed to elevated temperature for the stimulated muscle, and when a correction factor for temperature was considered, the mean rate of pH decline from 6.3 to 5.7 in pH units per hour was not statistically different due to stimulation. In agreement, Goll (1968) reported that ATP levels are higher in bovine muscle at the time of rigor onset (inextensible) for carcasses held at 1°C than those held at 37°C.

During the last decade the interest and subsequent number of publications concerning the use of electrical current to stimulate broiler carcasses has increased. As with the red meat publications cited, the emphasis for the research was the desire by poultry processors to eliminate any postchill whole carcass or front-half ageing prior to muscle removal. In Europe, the welfare of the bird seems to have been the driving force, but regardless of the reason for initiating the research, the PM muscle biochemistry, sarcomere length and ultimate tenderness of the cooked meat are the major measures of the ability to alter processing procedures that equate to less ageing time prior to boning and optimum tenderness in the cooked fillets.

Froning and Uijttenboogaart (1988) subjected carcasses to intermittent electrical stimulation at 100 V for 1 min (1 s on, 0.5 s off) after bleeding and compared them to a non-stimulated group. At various times after evisceration (0, 15, 30, 60, 120, 180, 240 min), one breast fillet was boned, and the remaining fillet was left on the carcass. To minimize cold shortening, carcasses were held at 15°C until fillets were boned. Stimulation resulted in lower fillet pH at all boning times, and a tenderizing effect (W-B shear values) at 120 and 240 min posteviseration, but not at 180 min. Electrical stimulation also increased redness measured objectively as 'a*' values at all boning times except 30 min. Cooking losses and expressible moisture were also increased due to electrical stimulation. Elevated R values have been reported after electrical stimulation at higher voltages as were lower pH and shear values, but greater cook loss for fillets boned at 2 h PM (Lyon et al., 1989; Walker et al., 1995). Birkhold and Sams (1993) applied electrical stimulation at 440 V for 15 s (2 s on, 1 s off) to broiler carcasses and reported that boning after chilling (1 h PM) resulted in lower pH and longer sarcomeres. After ageing for 24 h, A-K shear values from stimulated carcasses were significantly lower than from non-stimulated carcasses, and would be considered slightly tender (8.52 and 12.55 kg g^{-1}, respectively). Lyon and Dickens (1993) stimulated broiler carcasses at 200 V (138 mA) for 1 min during bleeding (2 s on, 1 s off) and reported lower pH and higher R values at 75 min PM, but no difference in sarcomere lengths. All the fillets were boned immediately after chilling (75 min PM) and held as fillets for 24 h prior to cooking and texture analysis. There were no significant differences noted in tenderness, W-B shear values were 9.31 kg for stimulated and 9.88 kg for control.

The difference between the Birkhold and Sams (1993) and Lyon and Dickens (1993) studies appears to be related to sarcomere length which may have resulted from sampling opposite ends of the fillet. Filleting immediately PM (without scalding or picking) and ageing for 24 h resulted in shorter sarcomeres for the anterior than the middle or posterior portion of the fillet (Papa and Fletcher, 1988b). Fillets removed after ageing 24 h did not vary in sarcomere length among locations. Smith et al. (1988) reported small changes in shear force for hot and cold boned fillets from the posterior (caudal) fillets (9.3 and 9.5 kg g^{-1}) but large differences for anterior (cranial) fillets (14.2 and

6.7 kg g^{-1}) samples. In addition, the duration of the stimulation period differed, 15 s (Birkhold and Sams, 1993) compared to 60 s (Lyon and Dickens, 1993). However, Birkhold *et al.* (1992) had earlier reported that stimulation durations of 15, 45 or 75 s did not significantly affect shear values or sarcomere lengths of fillets boned 1 h PM. Electrical stimulation to exhaustion (15 or 30 min) of fillets boned immediately PM consistently resulted in increased toughness (41% after 24 h ageing) compared to non-stimulated fillets (de Fremery and Pool, 1960). Electrical stimulation in combination with extended chilling for 2 or 3 h resulted in significantly lower W-B shear values (50 and 29%, respectively) than non-stimulated carcasses (Dickens and Lyon, 1995).

Thompson *et al.* (1987) reported on the effects of PM electrical stimulation on tenderness and physical characteristics of broiler fillets boned after feather removal (hot-boning); after immersion chilling in unagitated ice slush at 1°C for 1 h (chill boning); or after 48 h ageing (aged boning). A knife stunner (Cervin Electrical Systems) was used to immobilize the broilers and then stimulate the carcasses after bleeding for 90 s. Carcasses were stimulated for 15 s (2 s on, 1 s off, total of five cycles) at either 0, 240, 530 or 820 V. In a separate experiment, the effects of low voltage stimulation (45 V) for 9 or 18 s (2 s on, 1 s off) were compared to a group of carcasses not stimulated. Current flowed from the knife blade touching the neck of the carcass to the shackle line which served as the ground. Sarcomere length, pH, R value and A-K shear values were used to determine the effects of the electrical treatments on physical, biochemical and textural properties. Low voltage stimulation at both durations significantly decreased shear values compared to the non-stimulated carcasses when muscles were boned after picking, possibly because stimulation caused contractions which lowered the glycogen level. Electrical stimulation increased R values and decreased pH of hot boned and chill boned muscles, but had no effect on aged boned muscles. The 820 V treatment significantly decreased shear values (6.5 kg g^{-1}) of chill boned muscles to an acceptable level of tenderness. Thompson *et al.* (1987) noted that the tenderness response was more highly related to myofibrillar disruption and greater sarcomere length than to pH or ATP depletion. These findings are in agreement with the result of Sams *et al.* (1989) who reported that electrical stimulation lowered shear force at 2, 3 and 4 h PM but did not change R values. Location of the stimulation current resulted in different A-K shear values for neck application (8.6 kg g^{-1}) compared to application at the cranial end of the breast (6.3 kg g^{-1}; Sams *et al.*, 1992). The lower shear value attained when stimulation current was applied directly to the breast was assumed to result from a greater current flow through the fillets, resulting in more extensive contractions and fragmentation, compared to when stimulation current was applied to the neck.

The results of lower voltage levels for longer periods of time during bleeding have also been reported. Lyon *et al.* (1989) noted that a threshold level had to be obtained before any benefit was noted due to stimulation. Voltage levels of 50, 200 and 350 were evaluated using 20 cycles of 2 s on, 1 s off. Breast meat pH was noted at 10 min and 1 h PM, and R values at 2 h PM. Cooked yield, fluids and solids lost during heating, A-K shear values and TPA data were collected. Stimulation at 200 and 350 V resulted in lower pH values at both PM times and higher R values at 2 h PM. Stimulation at 350 V resulted in lower cook yields and higher percentages of fluids and solids lost suggesting a loss of functional properties and muscle integrity. Similar results were noted by Froning and Uijttenboogaart (1988).

Sams and Hirschler (1997) and Lyon *et al.* (1997a) conducted experiments under commercial conditions and reported that the combination of carcass stimulation during or immediately after bleeding and fillet marination in a phosphate solution resulted in tender broiler breast meat without any carcass ageing past the chiller (45–60 min). Sams and Hirschler (1997) also indicated that fillet yields increased 2% when the breasts were manually boned out of the chiller compared to 24 h later with the difference due to postchill drip loss.

Mechanical

Mechanical tenderization by flattening, pounding, cubing and chopping all break down connective tissue and improve tenderness. Mechanical application for whole muscle or carcasses are limited by final product appearance. Mechanical picking or beating and over-scalding cause more rapid drops in pH and ATP depletion resulting in increased fillet toughness at 2.5 h PM (de Fremery, 1966). However, delaying picking (30 min) accompanied by high temperature conditioning (32 vs. 0°C water baths) had no effect on cold boned (24 h) fillets (Uijttenboogaart and Fletcher, 1989). However, hot boning fillets at 45 min PM from broilers that had been delay picked resulted in increased A-K shear values (14.5 kg) compared to picking after scalding (12.5 kg; all fillets were cooked after 24 h ageing in ice). In the same report, hot boning fillets that had been high temperature conditioned at 32°C for 30 min resulted in lowered shear values (12.5 kg) compared to conditioning at 0°C (14.6 kg). Delayed picking mechanically stimulated prerigor muscle contractions resulting in greater degree of rigor shortening and toughening in hot boned fillets. High temperature conditioning accelerated ATP and glycogen utilization resulting in lower energy reserves and therefore less rigor shortening and toughening in hot boned fillets.

Extended chilling for 2 or 3 h had greater effects than belt flattening of fillets boned after chilling (Lyon *et al.*, 1997b). The authors reported a decrease in thickness as the main factor lowering shear values of belt flattened fillets, which was associated with structural damage to the fibres and sarcomeres. However, when flattened fillets were cooked they shortened which resulted in only marginally lower W-B shear values (Lyon and Lyon, 1991).

CONCLUSIONS

The biochemical basis for the conversion from muscle to meat is well documented in the scientific literature and many of these citations are as relevant today as when they were first reported. What is rapidly changing is the use of innovative treatments to alter the rate of these biochemical reactions and thus optimize processing efficiency. To successfully orchestrate these changes and ensure optimum properties for the finished meat product, a background in several disciplines will be needed (biochemistry, muscle biology, animal anatomy–physiology and food science). In addition, the ability to transfer basic knowledge to practical applications will be critical.

REFERENCES

Abbott, M.T., Pearson, A.M., Price, J.F. and Hooper, G.H. (1977) Ultrastructural changes during autolysis of red and white porcine muscle. *Journal of Food Science* 42, 1185–1188.

Ashgar, A. and Henrickson, R.L. (1982) Post-mortem stimulation of carcasses: effects on biochemistry, biophysics, microbiology, and quality of meat. *CRC Critical Reviews in Food Science and Nutrition* 18, 1–58.

Bate-Smith, E.C. and Bendall, J.R. (1949) Factors determining the time course of rigor mortis. *Journal of Physiology* 110, 47–65.

Bendall, J.R. (1980) The electrical stimulation of carcasses of meat animals. In: Lawrie, R.A. (ed.) *Developments in Meat Science*, 1. Applied Science, London, pp. 37–59.

Bendall, J.R., Ketteridge, C.C. and George, A.R. (1976) The electrical stimulation of beef carcasses. *Journal of the Science of Food and Agriculture* 27, 1123–1131.

Bilgili, S.F., Egbert, W.R. and Huffman, D.L. (1989) Research note: effect of postmortem aging temperature on sarcomere length and tenderness of broiler *Pectoralis major*. *Poultry Science* 68, 1588–1591.

Birkhold, S.G. and Sams, A.R. (1993) Fragmentation, tenderness, and post-mortem metabolism of early-harvested broiler breast fillets from carcasses treated with electrical stimulation and muscle tensioning. *Poultry Science* 72, 577–582.

Birkhold, S.G., Janky, D.M. and Sams, A.R. (1992) Tenderization of early-harvested broiler breast fillets by high-voltage post-mortem electrical stimulation and muscle tensioning. *Poultry Science* 71, 2106–2112.

Bratzler, L.J. (1932) Measuring the tenderness of meat by use of the Warner–Bratzler method. MSc thesis, Kansas State College, Manhattan.

Buege, D.R. and Marsh, B.B. (1975) Mitochondrial calcium and *post-mortem* muscle shortening. *Biochemical and Biophysical Research Communications* 65, 478–482.

Cason, J.A., Lyon, C.E. and Papa, C.M. (1997) Effect of muscle opposition during rigor on development of broiler breast meat tenderness. *Poultry Science* 76, 785–787.

Chrystall, B. (1994) Meat texture measurement. In: Pearson, A.M. and Dutson, T.R. (eds) *Quality Attributes and their Measurement in Meat, Poultry and Fish Products*, Blackie Academic and Professional, London, pp. 316–336.

Cooper, C.C., Cassens, R.G. and Briskey, E.J. (1969) Capillary distribution and fiber characteristics in skeletal muscle of stress-susceptible animals. *Journal of Food Science* 34, 299–302.

Cross, H.R., West, R.L. and Dutson, T.R. (1980) Comparison of methods for measuring sarcomere length in beef *Semitendinosus* muscle. *Meat Science* 5, 261–266.

Currie, R.W. and Wolfe, F.H. (1980) Rigor related changes in mechanical properties (tensile and adhesive) and extracellular space in beef muscle. *Meat Science* 4, 123–143.

Davey, C.L. (1984) The structure of muscle and its properties as meat. In: Bailey, A.J. (ed.) *Recent Advances in the Chemistry of Meat*. The Royal Society of Chemistry, London, pp. 1–21.

Davey, C.L. and Dickson, M.R. (1970) Studies in meat tenderness. Ultra-structural changes in meat during ageing. *Journal of Food Science* 35, 56–60.

Davidek, J. and Velisek, J. (1973) A quick method for examining rigor mortis. *Fleischwirtschaft* 53, 1285–1286, 1289–1290.

Dawson, P.L., Janky, D.M., Dukes, M.G., Thompson, L.D. and Woodward, S.A. (1987) Effect of post-mortem boning time during simulated commercial processing on the tenderness of broiler breast meat. *Poultry Science* 66, 1331–1333.

Dayton, W.R., Schollmeyer, J.V., Lepley, R.A. and Cortes. L.R. (1981) A calcium-activated protease possibly involved in myofibrillar protein turnover. Isolation of a low-calcium-requiring form of the protease. *Biochimica et Biophysica Acta* 659, 48–61.

de Fremery, D. (1966) Relationship between chemical properties and tenderness of poultry muscle. *Journal of Agricultural and Food Chemistry* 14, 214–217.

de Fremery, D. and Lineweaver, H. (1962) Early post-mortem chemical and tenderness changes in poultry. In: Leitch, J.M. (ed.) *Chemical and Physical Aspects of Food,* 1. Gordon and Breach, New York, pp. 13–21.

de Fremery, D. and Pool, M.F. (1960) Biochemistry of chicken muscle as related to rigor mortis and tenderization. *Food Research* 25, 73–87.

Dickens, J.A. and Lyon, C.E. (1993) Effect of two stunning voltages on blood loss and objective texture of meat deboned at various post-mortem times. *Poultry Science* 72, 589–593.

Dickens, J.A. and Lyon, C.E. (1995) The effects of electric stimulation and extended chilling times on the biochemical reactions and texture of cooked broiler breast meat. *Poultry Science* 74, 2035–2040.

Dodge, J.W. and Peters, F.E. (1960) Temperature and pH changes in poultry breast muscles at slaughter. *Poultry Science* 39, 765–768.

Dunn, A.A., Tolland, E.L.C., Kilpatrick, D.J. and Gault, N.F.S. (1993) Effect of *post-mortem* temperature on chicken M. *Pectoralis major*: isometric tension and pH profiles. *British Poultry Science* 34, 677–688.

Erdos, T. (1943) Rigor contracture and ATP. *Studies from the Institute of Medical Chemistry, University of Szeged* 4, 51.

Fleming, B.K., Froning, G.W., Beck, M.M. and Sosnicki, A.A. (1991) The effect of carbon dioxide as a preslaughter stunning method for turkeys. *Poultry Science* 70, 2201–2206.

Fletcher, D.L. (1993) Effects of stunning on poultry meat quality. Quality of poultry products. 1. Quality of poultry meat. *Proceedings of 11th European Symposium on the Quality of Poultry Meat and of 5th European Symposium on the Quality of Eggs and Egg Products.* World's Poultry Science Association, Tours, France, pp. 172–178.

Froning, G.W. and Uijttenboogaart, T.G. (1988) Effect of post-mortem electrical stimulation on color, texture, pH, and cooking losses of hot and cold deboned chicken broiler breast meat. *Poultry Science* 67, 1536–1544.

Goll, D.E. (1968) The resolution of rigor mortis. *Proceedings of the 21st Reciprocal Meat Conference,* Chicago, Illinois, pp. 16–46.

Goll, D.E., Arakawa, N., Stromer, M.H., Busch, W.A. and Robson, R. M. (1970) Chemistry of muscle proteins as a food. In: Briskey, E.J., Cassens, R.G. and Marsh, B.B. (eds) *The Physiology and Biochemistry of Muscle as a Food,* 2. The University of Wisconsin Press, Madison, pp. 755–800.

Goll, D.E., Otsuka, Y., Nagainis, P.A., Shannon, J.D., Sathe, S.K. and Muguruma, M. (1983) Role of muscle proteinases in maintenance of muscle integrity and mass. *Journal of Food Biochemistry* 7, 137–177.

Greaser, M.L. (1968) Ultrastructural and biochemical properties of isolated sarcoplasmic reticulum from skeletal muscle. PhD dissertation, University of Wisconsin, Madison.

Greaser, M.L., Cassens, R.G., Briskey, E.J. and Hoekstra, W.G. (1969) Post-mortem changes in subcellular fractions from normal and pale, soft, exudative porcine muscle. 1. Calcium accumulation and adenosine triphosphatase activities. *Journal of Food Science* 34, 120–124.

Hamm, R. (1960) Biochemistry of meat hydration. In: Chichester, C.O., Mrak, E.M. and Stewart, G.F. (eds) *Advances in Food Research*, 10. Academic Press, New York, pp. 355–463.

Hamm, R. (1970) Influence of salting beef immediately after slaughter on the water-holding capacity of meat and sausage mixtures. *British Food Manufacturing Industries Research Association Technical Circular* no. 447.

Hay, J.D., Currie, R.W., Wolfe, F.H. and Sanders, E.J. (1973) Effect of postmortem aging on chicken muscle fibrils. *Journal of Food Science* 38, 981–986.

Heath, G.B.S., Watt, D.J., Waite, P.R. and Meakins, P.A. (1983) Further observations on the slaughter of poultry. *British Veterinary Journal* 139, 285–290.

Heath, J.L. and Owens, S.L. (1997) Measurement of broiler breast meat shear values. *Journal of Applied Poultry Research* 6, 185–190.

Herring, H.K., Cassens, R.G. and Briskey, E.J. (1965) Further studies on bovine muscle tenderness as influenced by carcass position, sarcomere length, and fiber diameter. *Journal of Food Science* 30, 1049–1054.

Honikel, K.O. and Fischer, C. (1977) A rapid method for the detection of PSE and DFD porcine muscles. *Journal of Food Science* 42, 1633–1636.

Huxley, H.E. and Brown, W. (1967) The low-angle X-ray diagram of vertebrate striated muscle and its behavior during contraction and rigor. *Journal of Molecular Biology* 30, 383–434.

Janky, D.M., Dukes, M.G. and Sams, A.R. (1992) Research note: the effects of post-mortem wing restraint (muscle tensioning) on tenderness of early-harvested broiler breast meat. *Poultry Science* 71, 574–576.

Jeacocke, R.E. (1984) The control of post-mortem metabolism and the onset of *rigor mortis*. In: Bailey, A.J. (ed.) *Recent Advances in the Chemistry of Meat*. The Royal Society of Chemistry, London, pp. 41–57.

Kastenschmidt, L.L. (1970) The metabolism of muscle as a food. In: Briskey, E.J., Cassens, R.G. and Marsh, B.B. (eds) *The Physiology and Biochemistry of Muscle as a Food*, 2. The University of Wisconsin Press, Madison, pp. 735–753.

Khan, A.W. (1974) Relation between isometric tension, postmortem pH decline and tenderness of poultry breast meat. *Journal of Food Science* 39, 393–395.

Khan, A. W. (1975) Effect of chemical treatments causing rapid onset of rigor on tenderness of poultry breast meat. *Journal of Agricultural Food Chemistry* 23, 449–451.

Khan, A.W. and Frey, A.R. (1971) A simple method for following rigor mortis development in beef and poultry meat. *Canadian Institute of Food Technology Journal* 4, 139–142.

Khan, A.W. and Nakamura, R. (1970) Effects of pre- and postmortem glycolysis on poultry tenderness. *Journal of Food Science* 35, 266–267.

Kijowski, J., Niewiarowicz, A. and Kujawska-Biernat, B. (1982) Biochemical and technological characteristics of hot chicken meat. *Journal of Food Technology* 17, 553–560.

Kim, L.W., Fletcher, D.L. and Campion, D.R. (1988) Research note: Effect of electrical stunning and hot boning on broiler breast meat characteristics. *Poultry Science* 67, 674–676.

Koohmaraie, M. (1988) The role of endogenous proteases in meat tenderness, *Proceedings of the 41st Annual Reciprocal Meat Conference*. University of Wyoming, Laramie, pp. 89–100.

Koohmaraie, M. (1992) The role of Ca^{2+}-dependent proteases (calpains) in post mortem proteolysis and meat tenderness. *Biochimie* 74, 239–245.

Kramer, A., Aamlid. K., Guyer, R.B. and Rogers, H. (1951) New shear press predicts quality of canned limas. *Food Engineering* 23, 112–113.

Lee, Y.B., Hargus, G.L., Webb, J.E., Rickansrud, D.A. and Hagberg, E.C. (1979) Effect of electrical stunning on postmortem biochemical changes and tenderness in broiler breast muscle. *Journal of Food Science* 44, 1121–1128.

Li, Y., Siebenmorgen, T.J. and Griffis, C.L. (1993) Electrical stimulation in poultry: a review and evaluation. *Poultry Science* 72, 7–22.

Lister, D., Sair, R.A., Will, J.A., Schmidt, G.R., Cassens, R.G., Hoekstra, W.G. and Briskey, E.J. (1970) Metabolism of striated muscle of 'stress-susceptible' pigs breathing oxygen or nitrogen. *American Journal of Physiology* 218, 102–107.

Locker, R.H. (1960) Degree of muscular contraction as a factor in tenderness of beef. *Food Research* 25, 304–307.

Locker, R.H. and Hagyard, C.J. (1963) A cold shortening effect in beef muscles. *Journal of the Science of Food and Agriculture* 14, 787–793.

Locker, R.H. and Wild, D.J.C. (1982) Myofibrils of cooked meat are a continuum of gap filaments. *Meat Science* 7, 189–192.

Locker, R.H., Daines, G.J., Carse, W.A. and Leet, N.G. (1977) Meat tenderness and the gap filaments. *Meat Science* 1, 87–104.

Lopez, C.A. and Herbert, E.W. (1975) *The Private Franklin, The Man and His Family*, 1st edn. W.W. Norton, New York, pp. 44–45.

Lowe, B. (1948) Factors affecting the palatability of poultry with emphasis on histological post-mortem changes. *Advances in Food Research* 1, 203–256.

Lyon, C.E. and Dickens, J.A. (1993) Effects of electric treatments and wing restraints on the rate of post-mortem biochemical changes and objective texture of broiler *Pectoralis major* muscles deboned after chilling. *Poultry Science* 72, 1577–1583.

Lyon, B.G. and Lyon, C.E. (1990a) Texture profile of broiler *Pectoralis major* as influenced by post-mortem deboning time and heat method. *Poultry Science* 69, 329–340.

Lyon, C.E. and Lyon, B.G. (1990b) The relationship of objective shear values and sensory tests to changes in tenderness of broiler breast meat. *Poultry Science* 69, 1420–1427.

Lyon, B.G. and Lyon, C.E. (1991) Research note: shear value ranges by Instron Warner-Bratzler and single-blade Allo-Kramer devices that correspond to sensory tenderness. *Poultry Science* 70, 188–191.

Lyon, C.E. and Lyon, B.G. (1994) The location of wing restraints and the incidence of residual blood in broiler breast meat. *Journal of Applied Poultry Research* 3, 355–361.

Lyon, B.G. and Lyon, C.E. (1997) Sensory descriptive profile relationships to shear values of deboned poultry. *Journal of Food Science* 62, 885–897.

Lyon, C.E., Lyon, B.G. and Hudspeth, J.P. (1973) The effect of different cutting procedures on the cooked yield and tenderness of cut-up broiler parts. *Poultry Science* 53, 1103–1111.

Lyon, C.E., Hamm, D. and Thomson, J.E. (1985) pH and tenderness of broiler breast meat deboned various times after chilling. *Poultry Science* 64, 307–310.

Lyon, C.E., Davis, C.E., Dickens, J.A., Papa, C.M. and Reagan, J.O. (1989) Effects of electrical stimulation on the post-mortem biochemical changes and texture of broiler pectoralis muscle. *Poultry Science* 68, 249–257.

Lyon, C.E., Papa, C.M. and Wilson, R.L.Jr (1991) Effect of feed withdrawal on yields, muscle pH, and texture of broiler breast meat. *Poultry Science* 70, 1020–1025.

Lyon, C.E., Lyon, B.G., Papa, C.M. and Robach, M.C. (1992a) Broiler tenderness: effects of postchill deboning time and fillet holding time. *Journal of Applied Poultry Research* 1, 27–32.

Lyon, C.E., Robach, M.C., Papa, C.M. and Wilson, R.L. Jr (1992b) Research note: effects of wing restraints on the objective texture of commercially processed broiler breast meat. *Poultry Science* 71, 1228–1231.

Lyon, C.E., Lyon, B.G. and Dickens, J.A. (1997a) Effects of carcass stimulation, deboning time and marination on color and texture of broiler breast meat. *Poultry Science* 76 (Suppl. 1), 50 (Abstract).

Lyon, C.E., Bilgili, S.F. and Dickens, J.A. (1997b) Effects of chilling time and belt flattening on physical characteristics, yield, and tenderness of broiler breasts. *Journal of Applied Research* 6, 39–47.

MacNaughtan, A. F. (1978) A histological study of post mortem changes in the skeletal muscle of the fowl (*Gallus domesticus*). 1. The muscle fibers. *Journal of Anatomy* 126, 461–476.

Marsh, B.B. (1954) *Rigor mortis* in beef. *Journal of the Science of Food and Agriculture* 5, 70–75.

Marsh, B.B. and Carse, W.A. (1974) Meat tenderness and the sliding-filament hypothesis. *Journal of Food Technology* 9, 129–139.

Maruyama, K., Kimura, S., Ohashi, K. and Kuwano, Y. (1981) Connectin, an elastic protein of muscle. Identification of 'titin' with connectin. *Journal of Biochemistry (Tokyo)* 89, 701–709.

Matsukura, U., Okitani, A., Nishimuro, T. and Kato, H. (1981) Mode of degradation of myofibrillar proteins by an endogenous protease, cathepsin L. *Biochimica et Biophysica Acta* 662, 41–47.

McGinnis, J.P., Fletcher, D.L., Papa, C.M. and Buhr, R.J. (1989) Early post-mortem metabolism and muscle shortening in the *Pectoralis major* muscle of broiler chickens. *Poultry Science* 68, 386–392.

Meullenet, J.-F.C., Carpenter, J.A., Lyon, B.G., and Lyon, C.E. (1997) Bi-cyclical instrument for assessing texture profile parameters and its relationship to sensory evaluation of texture. *Journal of Texture Studies* 28, 101–118.

Murachi, T. (1983) Calpain and calpastatin. *Trends in Biochemical Sciences* 8, 167–169.

Newbold, R.P. (1966) Changes associated with rigor mortis. In: Briskey, E.J., Cassens, R.G. and Trautman, J.C. (eds) *The Physiology and Biochemistry of Muscle as a Food.* University of Wisconsin Press, Madison, pp. 213–224.

Nichols. J.E. and Cross, H.R. (1980) Effects of electrical stimulation and early postmortem muscle excision on pH decline, sarcomere length and color in beef muscles. *Journal of Food Protection* 43, 514–519.

Papa C.M. and Fletcher, D.L. (1988a) Effect of wing restraint on postmortem muscle shortening and the textural quality of broiler breast meat. *Poultry Science* 67, 275–279.

Papa, C.M. and Fletcher, D.L. (1988b) *Pectoralis* muscle shortening and rigor development at different locations within the broiler breast. *Poultry Science* 67, 635–640.

Papa, C.M., Lyon, C.E. and Fletcher, D.L. (1989) Effects of post-mortem wing restraint on the development of rigor and tenderness of broiler breast meat. *Poultry Science* 68, 238–243.

Papinaho, P.A. and Fletcher, D.L. (1996) The effects of stunning amperage and deboning time on early rigor development and breast meat quality of broilers. *Poultry Science* 75, 672–676.

Papinaho, P.A., Fletcher, D.L. and Buhr, R.J. (1995) Effect of electrical stunning amperage and peri-mortem struggle on broiler breast rigor development and meat quality. *Poultry Science* 74, 1533–1539.

Paul, P.C., Bratzler, L.J., Farwell, E.D. and Knight, K. (1952) Studies on tenderness of beef. I. Rate of heat penetration. *Food Research* 17, 504–510.

Pool, M.F., de Fremery, D., Campbell, A.A. and Klose, A.A. (1959) Poultry tenderness. II. Influence of processing on tenderness of chickens. *Food Technology* 13, 25–29.

Poole, G.H. (1997) Evaluation of modified atmosphere stunning and killing (mask) systems for broilers, PhD dissertation, University of Georgia, Athens, p. 58.

Poole, G.H. and Fletcher, D.L. (1995) A comparison of argon, carbon dioxide, and nitrogen in a broiler killing system. *Poultry Science* 74, 1218–1223.

Raj, A.B.M. (1994) Effect of stunning method, carcase chilling temperature and filleting time on the texture of turkey breast meat. *British Poultry Science* 35, 77–89.

Raj, A.B.M. and Nute, G.R. (1995) Effect of stunning method and filleting time on sensory profile of turkey breast meat. *British Poultry Science* 36, 221–227.

Raj, A.B.M., Grey, T.C., Audsely, A.R. and Gregory, N.G. (1990) Effect of electrical and gaseous stunning on the carcase and meat quality of broilers. *British Poultry Science* 31, 725–733.

Raj, A.B.M., Wilkins, L.J., Richardson, R.I., Johnson, S.P. and Wotton, S.B. (1997) Carcase and meat quality in broilers either killed with a gas mixture or stunned with an electric current under commercial processing conditions. *British Poultry Science* 38, 169–174.

Ramsbottom, J.M. and Strandine, E.J. (1949) Initial physical and chemical changes in beef as related to tenderness. *Journal of Animal Science* 8, 398–410.

Ruddick, J.E. and Richards, J.F. (1975) Comparison of sarcomere length measurement of cooked chicken and pectoralis muscle by laser diffraction and oil immersion microscopy. *Journal of Food Science* 40, 500–501.

Sair, R.A., Lister, D., Moody, W.G., Cassens, R.G., Hoekstra, W.G. and Briskey, E.J. (1970) The action of curare and magnesium on the striated muscle of stress-susceptible pigs. *American Journal of Physiology* 218, 108–114.

Sams, A.R. (1990) Electrical stimulation and high temperature conditioning of broiler carcasses. *Poultry Science* 69, 1781–1786.

Sams, A. (1996) Stunning basics. *Broiler Industry*. December, pp. 36–38.

Sams, A.R. (1997) Recent advances in electrical stimulation. Symposium: Recent advances in poultry slaughter technology. *Poultry Science Association 86th Annual Meeting,* 3–6 August, 1997.

Sams, A.R. and Hirschler, E.M. (1997) Commercial-scale electrical stimulation of poultry: the effects on tenderness, breast meat yield, and production costs. *Institute of Food Technology Meeting Abstracts,* p. 236.

Sams, A.R. and Janky, D.M. (1991) Characterization of rigor mortis development in four broiler muscles. *Poultry Science* 70, 1003–1009.

Sams, A.R., Janky, D.M. and Dukes, M.G. (1992) Research note: anatomical location of application influences the tenderizing effectiveness of electrical stimulation of broiler carcasses. *Poultry Science* 71, 1564–1567.

Sams, A.R., Janky, D.M. and Woodward, S.A. (1989) Tenderness and R-value changes in early harvested broiler breast tissue following post-mortem electrical stimulation. *Poultry Science* 68, 1232–1235.

Sams, A.R., Janky, D.M. and Woodward, S.A. (1990) Comparison of two shearing methods for objective tenderness evaluation and two sampling times for physical-characteristic analyses of early-harvested broiler breast meat. *Poultry Science* 69, 348–353.

Savell, J.W., Dutson, T.R., Smith, G.C. and Carpenter, Z.L. (1978) Structural changes in electrically stimulated beef muscle. *Journal of Food Science* 43, 1606–1609.

Sayre, R.N. (1970) Chicken myofibril fragmentation in relation to factors influencing tenderness. *Journal of Food Science* 35, 7–10.

Smith, D.P. and Fletcher, D.L. (1988) Compositional and biochemical variations within broiler breast muscle subjected to different processing methods. *Poultry Science* 67, 1702–1707.

Smith, D.P. and Fletcher, D.L. (1990) Allo-Kramer shear values of diced and intact samples of broiler breast meat. *Poultry Science* 69, 127 (abstract).

Smith, D.P., Lyon, C.E. and Fletcher, D.L. (1988) Comparison of the Allo-Kramer shear and texture profile methods of broiler breast meat texture analysis. *Poultry Science* 67, 1549–1556.

Solomon, L.W. and Schmidt, G.R. (1980) Effect of vacuum and mixing time on the extractability and functionality of pre- and postrigor beef. *Journal of Food Science* 45, 283–287.

Stewart, M.K., Fletcher, D.L., Hamm, D. and Thomson, J.E. (1984) The influence of hot boning broiler breast muscle on pH decline and toughening. *Poultry Science* 63, 1935–1939.

Takahashi, K., Fukazawa, T. and Yasui, T. (1967) Formation of myofibrillar fragments and reversible contraction of sarcomeres in chicken pectoral muscle. *Journal of Food Science* 32, 409–413.

Thomson, J.E., Lyon, C.E., Hamm, D., Dickens, J.A., Fletcher, D.L. and Shackelford, A.D. (1986) Effects of electrical stunning and hot deboning on broiler breast meat quality. *Poultry Science* 65, 1715–1719.

Thompson, L.D., Janky, D.M. and Woodward, S.A. (1987) Tenderness and physical characteristics of broiler breast fillets harvested at various times from post-mortem electricially stimulated carcasses. *Poultry Science* 66, 1158–1167.

Uijttenboogaart, T.G. and Fletcher, D.L. (1989) The effects of delayed picking and high-temperature conditioning on the texture of hot- and cold-boned broiler breast meat. *Journal of Muscle Foods* 1, 37–44.

Voyle, C.A. (1969) Some observations on the histology of cold-shortened muscle. *Journal of Food Technology* 4, 275–281.

Voyle, C.A. (1979) Meat. In: Vaughan, J.G. (ed.) *Food Microscopy,* Academic Press, London, pp. 193–232.

Walker, L.T., Shackelford, S.D., Birkhold, S.G. and Sams, A.R. (1995) Biochemical and structural effects of rigor mortis-accelerating treatments in broiler *Pectoralis. Poultry Science* 74, 176–186.

Wang, K. (1981) Nebulin, a giant protein component of N_2-line of striated muscle. *Journal of Cell Biology* 91, 355 (abstract).

Welbourn, J.L., Harrington, R.B. and Stadelman, W.J. (1968) Relationships among shear values, sarcomere lengths and cooling procedures in turkeys. *Journal of Food Science* 33, 450–452.

Will, P.A., Henrickson, R.L., Morrison, R.D. and Odell, G.V. (1979) Effect of electrical stimulation on ATP depletion and sarcomere length in delay-chilled bovine muscle. *Journal of Food Science* 44, 1646–1648.

Williams, C.S., Williams, J.W. and Chung, R.A. (1986) Comparative microscopy and morphometry of skeletal muscle fibers in poultry. *Food Microstructure* 5, 207–217.

Young, L.L. and Buhr, R.J. (1997) Effects of stunning duration on quality characteristics of early deboned chicken fillets. *Poultry Science* 76, 1052–1055.

Young, L.L., Northcutt, J.K. and Lyon, C.E. (1996) Effect of stunning time and poly-phosphates on quality of cooked chicken breast meat. *Poultry Science* 75, 677–681.

Young, L.L., Papa, C.M., Lyon, C.E., George, S.M. and Miller M.F. (1990) Research note: comparison of microscopic and laser diffraction methods for measuring sarcomere length of contracted muscle fibers of chicken *Pectoralis major* muscle. *Poultry Science* 69, 1800–1802.

CHAPTER 5
Poultry meat flavour

L.J. Farmer

Food Science Division, Department of Agriculture for Northern Ireland and The Queen's University of Belfast, Newforge Lane, Belfast BT9 5PX, UK

INTRODUCTION

Flavour is one of the main eating quality attributes which, together with appearance and texture, dictates our choice and enjoyment of foods. Studies during recent years have helped to clarify what can be done to modify or improve the texture of poultry meat and to understand and avoid colour defects; these have been reviewed elsewhere in this book (Lyon and Buhr, Chapter 4; Fletcher, Chapter 6). However, it is still unclear how production techniques can be modified to achieve consistent and desirable poultry flavour; this chapter reviews the progress which has been made.

Flavour is a combination of the sensations perceived by the two chemical senses, taste and smell. Taste is perceived by the taste buds on the tongue and other parts of the mouth, and mainly detects the four principal tastes: sweet, sour/acid, salt and bitter. However, other sensations such as astringency, metallic, pain ('hot' and 'cooling' foods), and 'umami' (a Japanese term meaning 'deliciousness') can also be detected. The sense of smell detects certain chemicals which, because of their chemical structure, stimulate the olfactory receptors at the top of the nasal cavity. These odorous substances can be detected in the air above the food, before we eat it, and in some cases this odour may dictate whether we decide to consume the food or not. However, odour compounds are also detected during eating as they pass in the breath from the mouth, through the posterior nares at the back of the nose, into the nasal cavity (Fig. 5.1).

A review of the flavour of a foodstuff, such as poultry, could cover a variety of aspects. A considerable amount of work, especially by the flavour companies, has been conducted and reviewed on the production of artificial flavourings to imitate cooked meat flavour (MacLeod and Seyyedain-Ardebili, 1981). Other studies have sought to identify the compounds causing taints and their sources (Land and Hobson-Frohock, 1977; Reineccius, 1979; Gray and Pearson, 1994). Rather less definitive information is available on how desirable flavour is generated, although some reviews have been written (Thomas et al., 1971; Gordon, 1972; Shi and Ho, 1994). This chapter concentrates on this third area, the formation of the characteristic flavour of poultry meat.

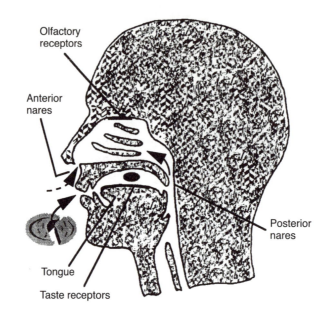

Fig. 5.1. Cross-section of the human head showing the position of the olfactory and taste receptors. The nasal and retro-nasal routes for odour detection are shown with dotted arrows.

FLAVOUR FORMATION IN POULTRY MEAT

Most research on the chemistry of flavour formation in poultry has been conducted on chicken (*Gallus domesticus*) and the remainder of this section will concentrate on these studies. Nevertheless, the principles behind the generation of flavour and, in all likelihood, many of the flavour compounds, will be common to all species of poultry. Substances contributing to flavour can be divided into aroma compounds and taste compounds.

Compounds Contributing to Taste

Taste compounds are non-volatile or water-soluble substances with taste or tactile properties. These can cause the sensations of salt, sour or acid, bitter, sweet, 'umami', etc. Most of the studies on taste compounds in meat have concerned red meats, but many of the same substances will contribute to the taste of poultry meat.

Salty tastes in meat are caused by sodium chloride and some other inorganic salts, together with monosodium glutamate and monosodium aspartate (MacLeod, 1986). While the concentration of salt in lean meat is likely to be consistent, in meat products the perception of saltiness can be affected by the amount of fat present (Wirth, 1988). Sweetness is caused by sugars and certain amino acids. In meat, sugars are formed by glycolysis which occurs after rigor mortis (Lawrie, 1992), but these are believed to be of little importance for taste in meat (Maga, 1994). Bitter tastes in meat are generally caused by amino acids and peptides (MacLeod, 1986). Sour or acid tastes are caused by acids, such as lactic acid, organic acids, amino acids and acidic phosphates (MacLeod, 1986).

Other taste sensations such as chemesthesis or the trigeminal response (the detection of 'hot' and 'cool' sensations) play little part in the flavour of unprocessed meat, but 'hot' sensations, from spices, chilli, pepper etc., are often used to contribute to the flavour of meat products. In contrast, flavour enhancers, such as monosodium glutamate, inosine monophosphate and guanosine monophosphate are natural components of meat and are believed to make a major contribution to meat flavour. They have been shown to improve flavour and have been used by the Japanese for many years to give 'umami' (Reineccius, 1994; Maga, 1994). The quantities present will be affected by glycolysis reactions and other processes occurring after death. Monosodium glutamate and the above nucleotides act synergistically, such that a 1:1 mixture gives a flavour intensity 30 times stronger than that of monosodium glutamate alone (Maga, 1994). It has been proposed that 'umami' or delicious taste may also be given by an octapeptide, known as 'beefy, meaty peptide' (Yamasaki and Maekawa, 1978) and various studies have investigated the taste of this substance (Spanier and Miller, 1993; Kuramitsu et al., 1993). However, other studies have reported that this peptide, once purified, does not possess a 'umami' taste (van Wassenaar et al., 1995), so the role of this substance is still unclear.

The taste compounds contributing to meat flavour have been reviewed (Baines and Mlotkiewicz, 1984; MacLeod, 1986; Maga, 1994). Again, most studies have concerned red meat, although similar results might be expected for poultry. It has been suggested that amino acids, peptides, proteins and nucleotides are most important for the taste of red meats. A study (Gasser et al., 1994) on the taste compounds contributing to the flavour of bouillon (minced lean beef boiled in water) has demonstrated that many amino acids, peptides, organic acids, salts and nucleotides have taste qualities. Most are present at below their taste thresholds (in meat extract as well as bouillon) suggesting that synergistic effects are of prime importance for the taste of meat. Of greatest importance for the bouillon-like taste (and salty taste) were the above-mentioned flavour enhancers, glutamic acid and inosine monophosphate. Also important was lactic acid, which increased the 'bouillon-like' character of the above compounds, and the potassium to sodium ratio. An imitation bouillon was prepared, containing the following compounds, which compared well sensorially with bouillon itself: aspartic acid, glutamic acid, adenosine monophosphate, inosine monophosphate, carnosine, anserine, carnitine, lactic acid, pyroglutamic acid, gelatin and salts containing sodium, potassium, calcium, magnesium, chloride and phosphate (Gasser et al., 1994). A series of studies have been conducted on the relative importance of individual taste compounds for chicken flavour. Fujimura et al. (1995, 1996) analysed the water-soluble components of cooked chicken extract (Table 5.1) and recombined the listed amino acids, metabolites of adenosine triphosphate

Table 5.1. Composition of chicken meat extract, indicating those components found to be important for taste (Fujimura *et al.*, 1995).

Compound	Conc.	Imp.[a]	Compound[b]	Conc.	Imp.
Amino acids (µg g^{-1})			*ATP metabolites (mg g^{-1})*		
Lysine	58	—	IMP	3.3	*
Glutamic acid	53	*	Inosine	0.15	—
Glycine	42	—	AMP	0.10	—
Threonine	40	—	ADP	0.033	—
Alanine	36	—	Hypoxanthine	0.014	—
Proline	34	—	ATP	0.012	—
Serine	33	—	*Inorganic ions (mg g^{-1})*		
Methionine	29	—	K$^+$	2.8	*
Arginine	24	—	PO$_4^{3-}$	2.0	—
Tyrosine	20	—	Cl$^-$	0.28	—
Aspartic acid	14	—	Na$^+$	0.27	—
Leucine	13	—	Mg^{2+}	0.045	—
Phenylalanine	10	—	Ca^{2+}	0.0003	—
Valine	7	—			
Histidine	5	—			
Isoleucine	5	—			

[a] Imp., importance: * = important for taste; — = not found to be important for taste.
[b] ATP = adenosine 5′-triphosphate, ADP = adenosine 5′-diphosphate, AMP = adenosine 5′-monophosphate, IMP = inosine 5′-monophosphate.

and inorganic ions to simulate the sensory properties of the chicken extract. By omitting individual compounds from this mixture the effect of each substance on taste was identified. Only inosine monophosphate, glutamic acid and potassium ions were found to have a detectable effect on the taste. Glutamic acid and inosine 5′-monophosphate conferred 'umami' and salty tastes, and the latter also caused sweetness. Potassium ions conferred sweet, salty and bitter tastes. The results were less statistically significant when these substances were added to the mixture, but similar effects were observed (Fujimura *et al.*, 1996).

A comparison of the concentrations of flavour enhancers in poultry with the red meats (Maga, 1994) indicates that cooked chicken has similar quantities of glutamic acid as rare-cooked beef, although greater quantities than lamb, pork or well-done beef. However, cooked chicken tends to have lesser concentrations of inosine monophosphate than beef. The relative importance of these taste substances for the flavour of meat from different species may be worthy of further study.

The compounds which contribute to taste in chicken (or other poultry) are generally present in the raw meat and do not require cooking for their generation. However, studies on red meats have shown that cooking may affect the concentrations of taste substances, and similar effects would be expected in poultry meat. Macy *et al.* (1964) analysed the water-soluble fraction of beef, pork and lamb before and after heating and found that the concentrations of many of the amino acids and sugars were depleted during heating. Analyses conducted on beef, pork and lamb meat showed similar results for reducing sugars (Macy et al., 1970c); reducing sugars were depleted by up to 20% during roasting. However, the concentrations of free amino acids increased during cooking of the meat itself (Macy et al., 1970c) and the authors presumed that this was due to the action of proteolytic enzymes. Cambero et al. (1992) also found that the levels of amino acids in beef broth increase on raising the cooking temperature from 55 to 95°C.

Macy et al. (1970a, 1970b) reported that the quantity of the flavour enhancer, inosine monophosphate, decreases, during cooking, to as little as 35% of the quantities in the uncooked meat. In contrast, Cambero et al. (1992) found that the concentration of inosine monophosphate increases as the cooking temperature of beef broth is increased from 55 to 95°C. However, this difference may be due to the considerable differences in methodology; Cambero et al. (1992) cooked minced beef for an hour at the selected temperature and then removed the solid matter by filtration and centrifugation before analysis, whereas Macy et al. (1970a) extracted the total nucleotides from the meat using perchloric acid. Both groups found increases in the concentrations of nucleosides, such as inosine, during cooking.

The changes in sugars, amino acids and nucleotides which occur during cooking will affect not only the taste of poultry meat but also its aroma and overall flavour, because many of these substances are also precursors for the chemical reactions responsible for the formation of odour compounds.

Compounds Contributing to Aroma

In contrast to the taste compounds in chicken, aroma compounds are largely formed during the cooking process. Indeed, raw meat has none of the aroma of cooked meat, and the characteristic aroma is largely generated during cooking (Crocker, 1948). The large quantities of volatiles released from roasted turkey, compared with the raw meat, reflect this fact (Siegl et al., 1995). During heating, chemical reactions occur which result in the formation of a range of aroma compounds which together contribute to the cooked chicken flavour which most of us find desirable.

Identification of the volatile compounds which give cooked poultry its desirable aroma may make it possible to determine which chemical reactions are responsible for forming these compounds during cooking. The many studies on the mechanisms of formation of volatile aroma compounds in simple model systems assist in this aim (for example, those reviewed by Vernin and Parkanyi, 1982). If these chemical reactions can be elucidated, then it should be possible to deduce which precursors are needed in raw meat to allow these reactions to take place during cooking to give the characteristic aroma of cooked poultry meat.

About 500 volatile aroma compounds have been reported in chicken (Schroll et al., 1988; Schliemann et al., 1988; Maarse and Visscher, 1989; Mottram, 1991; Ramarathnam et al., 1991; Ramarathnam et al., 1993; Werkhoff et al., 1993). Many of these have relatively high odour thresholds and make little contribution to the overall flavour. Others may be present at very low concentrations but, due to their very low odour thresholds, have a very large effect on the overall flavour. In recent years, efforts have focused on identifying the 'odour impact compounds', that is, those compounds which, due to a combination of their concentrations and odour thresholds, make a major contribution to the overall aroma and flavour of the meat. Over the last 10 years, developments in analytical instrumentation and methodology have allowed many of the compounds contributing to the aroma of cooked chicken to be identified despite the low concentrations of some of them. The compounds important for poultry meat flavour have been the subject of review (Shi and Ho, 1994).

The odour impact compounds are often identified by analysing very dilute aroma extracts by gas chromatography coupled with odour assessment; those volatile compounds whose odours are still detectable by nose at extreme dilution are taken to be the most important contributors to the odour (Gasser and Grosch, 1990). Other studies have identified many volatile components of meat flavour and evaluated the odour/flavour attributes and thresholds of individual compounds (Werkhoff et al., 1993). The odour impact compounds listed in Table 5.2 are those which are proposed as important by a range of workers using both of these methods. It is clear that different workers have reported different compounds to be important for flavour; this reflects the diversity of methods used for sample preparation, volatile extraction and odour assessment.

The compounds listed in Table 5.2 include a range of sulphur compounds (both heterocyclic and aliphatic), other heterocyclic compounds containing oxygen or nitrogen, and aldehydes and ketones. Individually, these compounds confer 'sulphurous', 'meaty', 'toasted', 'roasted', 'fatty', 'tallowy', 'fruity' or 'mushroom' aromas but together combine to give the characteristic aroma of cooked chicken. The odour impact compounds of cooked chicken differ from those important for the aroma of cooked beef in that bis(2-methyl-3-furyl)disulphide, methional and phenylacetaldehyde are of lesser importance, whereas certain lipid oxidation products, such as trans, trans-2,4-decadienal, γ-dodecadalactone and trans-undecenal (with 'fatty' characters), are of greater importance in the cooked chicken (Gasser and Grosch, 1990). The authors suggest that this difference may be related to the higher concentrations of linoleic acid in chicken than beef. An earlier study (Harkes and Begemann, 1974) also suggested that the aldehydes derived from n-6 fatty acids were responsible for the characteristic chicken flavour but suggested that arachidonic acid was particularly important.

The flavour and aroma of cooked chicken differs depending on the cooking method and it is, therefore, not surprising that differences are also observed in the range of volatile compounds detected from chicken heated in water (Ramarathnam et al., 1991, 1993), roasted chicken (Noleau and Toulemonde, 1986), fried chicken (Tang et al., 1983), chicken fat (Noleau and Toulemonde, 1987) and chicken broth (Gasser and Grosch, 1990). However, little attention has been given to the differences in key odour impact compounds between these different cooking methods.

Table 5.2. Compounds proposed as key odour compounds in cooked poultry meat.

Compound	Odour character	Ref.[a]	Probable origin[b]
S-containing			
(1) hydrogen sulphide	Sulphurous, eggy	1	From Strecker degradation reactions between cysteine and dicarbonyl compounds[6]
(2) dimethyltrisulphide	Gassy, metallic	5	From methionine by Strecker degradation[6]
(3) 3-mercapto-2-pentanone	Sulphurous	2	Reaction of H_2S (1) with carbonyl compound from Maillard reaction
(4) methional	Cooked potatoes	2, 4, 5	Strecker degradation of methionine[6]
Furanthiols and disulphides			
(5) 2-methyl-3-furanthiol	Meaty, sweet	2, 3, 5	Maillard reaction between cysteine and ribose or related compound,[7] or degradation of thiamine[8]
(6) 2,5-dimethyl-3-furanthiol	Meaty	2	Maillard reaction between cysteine and a hexose sugar
(7) 2-furanmethanethiol	Roasty	2	Maillard reaction between cysteine and ribose (or related compound),[9] or degration of thiamine[8]
(8) 2-methyl-3-(methylthio)furan	Meaty, sweet	3	As (5), followed by reaction with methanethiol from degradation of methionine
(9) 2-methyl-3-(ethylthio)furan	Meaty	3	As (5), followed by reaction with ethanethiol
(10) 2-methyl-3-methyldithiofuran	Meaty, sweet	3, 5	As (5), followed by reaction with methanethiol from degradation of methionine

continued overleaf

Table 5.2. Continued

Compound	Odour character	Ref.[a]	Probable origin[b]
(11) bis (2-methyl-3-furyl) disulphide	Meaty, roasted	3	As (5) followed by oxidation, or degradation of thiamine[8]

Other heteroocyclic compounds

Compound	Odour character	Ref.[a]	Probable origin[b]
(12) 2-formyl-5-methyl thiophene	Sulphurous	2	Reaction between dicarbonyl compounds and H_2S (both from Maillard reaction between amino acids and reducing sugars)[6]
(13) trimethylthiazole	Earthy	**2**	From 2,3-butanedione, ethanal, NH_3 and H_2S (all from Maillard reaction)[6]
(14) 2-acetyl-2-thiazoline	Roasty	2	From cysteamine and 2-oxopropanal, formed from Strecker degradation of cysteine and breakdown of sugars, respectively[10]
(15) 2,5(6)-dimethyl-pyrazine	Coffee, roasted	4	Strecker degradation of amino acids with dicarbony compounds(from Maillard reaction),and condensation of resulting amino-carbonyl compounds[6]
(16) 2,3-dimethyl-pyrazine	Meaty, roasted	4	As (15)
(17) 2-ethyl-3,5-dimethyl-pyrazine	Roasty	4	As (15)
(18) 3,5(2)-diethyl-2(6)-methyl-pyrazine	Sweet, roasted	4	As (15)

Table 5.2. Continued

Compound	Odour character	Ref.[a]	Probable origin[b]
(19) 2-acetyl-pyrroline	Popcorn	2	Maillard reaction between a reducing sugar and proline[11]

Aldehydes, ketones and lactones

Compound	Odour character	Ref.[a]	Probable origin[b]
(20) 1-octen-3-one	Mushrooms	2, 5	Thermal oxidation of *n*-6 fatty acids[12]
(21) *trans*-2-nonenal	Tallowy, fatty	2	Thermal oxidation of *n*-6 fatty acids[12]
(22) nonanal	Tallowy, green	**2**	Thermal oxidation of *n*-9 fatty acids[12]
(23) *trans, trans*-2,4-nonadienal	Fatty	2	Thermal oxidation of *n*-6 fatty acids[12]
(24) decanal	Green, aldehyde	4	Thermal oxidation of *n*-9 fatty acids[12]
(25) *Trans,trans*-2,4-decadienal (and an isomer)	Fatty, tallowy	**2, 4, 5**	Thermal oxidation of *n*-6 fatty acids[12]
(26) 2-undecenal	Tallowy, sweet	2	Thermal oxidation of *n*-9 fatty acids[12]
(27) γ-decalactone	Peach-like	2	Oxidation of triglyerides[12]
(28) γ-dodecalactone	Tallowy, fruity	2	Oxidation of triglyerides[12]

Other

Compound	Odour character	Ref.[a]	Probable origin[b]
(29) 2,3-butanedione	Caramel	5	Degradation of sugars in the Maillard reaction
(30) β-ionone	Violets	2	Oxidation reactions of β-carotene, from the diet[13]

continued overleaf

Table 5.2. Continued

Compound	Odour character	Ref.[a]	Probable origin[b]
(31) 14-methyl-pentadecanal	Fatty, tallowy, train-oil	3	Cleavage of plasmalogen phospholipids or from acetyl Co-A + acyl Co-A[3]
(32) 14-methyl-hexadecanal	Fatty, tallowy, orange-like	3	As (31)
(33) 15-methyl-hexadecanal	Fatty, tallowy	3	As (31)
(34) 4-methylphenol	Phenolic	2	From plant material or from the breakdown of the amino acid, tyrosine[14]

[a] References for the analysis of chicken aroma: 1 = Pippen and Mecchi (1969); 2 = Gasser and Grosch (1990); 3 = Werkhoff *et al.* (1993); 4 = Siegl *et al.* (1995); 5 = Farmer *et al.*, unpublished data (additional odour impact compounds are still being identified). References 1, 2, 3 and 5 studied chicken whereas reference 4 studied turkey. Gasser and Grosch (1990) reported those compounds of particular importance for the overall aroma in terms of the flavour dilution at which the compound was still detected; for those compounds with a flavour dilution of 128 or more the reference is indicated in **bold**.

[b] Additional references refer to the mechanisms of formation of the aroma compounds; 6 = Vernin and Parkanyi (1982); 7 = Güntert *et al.* (1992); 8 = van den Ouweland and Peer (1975); 9 = Farmer *et al.* (1989); 10 = Hofmann and Schieberle (1995); 11 = Tressl *et al.* (1985); 12 = Grosch (1982); 13 = Sanderson *et al.* (1971); 14 = Ha and Lindsay (1991).

The identities of these flavour compounds are of considerable importance to flavour companies wishing to synthesize a good chicken flavouring. However, of greater importance for the production of chicken with consistently good flavour is the elucidation of the chemical reactions and precursors which are important for their formation during cooking.

Chemical Reactions by which Chicken Aroma is Formed

Table 5.2 indicates, for each odour impact compound, which chemical reaction and precursors are needed for its formation. It is evident that the Maillard reaction, lipid oxidation and the degradation of thiamine are of particular importance.

Maillard reaction

The Maillard reaction contributes to the formation of flavour in most cooked foods. Even in its simplest form, between one amino acid and one reducing sugar, the Maillard reaction yields more than one hundred volatile products, and others remain to be identified (Salter *et al.*, 1988; Farmer *et al.*, 1989). It comprises a complex network of chemical reactions in which one or more amino acids (or peptides or proteins) react with reducing sugars by many pathways to yield many products. These include not only the volatile products which contribute to flavour, but also polymeric melanoidins, responsible for browning of baked products, certain antioxidative compounds and even some mutagenic compounds which may form under severe cooking conditions (Danehy, 1986). The main pathways of the Maillard reaction were elucidated by Hodge (1953) and have been reviewed by Mauron (1981).

Twenty of the key flavour compounds listed in Table 5.2 may be formed by the Maillard reaction. Hydrogen sulphide is formed by the reaction between the amino acid, cysteine and dicarbonyl Maillard products (by a reaction known as Strecker degradation; Schutte, 1974; Vernin and Parkanyi, 1982) and not only contributes to the overall meat flavour but is also an important and reactive intermediate in further reactions creating other sulphur-containing flavour compounds. Mecchi *et al.* (1964) showed that the H_2S derived from chicken muscle may be formed either from the cysteine and cystine present in protein or from glutathione; of these sources, protein was proposed as the main source of H_2S due to the greater quantities of this precursor. The reaction of H_2S with 5-methyl-4-hydroxy-3(2H)-furanone (another product of the Maillard reaction) yields 2-methyl-3-furanthiol, bis(2-methyl-3-furyl) disulphide and many related compounds (van den Ouweland and Peer, 1975). These compounds can also be formed from the reaction of ribose-5-phosphate and H_2S, in the absence of amino acids, by Maillard-type reactions (van den Ouweland and Peer, 1975). The mechanisms of formation of these and the other Maillard products listed in Table 5.2 have been reviewed by Mottram (1991, 1994) and Bailey (1994).

The precursors of the Maillard reaction present in raw meat are derived from the degradative reactions which occur in muscle after death. Free sugars and some sugar phosphates are formed by glycolysis and by the breakdown of ATP (Lawrie, 1992). The most reactive free sugar present in meat appears to be ribose, formed by the latter route. Ribose-5-phosphate is even more reactive (Mottram and Nobrega, 1997) but it is unclear whether sufficient quantities of this compound occur naturally in meat to contribute to flavour. Studies have indicated that these substances are more important for the formation of flavour in beef and pork than glucose and glucose-6-phosphate (Farmer *et al.*, 1996). As discussed earlier, under the effect of such compounds on taste, there is some evidence that the quantities of the precursors of the Maillard reaction are altered during cooking (Macy *et al.*, 1964).

Degradation of thiamine

Thiamine (vitamin B_1) is a bicyclic compound containing sulphur and nitrogen and its thermal degradation can yield a wide range of S- and N-containing volatile compounds many of which possess potent aromas (Buttery *et al.*, 1984;

Güntert *et al.*, 1992). Many of these are the same compounds which can also be formed by the Maillard reaction; for example 2-methyl-3-furanthiol, which is important for the 'meaty' aroma and flavour of chicken and beef (Gasser and Grosch, 1988, 1990), is one of the major products. This raises the question of which of these pathways is the more important for flavour formation in meats. Grosch *et al.* (1993) reported that small amounts of thiamine gave a much higher yield of 2-methyl-3-furanthiol than 20 times more ribose, when reacted with cysteine in an aqueous model system at pH 5.7. However, preliminary studies in our laboratory suggest that ribose may have more effect on the aroma than thiamine when added to raw poultry meat prior to cooking (Farmer, unpublished data).

Lipid oxidation

Lipid oxidation is well known as the cause of rancidity development, but it can also contribute to desirable food flavours. This complex series of reactions is ubiquitous in the natural world and has been extensively studied and reviewed (Grosch, 1982; Chan, 1987). When catalysed by endogenous enzymes it can result in the formation of many of the characteristic flavours of fruits and vegetables, whereas its occurrence at ambient temperatures in an uncontrolled fashion causes the formation of 'painty', 'cardboard' and 'rancid' odours in meat and other foods. However, when catalysed by heat, the thermal oxidation of lipids plays an important role in the generation of the desirable flavour of meat (Mottram, 1991). In all the above cases, lipid oxidation occurs via free radical mechanisms and the difference between them is in the balance of odour compounds produced.

Listed in Table 5.2 are nine compounds which are derived from the thermal oxidation of lipids and which are believed to contribute to the flavour of chicken. These comprise aldehydes, ketones, and lactones with individual odours described as 'green', 'fatty', 'mushrooms' and 'fruity'.

The reactivity of lipids in oxidation reactions is related to their degree of unsaturation; polyunsaturated lipids will be the most reactive both in the generation of desirable flavour and in the formation of off-flavours (Grosch, 1982), including the unpleasant flavour of reheated cooked meat, known as 'warmed-over-flavour' (Love and Pearson, 1971; Asghar *et al.*, 1988). Mottram and Edwards (1983) showed that, in beef and pork, the more saturated triacylglycerols played little part in the generation of volatile compounds or the characteristic odour of the cooked meat. The more unsaturated phospholipids, present as components of the muscle cell walls, were of much greater importance for flavour development. Although triacylglycerols are therefore not needed for flavour development, they can affect juiciness (Keeton, 1993) and the release of flavour (Chevance and Farmer, 1997), and therefore may influence how flavour is perceived.

Other reactions

Although the Maillard reaction and lipid oxidation reactions account for most of the compounds believed to contribute to the aroma of cooked chicken, some other reactions are also involved. The compound, β-ionone, which contributes a 'violet-like' aroma to most meats is derived from the oxidation of carotenoid compounds, probably derived from the diet (Sanderson *et al.*, 1971). The breakdown of plasmalogen phospholipids may be responsible for the formation of branched aldehydes (Werkhoff *et al.*, 1993). Phenolic compounds can be formed from the breakdown of plant material or from the amino acid, tyrosine (Ha and Lindsay, 1991).

The overall aroma and flavour of a food is the result of a balance between these various flavour forming reactions.

Precursors of Aroma-forming Reactions

Early studies on poultry flavour involved the use of dialysis, filtration and similar techniques to separate the uncooked meat into various fractions which, after heating, were subjected to sensory tests and analysis of flavour precursors (Koehler and Jacobson, 1967). These studies showed that the fraction which produced the most chicken and meaty flavour contained a range of carbohydrates, amino acids, purines and carbonyl compounds. Although this fraction was the only one which contained detectable amounts of ribose and lactic acid and which had a pH of 5.8, one can only speculate as to which of these might be of particular importance. Ishida and Yamamoto (1978) reported that, of a number of fractions, the strongest chicken flavour was derived from the water-soluble protein fraction. Schliemann *et al.* (1987) discussed the nature and concentrations of potential flavour precursors and also concluded that the aqueous components were responsible for the basic chicken flavour, but that the lipid contributed to the species flavour.

Other work has concentrated on creating a mixture of precursors which, when heated, gives the characteristic flavour of chicken. One such flavouring was patented by Tandy (1986), who reported that a mixture of amino acids, sulphur compounds and reducing disaccharides reacted together to give the species-specific flavour of chicken as long as the reaction mixture comprised about 50% of the amino acid, leucine. The amino acid serine was also suggested to be important.

More recent studies on the identities of key odour compounds allow a different approach which, nevertheless, leads to similar conclusions. Having identified many of the compounds contributing to flavour, and established some of the chemical reactions involved during cooking, it is possible to suggest which precursors are needed in the raw meat to give good chicken flavour. These are indicated in Table 5.2 and include a source of reducing sugars or related compounds, amino acids or peptides, especially those containing sulphur, lipids and polyunsaturated fatty acids. These broad classes of precursors include many individual sugars, amino acids, fatty acids etc. It is not known which or how much of these individual compounds are needed for optimum flavour formation. It is likely that some of the precursors needed are present in adequate concentrations in raw meat, whereas others may be limiting for aroma-forming reactions. The lack of such limiting precursors in some meat may explain its bland flavour. Current research in our laboratory is studying which of these potential precursors is limiting for beef and poultry flavour (Farmer *et al.*, 1996).

Factors Affecting Aroma-forming Reactions

The concentration of available precursors is only one factor which will affect the rate of aroma and flavour-forming reactions. Other physical and chemical factors will also influence the intensity and quality of the final flavour.

pH

Many of the reactions involved in flavour formation are pH dependent and the quantities of aroma compounds which contribute to poultry flavour will also be affected by pH. For instance, some of the furanthiols and their di- and trisulphides, important for the 'meaty' aroma of chicken, are formed in much greater quantities at low pH in model systems (Farmer and Mottram, 1990b) and in meat itself (Fig. 5.2a; Madruga and Mottram, 1995). In contrast, other compounds, such as pyrazines and thiazoles (Fig. 5.2b) increase with decreasing pH. These compounds are all products of the Maillard reaction but are formed by different pathways, which respond differently to pH changes. For instance 2-methyl-3-furanthiol is formed via the 1,2-enolization pathway, which is favoured by acidic conditions (Hicks and Feather, 1975). Similar results have been obtained for sulphur compounds in general from chicken meat adjusted to pH values over the range pH 2–10 (Rao *et al.*, 1977).

Lipid oxidation products are also affected by pH. The formation of unsaturated aldehydes tends to drop over the pH range 4–5.5 (Fig. 5.2c; Madruga and Mottram, 1995). Other compounds, including products of lipid oxidation and the Maillard reaction, show little effect of pH (Fig. 5.2d); these include the most abundant aldehydes, octanal and nonanal. Earlier studies (Rao *et al.*, 1977) indicated that higher pH values of 7–10 result in the formation of increasing quantities of 'carbonyl compounds', but that at a lower pH the concentrations remained approximately constant. As these carbonyl compounds probably mainly comprised the aldehydes, octanal and nonanal, these results seem to agree with those obtained by Madruga and Mottram (1995).

Temperature

Increased temperature of cooking favours both the Maillard reaction and lipid oxidation. Ang and Liu (1996a, b) have shown that the overall quantities of volatile products from both these reactions increase as the ultimate internal temperature of the chicken is raised from 60 to 80°C. Higher temperatures increase not only the rate of these chemical reactions but also the release of free amino acids and other precursors in the meat (Cambero *et al.*, 1992). Figure 5.3 compares the effect of temperature on the rates of increase of two products of the Maillard reaction and two products of lipid oxidation (Ang and Liu, 1996a), and it may be observed that, although the quantities of 2,3-butanedione and dimethyldisulphide increase at an approximately

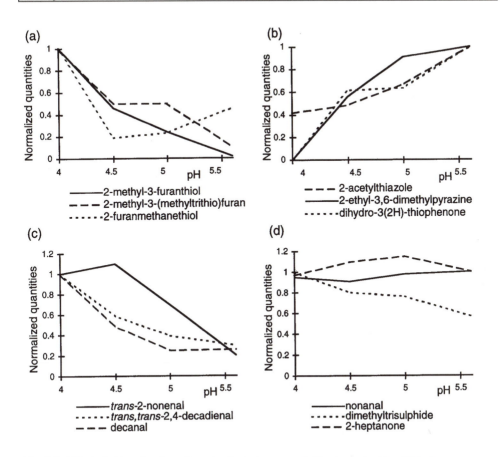

Fig. 5.2. Effect of pH on the formation of selected aroma volatiles in cooked beef (Madruga and Mottram, 1995).

constant rate over the temperature range, the quantities of the lipid oxidation products formed plateau after 70°C. Similar results were found in earlier experiments on the effect of temperature on the volatiles obtained from cooked beef (MacLeod and Ames, 1986). It has been suggested that the antioxidative effect of Maillard reaction products begins to inhibit the lipid oxidation reactions at temperatures higher than 77°C (Imafidon and Spanier, 1994). Thus, not only the intensity of flavour but also the balance of odour compounds will change as the temperature increases.

Other meat components

The different reactions contributing to aroma and flavour formation (the Maillard reaction, lipid oxidation, degradation of thiamine, etc.) do not occur in isolation. All meats are complex biological systems so it may be expected that the precursors and intermediates of these reactions, and indeed other meat components, would interact with each other. The interactions occurring between the Maillard reaction and the thermal oxidation of lipids have been demonstrated using both model systems and meat itself (Farmer and Mottram,

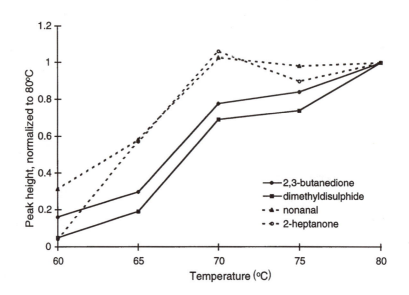

Fig. 5.3. Effect of temperature on the amounts of selected Maillard and lipid oxidation products, obtained from chicken breast meat using a dynamic headspace technique (Ang and Liu, 1996a).

1994; Whitfield and Mottram, 1996). Figure 5.4 shows the effect of such interactions in an aqueous model system on compounds which contribute to the characteristic chicken flavour. When phospholipid is heated alone, a quantity of lipid oxidation products is obtained; likewise, when cysteine and ribose are heated together, a range of Maillard products are produced. However, when these components are heated together, the presence of Maillard reactants decreases the formation of the aldehydes and the presence of phospholipid suppresses the formation of some of the furanthiols important for meaty flavours (Farmer and Mottram, 1990a, 1992). There is also evidence for the occurrence of such lipid–Maillard interactions in meat. First, long-chain heterocyclic compounds have been detected both in model systems (Farmer and Mottram, 1990a) and in chicken meat (Farmer and Mottram, 1994) which include either nitrogen and/or sulphur (from amino acids) and a long aliphatic chain (from fatty acids). Secondly, the addition of ribose (a Maillard precursor) to raw beef has been shown to reduce the formation of aliphatic aldehydes (Farmer *et al.*, 1996). Thus, the precursors and intermediates of each of these reactions will also affect the balance of flavour compounds produced by the others.

Thus, the characteristic flavour of poultry meat results from the combined effects of water-soluble taste compounds and volatile aroma compounds, derived from reactions occurring between the components of raw meat. The concentrations of these substances and the rate of the reactions between them are influenced by a range of parameters, and could, therefore, be affected by production or processing methods.

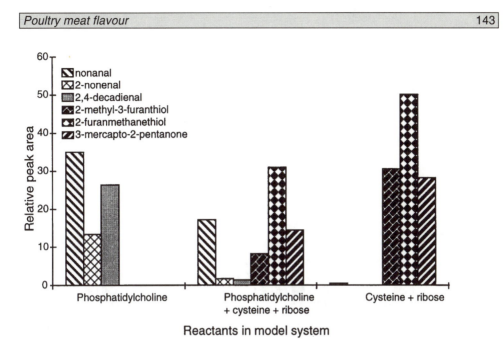

Fig. 5.4. Formation of selected volatile products from heated aqueous model systems containing a phospholipid, phosphatidylcholine, the Maillard reactants, cysteine and ribose or both lipid and Maillard reactants (Farmer and Mottram, 1990a, 1992).

EFFECT OF PRODUCTION AND PROCESSING FACTORS ON POULTRY FLAVOUR

Factors which *might* affect flavour include the production factors of age, sex, genotype, diet and stocking density, the method of slaughter, the postslaughter factors of time of evisceration, time and temperature of chilling and storage, and finally, cooking method. All of these factors could, in theory, affect either the composition of the raw meat, and therefore the availability of precursors, or the progress of flavour-forming reactions during cooking. Many studies have investigated the effect of production factors on the sensory quality of poultry and these investigations have been reviewed previously (Land and Hobson-Frohock, 1977; Poste, 1990; Ramaswamy and Richards, 1982).

Figure 5.5 gives a very general overview of a literature survey on factors affecting flavour intensity (or, in some cases, flavour preference) of cooked poultry meat. This overview is incomplete and the implied assumption that flavour intensity is related to preference is not necessarily valid. Nevertheless, Figure 5.5 illustrates the considerable disagreement between studies. For instance, whereas four studies found that slower growing strains give meat with more flavour, three others reported no significant difference. Some of these disagreements may be due to variations in rearing regime or sensory methodology. Nevertheless, they emphasize the difficulty of fully rationalizing the impact of production factors on flavour. The effects on flavour of the main production and processing factors are discussed below.

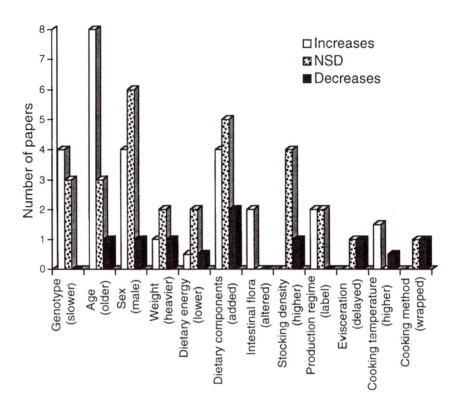

Fig. 5.5. Literature survey on the effect of production or processing factors on poultry meat flavour. Number of papers reporting an increase, decrease or no significant difference in intensity (or in a few cases, acceptability) of flavour.

Genotype

Studies on the effect of genotype or strain on poultry flavour have been conducted for many years and have yielded a range of results. Land and Hobson-Frohock (1977) reviewed a number of studies conducted from the 1950s onwards and found little evidence of statistical significance between different strains of chicken (e.g. New Hampshire crosses, Barred Plymouth Rock) or geese (Pilgrim, Hungarian and Chinese) although they suggested that some of the differences might have been statistically significant if more discriminating sensory methods had been used.

Most of the more recent work has been designed to ascertain whether there is a difference in flavour between modern strains of chicken with their rapid growth rates and slower growing birds. These studies have reported flavour differences for genotypes of differing growth rate and have variously attributed these to differences in age or weight. Touraille *et al.* (1981a) found significant increases in the intensity of flavour of breast and thigh meat from chickens of the slower of two genotypes when compared at the same weight but different ages (63 and 144 days). However, when slaughtered at the same age no significant differences were observed and the authors concluded that most of the observed differences were due to the difference in age. Farmer *et al.* (1997) found that the odour, but not flavour, differed between meat from 'Ross 1' birds (49 days) and that from the slower growing 'ISA 657' birds (84 days). This effect again appeared to be related to the difference in age, but in this case the stronger odour was detected in the younger birds; no differences in odour or flavour of breast meat were detected when both genotypes were grown to the same age. Differences in age may also explain the reputedly improved flavour of some local speciality breeds, such as the 'Palace Chicken' from China which has a growth period of 120 days (Qinghua, 1994). The 'Hinai-dori', a Japanese native chicken, is also a slower growing chicken and has been shown to be more palatable than conventional broilers (Fujimura *et al.*, 1994); this has been attributed to its higher concentration of the flavour enhancer, inosine monophosphate.

Chambers *et al.* (1989) studied four strains of chicken and reported that the flavour of the dark meat was significantly more intense in the modern strains (Hubbard or Ross × Arbor Acre stocks) than the slower growing chickens (experimental strains) when slaughtered at the same age (47 days). However, when the slower-growing birds were slaughtered at the same weight (i.e. at 75 or 103 days), these differences were not seen and, indeed, the older strains tended to give the more intense flavour ($P < 0.10$). In this case, the observed differences seem to be attributed to differences in body weight. Delpech *et al.* (1983) found no significant difference in the flavour of meat from slow growing *Label*-type chickens and a rapid growing strain.

Age

One of the few production factors which has an unambiguous effect on flavour is age. An increase in flavour in older birds was reported in the 1950s and 1960s, as reviewed by Land and Hobson-Frohock (1977) and Ramaswamy and Richards (1982). Most of the more recent studies addressing the effect of age on flavour have also reported a positive effect of age.

A series of studies by Touraille and co-workers demonstrated that the flavour intensity of male chickens from a slow-growing Label-Rouge strain increased up to 14 weeks; this they attributed to the fact that, at this time, the birds were reaching sexual maturity (Fig. 5.6; Touraille *et al.*, 1981a, b). A similar effect was not observed for female chickens (Ricard and Touraille, 1988). Scholtyssek and Sailer (1986) also reported flavour changes in male but not female chickens. They found that, for male birds, the meat from 6- and 8-week-old birds was preferred to that at 10 weeks with the 12 week birds in between. It is possible that a similar increase in flavour intensity was observed as that reported by Touraille *et al.* (1981b), but that it was not liked by the panel. In contrast, Tawfik *et al.* (1990) observed an increase in flavour acceptability from 4 to 12 weeks for both sexes analysed together. Sonaiya *et al.* (1990) found that the flavour of both breast and thigh from both male and female Lohmann chickens was generally more intense at 54 days than 34 days.

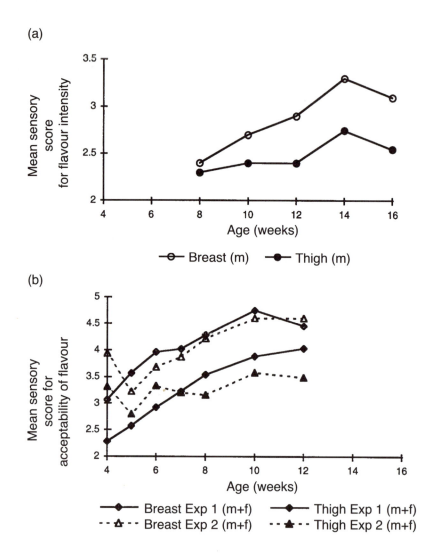

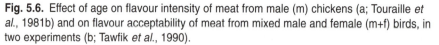

Fig. 5.6. Effect of age on flavour intensity of meat from male (m) chickens (a; Touraille *et al.*, 1981b) and on flavour acceptability of meat from mixed male and female (m+f) birds, in two experiments (b; Tawfik *et al.*, 1990).

Two studies have reported no effect of age on flavour. Rabot *et al.* (1996) reported no overall difference in flavour between chickens slaughtered at 11 and 55 weeks. However, their data indicate that for one genotype ('X33', a rapid growing strain, also used by Touraille and co-workers; Ricard and Touraille, 1988; Touraille *et al.*, 1981a, b) breast meat from the older birds did receive significantly higher scores for flavour. Mohan *et al.* (1987) found no flavour differences between chickens slaughtered at the rather younger ages of 6 and 8 weeks of age.

Chickens undergo physiological changes as they grow older and reach maturity, and these changes will have effects on the taste compounds and flavour precursors in the muscle. However, few of those papers which report flavour differences due to age propose a chemical explanation for their observations. Touraille *et al.* (1981b) found no correlation with any physicochemical measurements (e.g. pH, dry matter, lipid content) but suggested that the composition of the lipids may be of importance. In an early investigation of the differences in volatile odour compounds, Minor *et al.* (1965) reported that a greater concentration of volatiles was obtained from cooked meat from old hens (20 months) than from young pullets (12 weeks). However, this does not seem to arise from greater concentrations of reducing sugars as these, including ribose, seemed to be present in lower concentrations in older birds (Lilyblade and Peterson, 1962). Current studies in our own laboratories suggest that other precursors may be present at higher concentrations in older chickens (Farmer, unpublished data).

Sex

Reviews conducted 15 to 20 years ago (Land and Hobson-Frohock, 1977; Ramaswamy and Richards, 1982) reported that some studies had detected a difference in flavour between male and female chickens. In these cases, meat from the male birds tended to have a stronger flavour or to be preferred to that from the female birds. However, many of the investigations reviewed reported no effect of sex. More recent studies (Scholtyssek and Sailer, 1986) also found a difference between sexes; the leg and breast meat from the female birds was preferred. In contrast, Ristic (1993) found that breast meat from male birds received higher scores for flavour. Ricard and Touraille (1988) found that there was no difference in flavour between meat from the two sexes until the birds reached 14 weeks, at which time the male birds had meat (breast and thigh) with a stronger flavour. Many of the studies which had previously shown an effect of age on flavour (Land and Hobson-Frohock, 1977; Ramaswamy and Richards, 1982) had also used birds of approximately this age. It therefore seems likely that the observed effect of sex on flavour is related to age and the stronger flavour achieved when male birds reach maturity.

Diet

Previous reviews (Land and Hobson-Frohock, 1977; Ramaswamy and Richards, 1982; Poste, 1990) have summarized a large number of investigations on the effect of diet on flavour. It is evident that large changes can be made to the diet without great effect on the flavour (Land and Hobson-Frohock, 1977). Indeed, many studies are conducted in order to establish that a proposed new feed ingredient has no detrimental effect on quality; for example, the inclusion of hulless oats was found to have no effect on flavour (Poste *et al.*, 1996). However, some feeds can have a deleterious effect on flavour and highly unsaturated oils, especially fish oils, tend to cause a fishy taint in the resulting poultry meat (Land and Hobson-Frohock, 1977; Ramaswamy and Richards, 1982; Poste, 1990; Leskanich and Noble, 1997). Of all the diets examined, few were found to have a beneficial effect on flavour.

There is some indication that modification of the intestinal microflora by dietary means can affect flavour (Harris *et al.*, 1968; Mead *et al.*, 1983). Harris *et al.* (1968) reported that chickens reared under conventional conditions gave meat with a significantly different flavour compared with that from chickens reared in a germ-free environment; the flavour of the former was described as stronger and a more characteristic chicken flavour. However, birds reared with specific microflora designed to mimic the main natural species gave meat which was not different in flavour from that from the 'germ-free' chickens and showed little difference to that from conventional birds. Thus, although these data suggested an effect, they were not fully conclusive. The more recent study (Mead *et al.*, 1983) compared chickens which had been fed an increased proportion of whole wheat and fresh green vegetables and showed that these birds had higher counts of *Escherichia coli* and faecal streptococci, as well as other differences in microflora, in their intestines. These chickens also gave breast meat which was significantly different in flavour from that of controls and was described as 'richer', 'meatier', 'sweeter', 'more roast' but also sometimes 'gamey' and 'off'.

Several studies have investigated the effect of dietary vitamin E. However, in most cases the main interest was the possible positive effect of vitamin E on oxidative stability and the suppression of off-flavour formation during storage. Bartov *et al.* (1983) did not examine flavour as such, but found that additional vitamin E in the diet (40 mg kg^{-1}) increased the acceptability of turkey drumsticks after storage for 7 months at $-18°C$. Blum *et al.* (1992) found that vitamin E supplementation delayed flavour deterioration during 5 to 12 days storage as fresh birds. De Winne and Dirinck (1996) compared chickens fed diets containing vitamin E at 15–20 mg kg^{-1} and 200 mg kg^{-1} after frozen storage, thawing and subsequent storage at 4°C, and reported that the occurrence of off-flavours was significantly reduced in meat from vitamin E supplemented birds. The higher scores for off-flavour occurring in meat from the unsupplemented birds coincided with a higher susceptibility to oxidation and also greater quantities of aldehydes among the extracted volatile compounds. Thus, the vitamin E is clearly suppressing lipid oxidation, and thereby altering the balance of aroma and flavour compounds, in the stored samples. Interestingly, one study (Sheldon *et al.*, 1997) has found that vitamin E can confer an improvement on the flavour of cooked turkey, detectable by a trained panel, even after storage of the refrigerated raw sample for only one day.

Production Regime and Environment

A number of reports have considered the effect of aspects of the production regime, such as husbandry methods, environmental conditions or stocking density, on various aspects of eating quality, including flavour. Some of the early studies, reviewed by Land and Hobson-Frohock (1977), examined the effect of type or presence of litter, exposure to ammonia and free range versus intensive conditions. Except for one comment suggesting an adverse effect of using peanut-hull litter, no differences in flavour were observed.

The introduction of the *Label Rouge* and *Label Fermier* production regimes in France led to a number of papers comparing these chickens with those reared by conventional systems. Under these regimes, chickens are reared under strict standards requiring (for the *Label Rouge* system) the use of a slow-growing chicken, a low-fat, high-cereal diet, low stocking densities, a minimum rearing period of 81 days and strict processing and quality control conditions (King, 1984). In a study on chickens purchased at retail, 'Label' chicken was found to have the more intense odour and also, for the thigh meat, a more intense flavour; the *Label* meat was preferred overall (Lassaut *et al.*, 1984; Touraille *et al.*, 1985). These authors suggested that the increased age of the *Label* birds was responsible for this improvement in flavour. A later study, in which the chickens were grown under controlled conditions suggested that the flavour of *Label Fermier* chicken was more intense, albeit not significantly so (Culioli *et al.*, 1990). The effect was more pronounced for female birds.

Farmer *et al.* (1997) examined the effect of four of the factors which define *Label Rouge* chickens (diet, genotype, stocking density and age) on a range of sensory attributes. In terms of odour and flavour, the most pronounced differences were again due to age; the older birds tended to have a more intense odour and flavour, significantly so for some attributes. Significant differences in odour intensity were observed due to genotype; for example, overall odour intensity was higher in Ross than in 'ISA 657' birds. The effects of diet and stocking density on odour and flavour were few, although there was a non-significant tendency for the birds at low stocking density to give breast meat with greater 'flavour intensity' and more 'chicken flavour'. This study supports the assertion by Lassaut *et al.* (1984) that the improved flavour of *Label* chicken is largely due to its greater age at slaughter.

No effect of stocking density was observed by Skaarup (1983) who reported that confined birds had at least as much flavour as free range chickens. Likewise, Deroanne *et al.* (1983) found no significant difference between the flavour of intensively reared and free range chickens. However, Ristic (1993) reported that both breast and thigh meat from free range chickens had more desirable flavour than that from pen-reared birds.

Sonaiya *et al.* (1990) reported that a temperature on a diurnal cycle of 21–30°C gave chicken breast meat with a higher score for flavour than that obtained from birds reared at 21°C. These authors suggested that the more pronounced flavour of birds reared at the higher temperature may be related to the greater concentration of polyunsaturated fatty acids detected in the depot fat of these birds. However, in a related study, the same group reported that a consistently elevated rearing temperature had no direct effect on flavour (Tawfik *et al.*, 1990).

Slaughter and Postslaughter Treatment

Few studies have investigated the possible role of slaughter and postslaughter treatment on flavour. Mead *et al.* (1983) examined the effect of the time of evisceration on poultry flavour. Storage of the birds for 8 days before evisceration gave a significant difference in flavour compared with birds which had been eviscerated when fresh; the first group were judged to be 'stronger' and 'meatier' but also more 'gamey', 'livery', 'stale' and 'off'.

Denoyer *et al.* (1996) examined the flavour of duck livers obtained by hot evisceration, 35 min post-mortem and those obtained by cold evisceration after 24 h at 10°C. The former received higher sensory scores for overall odour intensity and yielded a greater number of volatiles derived from the Maillard reaction, when measured by gas chromatography–mass spectroscopy.

An increased conditioning period between slaughter and consumption can result in an increased 'brothy' taste (Kato and Nishimura, 1987). These authors examined the composition of the meat and reported that increased ageing reduced the concentration of IMP but increased the amounts of amino acids, including the flavour enhancer, glutamic acid and oligopeptides. They concluded that this increase in glutamate may be responsible for the increased brothy flavour of the conditioned chicken. A longer storage period has also been shown to increase the concentrations of reducing sugars (Lilyblade and Peterson, 1962) which may again affect flavour formation.

Cooking Method

A few studies have examined aspects of cooking method and their effect on flavour. Method of thawing, cleaning and trimming, wrapping in foil, oven bags or not wrapping were found not to affect the flavour, although texture was affected (McBride *et al.*, 1977). In contrast, results obtained in our laboratory indicate that open roasting (unwrapped) gives chicken with more roast flavour than cooking wrapped in foil or a roaster bag (Fig. 5.7; Farmer, unpublished data).

Joseph *et al.* (1996) examined the effect of final internal cooking temperature on the flavour (and other sensory attributes) of various species of poultry found in Nigeria. In all cases he found that the flavour improved from 65°C to 80°C and then declined slightly when cooked to 85°C. Chicken portions cooked at different oven temperatures gave some flavour differences; the higher oven temperature tended to give more chicken flavour (Farmer, unpublished data).

A comparison of chicken cooked by microwave and conventional ovens showed that conventional heating gave a preferable flavour for both breast and leg meat (Salama, 1993). This may be explained by the various effects of microwave cooking on flavour (Reineccius and Whorton, 1990); Maillard browning is reduced due to the absence of hot dry air around the food, the flavour-binding properties of the food constituents may be altered by the different heating characteristics and flavour can be lost due to steam distillation effects. Premarinading in sodium chloride or sodium tripolyphosphate tended to give increased scores for flavour for both cooking methods (Salama, 1993).

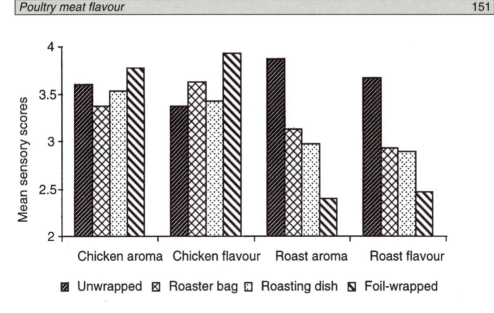

Fig. 5.7. Effect of cooking method on hedonic score for intensity of chicken and roasted aroma and flavour (Farmer, unpublished data).

CONCLUSIONS

The studies summarized in this and previous reviews indicate that production factors can affect flavour, but often they do so inconsistently. One exception is that older chickens, in particular males nearing maturity, give meat with more flavour. These changes in flavour must be related to the composition of the meat prior to cooking.

Many, but probably not all, of the important flavour compounds have now been identified and it is possible to deduce the reactions most likely to be responsible for their formation. It is then possible to suggest which precursors are required in the raw meat to give good flavour. It is not yet possible to fully explain why some chickens have more flavour in terms of the differences in their chemical composition. However, recent studies have narrowed the gap between our understanding of the mechanisms of flavour formation and the ability to use the information during production or processing of poultry to improve the ultimate flavour of the meat.

ACKNOWLEDGEMENTS

Support from Moy Park Ltd, Craigavon, Northern Ireland and the Industrial Research and Technology Unit, Department of Economic Development, Northern Ireland towards the author's poultry flavour research is gratefully acknowledged.

REFERENCES

Ang, C.Y.W. and Liu, F. (1996a) Influence of heating end-point temperature on volatiles from poultry meat – a review. *Journal of Muscle Foods* 7, 291–302.

Ang, C.Y.W. and Liu, F. (1996b) Static headspace capillary GC method for determining changes of volatiles from heated chicken breast meat. *Journal of Muscle Foods* 7, 131–138.

Asghar, A., Gray, J.I., Buckley, D.J., Pearson, A.M. and Booren, A.M. (1988) Perspectives on warmed-over flavor. *Food Technology* 42, 102–109.

Bailey, M.E. (1994) Maillard reactions and meat flavor development. In: Shahidi, F. (ed.) *Flavor of Meat and Meat Products.* Chapman & Hall, Glasgow, pp. 153–173.

Baines, D.A. and Mlotkiewicz, J.A. (1984) The chemistry of meat flavour. In: Bailey, A.J. (ed.) *Recent Advances in the Chemistry of Meat.* Royal Society of Chemistry, London, pp. 119–164.

Bartov, I., Basker, D. and Angel, S. (1983) Effect of dietary vitamin E on the stability and sensory quality of turkey meat. *Poultry Science* 62, 1224–1230.

Blum, J.C., Touraille, C., Salichon, M.R., Ricard, F.H. and Frigg, M. (1992) Effect of dietary vitamin E supplies in broilers, 2nd Report. Male and female growth rate, viability, immune response, fat content and meat flavour variations during storage. *Archiv für Geflügelkunde* 56, 37–42.

Buttery, R.G., Haddon, W.F., Seifert, R.M. and Turnbaugh, J.G. (1984) Thiamin odor and bis(2-methyl-3-furyl)disulphide. *Journal of Agricultural and Food Chemistry* 32, 674–676.

Cambero, M.I., Seuss, I. and Honikel, K.O. (1992) Flavor compounds of beef broth as affected by cooking temperature. *Journal of Food Science* 57, 1285–1290.

Chambers, J.R., Fortin, A., Mackie, D.A. and Larmond, E. (1989) Comparison of sensory properties of meat from broilers of modern stocks and experimental strains differing in growth and fatness. *Canadian Institute of Food Science and Technology Journal* 22, 353–358.

Chan, H.W.-S. (1987) *Autoxidation of Unsaturated Lipids.* Academic Press, London.

Chevance, F.F.V. and Farmer, L.J. (1997) Influence of fat on the flavour of an emulsified meat product. In: *Proceedings of Charalambous Memorial Symposium.* American Chemical Society, Washington, DC, Limnos, Greece, pp. 255–270.

Crocker, E.C. (1948) The flavor of meat. *Food Research* 13, 179–183.

Culioli, J., Touraille, C., Bordes, P. and Girard, J.P. (1990) Caractéristiques des carcasses et de la viande du poulet 'label fermier'. [Carcass and meat characteristics of 'Label Fermier' chickens]. *Archiv für Geflügelkunde* 53, 237–245.

Danehy, J.P. (1986) Maillard reactions: non-enzymic browning in food systems with special reference to the development of flavour. *Advances in Food Research* 30, 77–138.

Delpech, P., Dumont, B.L. and Nefzaoui, A. (1983) Influence du rationnement et du patrimone génétique de poulets sur les charactéristiques phisico-chimiques et sensorielles de la viande à différents âges. In: Lahellec, C., Ricard, F.H. and Colin, P. (eds) *Proceedings of European Symposium on Quality of Poultry Meat.* Ministère de l'Agriculture, Station Expérimentale d'Aviculture, Ploufragen, France, pp. 21–27.

Denoyer, C., Viallon, C., Renou, J.P., Frencia, J.P., Lorrain, P. and Berdagué, J.L. (1996) Incidence du mode d'éviscération sur la fraction volatile et la flaveur du foie gras de canard. [Effects of evisceration method on the volatile fraction and flavour of duck foie gras]. *Viandes Produits Carnés* 17, 179–184.

Deroanne, C., Castermant, B. and Despontin, J.P. (1983) Influence des conditions d'élevage sur la qualité de la viande de volaille. In: Lahellec, C., Ricard, F.H. and Colin, P. (eds) *Proceedings of European Symposium on Quality of Poultry Meat.*

Ministère de l'Agriculture, Station Expérimentale d'Aviculture, Ploufragen, France, pp. 28–36.

De Winne, A. and Dirinck, P. (1996) Studies on vitamin E and meat quality. 2. Effect of feeding high vitamin E levels on chicken meat quality. *Journal of Agricultural and Food Chemistry* 44, 1691–1696.

Farmer, L.J. and Mottram, D.S. (1990a) Interaction of lipid in the Maillard reaction between cysteine and ribose: effect of a triglyceride and three phospholipids on the volatile products. *Journal of the Science of Food and Agriculture* 53, 505–525.

Farmer, L.J. and Mottram, D.S. (1990b) Recent studies on the formation of meat-like aroma compounds. In: Bessière, Y. and Thomas, A.F. (eds) *Flavour Science and Technology.* Wiley, Chichester, pp. 113–116.

Farmer, L.J. and Mottram, D.S. (1992) Effect of cysteine and ribose on the volatile thermal degradation products of a triglyceride and three phospholipids. *Journal of the Science of Food and Agriculture* 60, 489–497.

Farmer, L.J. and Mottram, D.S. (1994) Lipid-Maillard interactions in the formation of volatile aroma compounds. In: Maarse, H. and van der Heij, D.G. (eds) *Trends in Flavour Research.* Elsevier, Amsterdam, pp. 313–326.

Farmer, L.J., Mottram, D.S. and Whitfield, F.B. (1989) Volatile compounds produced in Maillard reactions involving cysteine, ribose and phospholipid. *Journal of the Science of Food and Agriculture* 49, 347–368.

Farmer, L.J., Hagan, T.D.H. and Paraskevas, O. (1996) A comparison of three sugars and inosine monophosphate as precursors meat aroma. In: Taylor, A.J. and Mottram, D.S. (eds) *Flavour Science. Recent Developments.* Royal Society of Chemistry, Cambridge, pp. 225–230.

Farmer, L.J., Perry, G.C., Lewis, P.D., Nute, G.R., Piggott, J.R. and Patterson, R.L.S. (1997) Responses of two genotypes of chicken to the diets and stocking densities of conventional UK and *Label Rouge* production systems. II. Sensory attributes. *Meat Science* 47, 77–93.

Fujimura, S., Muramoto, T., Katsukawa, M., Hatano, T. and Ishibashi, T. (1994) Chemical analysis and sensory evaluation of free amino acids and 5′-inosinic acid in meat of Hinai-dori, Japanese native chicken. Comparison with broilers and layer pullets. *Animal Science and Technology (Japan)* 65, 610–618.

Fujimura, S., Kawano, S., Koga, H., Takeda, H., Kadowaki, M. and Ishibashi, T. (1995) Identification of taste-active components in the chicken meat extract by omission test. Involvement of glutamic acid, IMP and potassium ion. *Animal Science and Technology (Japan)* 66, 43–51.

Fujimura, S., Koga, H., Takeda, H., Tone, N., Kadowaki, M. and Ishibashi, T. (1996) Role of taste-active components, glutamic acid, 5′-inosinic acid and potassium ion in taste of chicken meat extract. *Animal Science and Technology (Japan)* 67, 423–429.

Gasser, U. and Grosch, W. (1988) Identification of volatile flavour compounds with high aroma values from cooked beef. *Zeitschrift für Lebensmittel Untersuchung und Forschung* 186, 489–494.

Gasser, U. and Grosch, W. (1990) Primary odorants of chicken broth – a comparative-study with meat broths from cow and ox. *Zeitschrift für Lebensmittel Untersuchung und Forschung* 190, 3–8.

Gasser, U., Warendorf, T., Grosch, W. and Belitz, H.-D. (1994) The flavour of bouillon. In: Birch, G.G. and Campbell-Platt, G. (eds) *Synergy.* Intercept Ltd, Andover, pp. 129–144.

Gordon, A. (1972) Meat and poultry flavour. *The Flavour Industry*, September, 445–453.

Gray, J.I. and Pearson, A.M. (1994) Lipid-derived off-flavors in meat – formation and inhibition. In: Shahidi, F. (ed.) *Flavor of Meat and Meat Products*. Chapman & Hall, Glasgow, pp. 116–143.

Grosch, W. (1982) Lipid degradation products and flavors. In: Morton, I.D. and MacLeod, A.J. (eds) *Food Flavors*. Elsevier, Amsterdam, pp. 325–398.

Grosch, W., Zeiler-Hilgart, G., Cerny, C. and Guth, H. (1993) Studies on the formation of odorants contributing to meat flavours. In: Schreier, P. and Winterhalter, P. (eds) *Progress in Flavour Precursor Studies*. Allured Publishing, Carol Stream IL, pp. 329–342.

Güntert, M., Brüning, J., Emberger, R., Hopp, R., Köpsel, H., Surburg, H. and Werkhoff, P. (1992) Thermally degraded thiamin. A potent source of interesting flavor compounds. In: Teranishi, R., Takeoka, G.R. and Güntert, M. (eds) *Flavor Precursors. Thermal and Enzymatic Conversions*. American Chemical Society, Washington, DC, pp. 140–163.

Ha, J.K. and Lindsay, R.C. (1991) Volatile alkylphenols and thiophenol in species-related characterizing flavors of red meats. *Journal of Food Science* 56, 1197–1202.

Harkes, P.D. and Begemann, W.J. (1974) Identification of some previously unknown aldehydes in cooked chicken. *Journal of the American Oil Chemists' Society* 51, 356–359.

Harris, N.D., Strong, D.H. and Sunde, M.L. (1968) Intestinal flora and chicken flavor. *Journal of Food Science* 33, 543–547.

Hicks, K.B. and Feather, M.S. (1975) Studies on the mechanism of formation of 4-hydroxy-5-methyl-3(2H)-furanone, a component of beef flavor. *Journal of Agricultural and Food Chemistry* 23, 957–960.

Hodge, J.E. (1953) Chemistry of browning reactions in model systems. *Journal of Agricultural and Food Chemistry* 1, 928–943.

Hofmann, T. and Schieberle, P. (1995) Studies on the formation and stability of the roast-flavor compound 2-acetyl-2-thiazoline. *Journal of Agricultural and Food Chemistry* 43, 2946–2950.

Imafidon, G.I. and Spanier, A.M. (1994) Unraveling the secret of meat flavor. *Trends in Food Science and Technology* 5, 315–321.

Ishida, K. and Yamamoto, A. (1978) Properties of the cooking flavors of chicken fractions. *Nippon Shokuhin Kogyo Gakkaishi* 25, 367–373.

Joseph, J.K., Awosanya, B., Adeniran, A.T. and Otagba, U.M. (1996) The effects of end-point internal cooking temperatures on the meat quality attributes of selected Nigerian poultry meats. *Flavour Quality and Preference* 8, 57–61.

Kato, H. and Nishimura, T. (1987) Taste components and conditioning of beef, pork and chicken. In: Kawamura, Y. and Kare, M.R. (eds) *Umami: a Basic Taste*. Marcel Dekker, New York, pp. 289–306.

Keeton, J.T. (1993) Low-fat meat products – technological problems with processing. *Meat Science* 36, 261–276.

King, R.B.N. (1984) The breeding, nutrition, husbandry and marketing of 'Label Rouge' poultry. A report for the ADAS agriculture overseas study tour programme for 1984/85. Ministry of Agriculture, Fisheries and Food, London.

Koehler, H.H. and Jacobson, M. (1967) Characteristics of chicken flavor-containing fraction extracted from raw muscle. *Journal of Agricultural and Food Chemistry* 15, 707–712.

Kuramitsu, R., Tamura, M., Nakatani, M. and Okai, H. (1993) New usage of aspartic acid and glutamic acid as food materials. In: Spanier, A.M., Okai, H. and Tamura, M. (eds) *Food Flavor and Safety, Molecular Analysis and Design*. American Chemical Society, Washington, DC, pp. 138–148.

Land, D.G. and Hobson-Frohock, A. (1977) Flavour, taint and texture in poultry meat. In:

Boorman, K.N. and Wilson, B.J. (eds) *Growth and Poultry Meat Production.* British Poultry Science Ltd, Edinburgh, pp. 301–334.

Lassaut, B., Sylvander, B., Touraille, C. and Sauvageot, F. (1984) L'évaluation comparée des propriétés sensorielles de deux produits, identiques par leurs caractéristiques d'usage mais différenciés et substituables lors de l'acte d'achat. *Sciences des Aliments* 4, 33–39.

Lawrie, R.A. (1992) *Meat Science,* 5th edn. Pergamon, Oxford.

Leskanich, C.O. and Noble, R.C. (1997) Manipulation of the n-3 polyunsaturated fatty acid composition of avian eggs and meat. *World's Poultry Science Journal* 53, 155–183.

Lilyblade, A.L. and Peterson, D.W. (1962) Inositol and free sugars in chicken muscle post-mortem. *Journal of Food Science* 27, 245–249.

Love, J.D. and Pearson, A.M. (1971) Lipid oxidation in meat and meat products – a review. *Journal of the American Oil Chemists' Society* 48, 547–549.

Maarse, H. and Visscher, C.A. (1989) *Volatile Compounds in Food — Qualitative and Quantitative Data,* 6th edn. TNO-CIVO Food Analysis Institute, Zeist, The Netherlands.

MacLeod, G. (1986) The scientific and technological basis of meat flavours. In: Birch, G.C. and Lindley, M.G. (eds) *Developments in Food Flavors.* Elsevier, London, pp. 191–223.

MacLeod, G. and Ames, J.M. (1986) The effect of heat on beef aroma: comparisons of chemical composition and sensory properties. *Flavour and Fragrance Journal* 1, 91–104.

MacLeod, G.M. and Seyyedain-Ardebili, M. (1981) Natural and simulated meat flavors (with particular reference to beef). *CRC Critical Reviews Food Science and Nutrition* 14, 309–437.

Macy, R.L., Naumann, H.D. and Bailey, M.E. (1964) Water-soluble flavor and odor precursors of meat. II Effects of heating on amino nitrogen constituents and carbohydrates in lyophilized diffusates from aqueous extracts of beef, pork, and lamb. *Journal of Food Science* 29, 142–148.

Macy, R.L., Naumann, H.D. and Bailey, M.E. (1970a) Water-soluble flavor and odor precursors of meat. 3. Changes in nucleotides, total nucleosides and bases of beef, pork and lamb during heating. *Journal of Food Science* 35, 78–80.

Macy, R.L., Naumann, H.D. and Bailey, M.E. (1970b) Water-soluble flavor and odor precursors of meat. 4. Influence of cooking on nucleosides and bases of beef steaks and roasts and their relationship to flavor, aroma and juiciness. *Journal of Food Science* 35, 81–83.

Macy, R.L., Naumann, H.D. and Bailey, M.E. (1970c) Water-soluble flavor and odor precursors of meat. 5. Influence of heating on acid-extractable non-nucleotide chemical constituents of beef, lamb and pork. *Journal of Food Science* 35, 83–87.

Madruga, M.S. and Mottram, D.S. (1995) The effect of pH on the formation of Maillard-derived aroma volatiles using a cooked meat system. *Journal of the Science of Food and Agriculture* 68, 305–310.

Maga, J.A. (1994) Umami flavor in meat. In: Shahidi, F. (ed.) *Flavor of Meat and Meat Products.* Chapman & Hall, Glasgow, pp. 98–115.

Mauron, J. (1981) The Maillard reaction in food: a critical review from the nutritional standpoint. In: Eriksson, C. (ed.) *Maillard Reactions in Food.* Pergamon Press, Oxford, pp. 3–35.

McBride, R.L., Kuskis, A. and Board, P.W. (1977) How should frozen chicken be roasted? *CSIRO Food Research Quarterly* 37, 49–53.

Mead, G.C., Griffiths, N.M., Impey, C.S. and Coplestone, J.C. (1983) Influence of diet on the intestinal microflora and meat flavour of intensively-reared broiler chickens. *British Poultry Science* 24, 261–272.

Mecchi, E.P., Pippen, E.L. and Line-Weaver, H. (1964) Origin of hydrogen sulfide in heated chicken muscle. *Journal of Food Science* 29, 393–399.

Minor, L.J., Pearson, A.M., Dawson, I.E. and Schweigert, B.S. (1965) Gas chromatographic analysis of volatile constituents from cooked carcasses of old and young chickens. *Poultry Science* 44, 535–543.

Mohan, B., Narahari, D., Venkatesan, E.S. and Alfred Jaya Prasad, I. (1987) The influence of age and sex on the chemical composition, tenderness and organoleptic characteristics of broiler meat. *Cheiron* 16, 145–151.

Mottram, D.S. (1991) Meat. In: Maarse, H. (ed.) *Volatile Compounds in Foods and Beverages.* Marcel Dekker, New York, pp. 107–177.

Mottram, D.S. (1994) Some aspects of the chemistry of meat flavor. In: Shahidi, F. (ed.) *Flavor of Meat and Meat Products.* Chapman & Hall, Glasgow, pp. 210–230.

Mottram, D.S. and Edwards, R.A. (1983) The role of triglycerides and phospholipids in the aroma of cooked beef. *Journal of the Science of Food and Agriculture* 34, 517–522.

Mottram, D.S. and Nobrega, I.C.C. (1997) Formation of volatile sulphur compounds in reaction mixtures containing cysteine and three different ribose compounds. In: *Proceedings of Charalambous Memorial Symposium.* American Chemical Society, Washington DC, Limnos, Greece, pp. 483–492.

Noleau, I. and Toulemonde, B. (1986) Quantitative study of roast chicken flavor. *Lebensmittel Wissenschaft und Technologie* 19, 122–125.

Noleau, I. and Toulemonde, B. (1987) Volatile components of roast chicken fat. *Lebensmittel Wissenschaft und Technologies* 20, 37–41.

Pippen, E.L. and Mecchi, E.P. (1969) Hydrogen sulfide, a direct and potentially indirect contributor to cooked chicken aroma. *Journal of Food Science* 34, 443–446.

Poste, L.M. (1990) A sensory perspective of effect of feeds on flavor in meats: poultry meats. *Journal of Animal Science* 68, 4414–4420.

Poste, L.M., Butler, G., Cave, N.A. and Burrows, V.D. (1996) Sensory analysis of meat from broiler chickens fed diets containing hulless oats (*Avena nuda*). *Canadian Journal of Animal Science* 76, 313–319.

Qinghua, Z. (1994) 'Palace chicken' – a superior Chinese breed. *Misset World Poultry* 10, 47.

Rabot, C., Rousseau, F., Dumont, J.P., Remignon, H. and Gandemer, G. (1996) Poulets de chair: effets respectifs de l'âge et du poids d'abbatage sur les caractéristiques lipidiques et sensorielles des muscles [Chicken meat: effects of age and slaughter weight on lipid composition and organoleptic qualities]. *Viandes Produits Carnés* 17, 17–43.

Ramarathnam, N., Rubin, L.J. and Diosady, L.L. (1991) Studies on meat flavor. 2. A quantitative investigation of the volatile carbonyls and hydrocarbons in uncured and cured beef and chicken. *Journal of Agricultural and Food Chemistry* 39, 1839–1847.

Ramarathnam, N., Rubin, L.J. and Diosady, L.L. (1993) Studies on meat flavor. 4. Fractionation, characterization, and quantitation of volatiles from uncured and cured beef and chicken. *Journal of Agricultural and Food Chemistry* 41, 939–945.

Ramaswamy, H.S. and Richards, J.F. (1982) Flavour of poultry meat — a review. *Canadian Institute of Food Science and Technology Journal* 15, 7–18.

Rao, C.S., Day, E.J. and Chen, T.C. (1977) Effects of pH on the flavor volatiles of poultry meat during cooking. *Poultry Science* 56, 1034–1035.

Reineccius, G. (ed.) (1994) *Source Book of Flavors*, 2nd edn. Chapman & Hall, New York.

Reineccius, G.A. (1979) Off-flavors in meat and fish – a review. *Journal of Food Science* 44, 12–21, 24.

Reineccius, G.A. and Whorton, C. (1990) Flavor problems associated with the microwave cooking of food products. In: *The Maillard Reaction*. Birkhauser Verlag, Basel, pp. 197–208.

Ricard, F.H. and Touraille, C. (1988) Influence du sexe sur les caractéristiques organoleptiques de la viande de poulet. *Archiv für Geflügelkunde* 52, 27–30.

Ristic, M. (1993) Schlachtköerperwert von Broilern verschiedener Herkünfte aus herkömmlichen und alternativen Mastverfahren. [Carcass quality of broilers of various strains from conventional and alternative rearing methods]. *Mitteilungsblatt der Budesanstalt für Fleischforschung, Kulmbach* 32, 295–301.

Salama, N.A. (1993) Evaluation of two cooking methods and precooking treatments on characteristics of chicken breast and leg. *Grasas y Aceites* 44, 25–29.

Salter, L.J., Mottram, D.S. and Whitfield, F.B. (1988) Volatile compounds produced in Maillard reactions involving glycine, ribose and phospholipid. *Journal of the Science of Food and Agriculture* 46, 227–242.

Sanderson, G.W., Co, H. and Gonzalez, J.G. (1971) Biochemistry of tea formation: the role of carotenes in black tea aroma formation. *Journal of Food Science* 36, 231–236.

Schliemann, J., Wölm, G., Schrödter, R. and Rutloff, H. (1987) Hühnerfleischaroma – Bildung, Zusammensetzung und Gewinnung. 1. Mitt. Aromavorläufer. [Chicken flavour – Formation, composition and production. 1. Flavour precursors]. *Die Nahrung* 31, 47–56.

Schliemann, J., Wölm, G., Schrödter, R. and Rutloff, H. (1988) Hühnerfleischaroma – Bildung, Zusammensetzung und Gewinnung. 2. Mitt. Aromastoffe. [Chicken flavour – Formation, composition and production. 2. Flavour substances]. *Die Nahrung* 32, 595–607.

Scholtyssek, S. and Sailer, K. (1986) Geschmacksunterschiede im Geflügelfleisch. *Archiv für Geflügelkunde* 50, 49–54.

Schroll, W., Nitz, S. and Drawert, F. (1988) Untersuchungen zum Kocharoma von Hühnerfleisch und -hydrolysaten. [Detection of aroma compounds in cooked chicken meat and hydrolysate]. *Zeitschrift für Lebensmittel Untersuchung und Forschung* 187, 558–560.

Schutte, L. (1974) Precursors of sulfur-containing flavor compounds. *Critical Reviews in Food Science and Nutrition* 4, 457–505.

Sheldon, B.W., Curtis, P.A., Dawson, P.L. and Ferket, P.R. (1997) Effect of dietary vitamin E on the oxidative stability, flavor, color and volatile profiles of refrigerated and frozen turkey breast meat. *Poultry Science* 76, 634–641.

Shi, H. and Ho, C.-T. (1994) The flavour of poultry meat. In: Shahidi, F. (ed.) *Flavor of Meat and Meat Products*. Chapman & Hall, Glasgow, pp. 52–70.

Siegl, H., Leitner, E. and Pfannhauser, W. (1995) Characterisation of flavour compounds in roasted turkey. In: *Proceedings of Current Status and Future Trends. Proceedings of EuroChem VIII*. Vienna, Austria, pp. 490–493.

Skaarup, T. (1983) The quality of meat from free range chickens versus chickens in confinement. In: Lahellec, C., Ricard, F.H. and Colin, P. (eds.) *Proceedings of European Symposium on Quality of Poultry Meat*. Ministère de L'Agriculture, Station Expérimentale d'Aviculture, Ploufragen, France, pp. 37–45.

Sonaiya, E.B., Ristic, M. and Klein, F.W. (1990) Effect of environmental temperature, dietary energy, age and sex on broiler carcase portions and palatability. *British Poultry Science* 31, 121–128.

Spanier, A.M. and Miller, J.A. (1993) Roles of proteins and peptides in meat flavor. In: Spanier, A.M., Okai, H. and Tamura, M. (eds.) *Food Flavor and Safety, Molecular Analysis and Design.* American Chemical Society, Washington, DC, pp. 78–97.

Tandy, J.S. (1986) Chicken flavorants and processes for preparing them. United States Patent no. 4592917.

Tang, J., Jin, Q.Z., Shen, G.H., Ho, C.T. and Chang, S.S. (1983) Isolation and identification of volatile compounds from fried chicken. *Journal of Agricultural and Food Chemistry* 31, 1287–1292.

Tawfik, E.S., Osman, A.M.A., Ristic, M., Hebeler, W. and Klein, F.W. (1990) Einfluss der Stalltemperatur auf Mastleistung, Schlachtkörperwert und Fleischbeschaffenheit von Broilern unterschiedlichen Alters und Geschlechts. 4. Mitteilung: sensorische bewertung der Fleischbeschaffenheit. [Effect of environmental temperature and growth, carcass traits and meat quality of broilers of both sexes and different ages. 4. Report: sensoric test of meat quality]. *Archiv für Geflügelkunde* 54, 14–19.

Thomas, C.P., Dimick, P.S. and MacNeil, J.H. (1971) Sources of flavour in poultry skin. *Food Technology* 25, 109–115.

Touraille, C., Kopp, J., Valin, C. and Ricard, F.H. (1981a) Qualité du poulet. 1. Influence de l'âge et de la vitesse de croissance sur les caractéristiques physico-chimiques et organoleptiques de la viande. *Archiv für Geflügelkunde* 45, 69–76.

Touraille, C., Kopp, J., Valin, C. and Ricard, F.H. (1981b) Qualité du poulet. 2. Evolution en fonction se l'âge des caractéristiques physico-chimiques et organoleptiques de la viande. *Archiv für Geflügelkunde* 45, 97–104.

Touraille, C., Lassaut, B. and Sauvageot, F. (1985) Qualités organoleptiques de viandes de poulets label. *Viandes Produits Carnés* 6, 67–72.

Tressl, R., Helak, B., Martin, N. and Rewicki, D. (1985) Formation of flavour compounds from 1-proline. In: Berger, R., Nitz, S. and Schreier, P. (eds) *Topics in Flavour Research.* Verlag Hangenham, Freising, Germany, pp. 139–160.

van den Ouweland, G.A.M. and Peer, H.G. (1975) Components contributing to beef flavor. Volatile compounds produced by the reaction of 4-hydroxy-5-methyl-3(2H)-furanone and its thio analog with hydrogen sulfide. *Journal of Agricultural and Food Chemistry* 23, 501–505.

van Wassenaar, P.D., van den Oord, A.H.A. and Schaaper, W.M.M. (1995) Taste of 'delicious' beefy meaty peptide. Revised. *Journal of Agricultural and Food Chemistry* 43, 2828–2832.

Vernin, G. and Parkanyi, C. (1982) Mechanisms of formation of heterocyclic compounds in Maillard and pyrolysis reactions. In: Vernin, G. (ed.) *Chemistry of Heterocyclic Compounds in Flavors and Aromas.* Ellis Horwood, Chichester, pp. 151–207.

Werkhoff, P., Brüning, J., Emberger, R., Güntert, M. and Hopp, R. (1993) Flavor chemistry of meat volatiles: New results on flavor components from beef, pork and chicken. In: Hopp, R. and Mori, K. (eds) *Recent Developments in Flavor and Fragrance Chemistry.* VCH, Weinheim, pp. 183–213.

Whitfield, F.B. and Mottram, D.S. (1996) Maillard lipid interactions in low moisture systems. In: Pickenhagen, W., Ho, C.T. and Spanier, A.M. (eds) *Contribution of Low and Non-volatile Materials to the Flavor of Foods.* Allured Publishing, Carol Stream IL, pp. 149–182.

Wirth, F. (1988) Technologies for making fat-reduced meat products. *Fleischwirtschafte* 68, 1153–1156.

Yamasaki, Y. and Maekawa, K. (1978) A peptide with a delicious taste. *Agricultural and Biological Chemistry* 42, 1761–1765.

CHAPTER 6
Poultry meat colour

D.L. Fletcher

Department of Poultry Science, University of Georgia, Athens, GA 30602, USA

INTRODUCTION

One of the most important quality attributes of a food product is appearance. Appearance is often critical for both the initial selection of a product as well as for final sensory evaluation. The major contributing factor to the appearance of many foods is colour, whose importance in our everyday lives is now recognized to be extremely important. However, it is often difficult to comprehend let alone to apply economic value to the colour of foods such as poultry.

Although the importance of colour, especially in art, has long been appreciated, the scientific basis for the study of colour is relatively young and often poorly understood. Colour is more complex than can be defined in purely physical or chemical means, and indeed depends on a fundamental knowledge of both human physiology and psychology.

In poultry, colour is an extremely important quality attribute for eggshell, yolk, skin, meat and bone. Consumers are often willing to pay a premium price for poultry products based on eggshell colour, yolk colour or broiler skin colour. Factors influencing these attributes have major economic importance for producers wishing to establish a premium price or to improve market share. In addition, 'red' or 'pink' fully cooked poultry meat is often considered to be a major defect. Successful manipulation of these colour attributes involves an understanding of colour and colour measurement systems, factors affecting pigment levels in the skin and tissues, processing factors which influence final product colour, and the source of potential colour-related defects.

THE IMPORTANCE OF COLOUR TO POULTRY PRODUCTS

Of the three major food quality attributes, colour, flavour and texture, colour may be the most critical. Colour is the main visual or appearance factor involved in the selection of a food. If colour is deemed unacceptable, the product will not be considered further. Once selected, colour is also important to the ultimate acceptance or rejection of the food on consumption and can indeed affect perceptions of the other major sensory attributes. As important as colour is in the selection and acceptance of a food, there are surprisingly wide variations in colour which fit preconceived ideas of what the most acceptable colour should be for a particular food product (Francis and Clydesdale, 1975).

The wide variations in acceptable poultry colours are exemplified by the regional preferences for broiler skin and egg yolk colour that exist throughout different parts of the world. Differences in the regional preferences for the degree of pigmentation, both in chickens and egg yolks, were reported as early as 1915 by Palmer. Although regional preferences are well established, consumer surveys have often been contradictory. Since most of the surveys were conducted in relatively small geographical sample areas, these contradictions appear to be regional as well.

Even in market areas where the degree of skin pigmentation is not critical, quality control pressures are such that producers must be concerned with product uniformity. Therefore, it is common to see poultry producers who do not feed for any specific level of pigmentation to monitor the source of feeds and the concentration of xanthophyll within the final feed formulation.

With regard to the actual meat colour, the primary issues are muscle type (light and dark meat), colour variation and colour defects. As a general rule, preferences for light meat or dark meat are based on factors other than just colour and the two are generally assessed separately as opposed to being compared directly. Few, if any studies have been conducted to determine the optimum colour of poultry white or dark meat for any particular market. Most colour problems associated with breast meat relate to extremes of paleness (PSE like condition) and darkness which appear as defects when viewed in the context of or in direct comparison with other products. Variations in breast meat colour in multiple-fillet packages is an example of how muscle colour variation can be important. Mottling, or uniformity of colour within a muscle or fillet is almost always considered to be a defect regardless of actual colour preference. In addition, numerous problems and processing defects can occur which cause appearance problems in some products. Bruises, poor bleeding, haemorrhages, bone darkening, and other blood-related problems are not uncommon.

COLOUR MEASUREMENT

Colour itself is not easily defined. The American Heritage College Dictionary (1993) defines colour as, 'that aspect of things that is caused by differing qualities of the light reflected or emitted by them, definable in terms of the observer or the light . . .'. In fact, colour cannot be defined by purely physical or chemical means. For colour, three components must exist: a light source, a detector (or observer) and an object. Whereas light sources can be well defined in physical terms, the detector, either objective (instrumental) or subjective (human), must ultimately be based on sensory data. Colour measurement systems are therefore predicated on the consistent and well-defined conditions of light source and sample presentation.

Determination of colour originally was simply a subjective matter of using colour names and descriptors to describe a specific colour. Such terms as 'bright yellow', 'deep yellow', 'golden yellow' or 'pale yellow' were used to describe poultry products. However, people differ in their ability to see, to visualize and to describe colour accurately. Also, prior to the understanding of light sources, problems in colour matching were widespread. To reduce this problem, visual colour standards were developed to aid in making colour matches. These systems are still very popular today and permeate our society in such simple application as the use of fabric swatches and paint chips. Major efforts have been made in the past century to describe and measure colour in chemical terms. By understanding pigments and their blending properties, it was hoped that colour could be described and manipulated in purely chemical terms. Thus, in some areas, the term pigmentation and colour are often used synonymously, often with confusing and contradictory results. During the past 60 years, instrumental methods have become widespread which use basic principles of standardized light sources, sample presentations, and light detectors to measure colour.

METHODOLOGY

Since methodologies vary, any meaningful discussion of poultry colour must first begin with a definition of colour in terms of how it is measured and described. One of the more confusing aspects of poultry pigmentation has been the inconsistent application of terminology and use of established procedures. As previously noted, the terms pigmentation and colour are not synonymous. Also, it has not been uncommon to find examples in which colour evaluations and pigment assays have been used interchangeably. In other words, colour evaluations have been used to make inferences about pigment utilization or biological availability. Since the chemistry of the pigment determines much about its biological activity in terms of absorption and deposition, and since the colour produced by the pigment may be independent of such biological considerations, it is not surprising that much confusion and contradiction has arisen concerning the evaluation of pigments and colour.

In essence, the procedures that are most commonly used in evaluating product colour or pigment content can be classified into three general categories; visual, chemical-spectrophotometric (including direct pigment analyses) and reflectance colorimetry. In addition, the procedures used to evaluate the pigment content of feedstuffs should also be considered. It should also be noted that this method of classification is not exclusive and some methods may actually be classified under more than one class. Examples of this overlap will be most apparent in descriptions of the chemical-spectrophotometric procedures which can include direct pigment analysis.

Visual

A major problem in studying pigmentation and colour has been in the establishment of colour standards. Although the human eye is capable of discerning very minor differences in colour, problems associated with the subjective nature of describing and quantifying these colour differences reduce the desirability of using subjective scoring systems. To overcome the inherent inaccuracies associated with descriptive colour terms, colour standards were developed against which an egg yolk, poultry product or meat sample could be compared and assigned a more consistent score. An excellent review of the development of visual standards for use with egg yolk colour determinations has been presented by Vuilleumier (1969). Many of these methods were then further developed for use with chicken skin or meat.

Most of the visual standards which have been developed share common attributes. Egg yolk, skin or meat colour ranges are first developed and then matched with a series of pigments, paints or other colour standards. The series is then numbered and colours are expressed against a linear scale. Parker *et al.* (1925) described an 'arbitrary' set of standards developed by matching painted transparencies to match a set of 10 'typical' eggs chosen to represent the range of yolks from 'practically invisible' to 'distinct reddish' on a scale from 1 to 10.

Heiman and Carver (1935) developed a rotor with 24 convex glass discs painted to range in colour from white to brick red by using a mixture of white, Chinese yellow, orange and rich red Duco paints. An egg was placed on a black background and compared to the 24 coloured disks at a 20° presentation angle under a standard light source.

The next major development in visual standards came with the development of the Hoffman–LaRoche yolk colour fan in 1956. The history, development and use of the Roche yolk colour fan was reviewed by Vuilleumier (1969). The Roche colour fan has probably been the most enduring and successful of the visual standards, not only for yolk colour, but also, extensively, for broiler skin colour analysis.

Numerous other visual methods of evaluating egg yolk or skin colour have been developed. Some of these methods pay special attention to presentation, surface gloss, shape, texture and degree of colour possibilities (Fletcher, 1989).

Twining *et al.* (1971) used an arbitrary visual broiler skin pigmentation scale ranging from 1 to 5, where 1 was maximum pigmentation and 5 was nearly devoid of pigmentation. Similar subjective scoring systems have been widely used by commercial producers to evaluate xanthophyll product performance and for routine quality control applications.

Chicken shank colour visual standards have often relied on methods and standards developed for egg yolk colour analyses. Brown (1930) used the Milton Bradley colour top to evaluate yolk colour and shank colour. Ringrose *et al.* (1939) used a series of colour tubes originally developed to measure egg yolk colour to determine the intensity of chick shank colour. Culton and Bird (1941) and Bird (1943) used the Heiman and Carver Yolk Colour Rotor to score chicken shank colour. Marusich (1970) proposed the use of beta-apo-8'-

carotenoic acid ethyl ester as a visual reference standard for broiler pigmentation analyses using the Roche colour fan.

As previously mentioned, the most widely used visual standard for evaluating broiler skin or shank colour has been the Roche colour fan. Other visual standards have also been developed. The Ralston Purina Co. (St Louis, Missouri) produced and distributed a Purina Skin Colour Guide which was a series of colour plates with a textured surface to simulate that of chicken skin. Harms *et al.* (1971) and Twining *et al.* (1971) reported on the use of the Purina Skin Colour Guide. A seven-point scale broiler skin colour standard has also been produced and distributed by American Hoechst. Numerous other 'in-house' or proprietary standards have also been developed and used in limited application.

Waldroup and Johnson (1974) described the lack of agreement between persons using the Roche colour fan to evaluate broiler shank colour. The authors supported the recommendation of Vuilleumier (1969) that colour evaluations using the Roche colour fan should be performed by the same observer or if different observers are used, to test the individuals for colour agreement.

Similar visual standards have also been developed for red meat colour evaluation. Meat colour charts for pork and beef have been produced and distributed for use in localized markets. However, similar colour charts have not been forthcoming for use in poultry meat colour evaluations. The main exception is that many companies have developed proprietary quality control charts for in-house use. Such colour charts are mainly used for process control and enforcement of product specifications in procurement.

More common than strict colour evaluation standards has been the development of visual standards for poultry carcass or meat defects, many of which are colour related. For example, the development of a classification system for broiler carcasses developed by the Commodity Board for Poultry and Eggs in the Netherlands used numerous colour plates for evaluation of defects (Daniëls *et al.,* 1989).

Chemical–spectrophotometric and Direct Pigment Analyses

The subjective nature of visual evaluations, with or without the use of standards, resulted in the need to develop more objective means of colour description. Early attempts to create a more objective means of evaluating colour were based on the chemical extraction and quantification of the carotenoid pigments responsible for colour in skin and the haem pigments found in meat.

Chemical–spectrophotometric procedures have also been applied to broiler skin pigmentation analyses. Heiman and Tighe (1943) developed a method in which a 5/8 inch shank skin punch was extracted in acetone and pigment concentration was determined using a Klett-Summerson photo-electric colorimeter with a blue light filter no. 42. Potter *et al.* (1956) used a similar method to evaluate broiler skin samples removed with a cork borer and extraction with acetone. Determination of carotenoid concentration was made with an Evelyn colorimeter with filter 440. Day and Williams (1958) used a modification of the procedure reported by Heiman and Tighe in which the acetone extracted samples were read on a Coleman Junior spectrophotometer at a wavelength of 436 nm.

Stone *et al.* (1971) compared subjective measurements of shank pigmentation to objective measures of carotenoid concentrations in various tissues of the chicken. They concluded that blood carotenoid concentration (as compared to skin, fat or liver) was the best objective measure to relate to subjective shank scores because of its high repeatability and because blood samples could be used without killing the bird. The work of Twining *et al.* (1971) appears to confirm this observation.

In both red meat and poultry meat, extraction and quantification of the primary muscle pigment myoglobin has been used to evaluate meat colour potential. Since meat colour depends on the chemical state of the myoglobin, evaluation of its content in meat is often only a relative estimate of its potential and is often less important than the reaction state in regard to final meat colour. Procedures to extract and to quantify total haem pigments (myoglobin and haemoglobin) have been well described for red meat (Ginger *et al.* 1954; Fleming *et al.*, 1960) and for poultry (Froning *et al.*, 1968; Saffle, 1973). The extraction and quantification of cytochrome *c*, suspected of contributing to pinkness in cooked turkey meat, was described by Ngoka and Froning (1982).

Problems with both visual scoring systems as well as chemical-spectrophotometric and direct pigment analyses are encountered when these results are assumed to be directly or linearly associated with final product colour. In actuality, this is rarely the case. For example, the Roche Colour Fan and the AOAC methods use what appears to be linear scales to describe non-linear colour values. This becomes most apparent in that egg yolk or skin colour values do not respond in a linear fashion with increasing feed pigment content, specially in the range from yellow to orange. This is also true for the relationship between haem pigment concentrations to final meat colour values where the chemical state of the haem is more critical to final product colour than the absolute amount of haem in the tissue.

Reflectance Colorimetry

The use of reflectance colorimetry to evaluate food colour has been widespread. An excellent review of the principles and uses of colorimetry in foods has been presented by Francis and Clydesdale (1975).

Fry *et al.*, (1969) described the use of reflectance colorimetry to determine skin and shank pigmentation of broilers. The authors used an IDL Colour-Eye with skin and shank samples first removed from the carcass and placed on white backgrounds for colour analyses. Davies *et al.* (1969) reported on the use of a Hunterlab D-20 colour difference meter to measure foot pad, shank, leg and breast skin colour directly on the carcass. In a later work by the same authors (Yacowitz *et al.*, 1978) the actual data in Hunter L, a, b units were presented. Dansky (1971) used a Hunterlab D-20 colour difference meter to evaluate and compare alfalfa meal, alfalfa concentrate, marigold or corn gluten meal on processed broilers. Scholtyssek (1977) described the use of a Hunterlab D23D3 colour difference meter to evaluate broiler colour on a triangular piece of back skin.

Twining *et al.* (1971) used the Hunterlab D-25-A in measuring broiler skin colour and comparing the results to those obtained by visual scoring and plasma carotenoids. Shank visual scoring with the Roche colour fan, skin visual scoring with the Purina skin colour guide, breast skin colour using the Hunter colour difference meter, visual scoring using a five point arbitrary scale and plasma carotenoid concentration were compared. Significant correlations were found between all of the methods when using individual bird data, but when the methods were compared on a treatment basis, only two combinations were significantly correlated: shank scores (Roche colour fan) with visual skin scores (arbitrary scale) and plasma carotenoid concentration with visual skin scores.

Hinton *et al.* (1973) compared both subjective scoring with a Roche colour fan and colorimetric evaluations of both natural and synthetic pigments in broiler diets. The authors reported good correlation between shank and skin colour evaluations and that colorimetric evaluations were more critical in colour differentiation than was visual scoring.

The use of a portable Minolta colorimeter for broiler skin colour has also been evaluated. Janky (1986) reported that use of the Minolta colorimeter would not be applicable for measurements of colour from intact broiler shanks from either live or dead birds. The author also concluded that due to the small sampling area of the Minolta colorimeter, choosing the sample area would have to be carefully controlled or a larger number of samples evaluated in order to obtain meaningful correlations with visual scores. Twining *et al.* (1986) reported high correlations (0.87, 0.91, 0.92 and 0.92) between colour difference measurements with the Minolta colorimeter and the Roche colour fan using live birds.

The major advantages of reflectance colorimetry are its objectivity, accuracy and reproducibility. Major disadvantages are the dependence on equipment which is usually expensive and the abstract nature of colour description systems. Reflectance colorimetric data are difficult to relate to problems associated with feed formulation and consumer acceptance. Where reflectance colorimetry is very well suited for egg yolk colour measurements, it is less applicable for broiler skin colour evaluation due to the non-homogeneity of the skin surface and the small sample area. It is estimated that colorimeters only measure from about 0.03% up to 0.13% of the entire surface of a broiler (Fletcher, 1988).

Although reflectance colorimetry has been widely used in meat colour determinations and extensive references attest to its use, it is of questionable application. Since most reflectance colorimeters are designed to determine colour of opaque surfaces it is assumed that most or all of the light is either reflected or absorbed. Translucent materials, such as meat, often scatter much of the light resulting in poor reproducibility and comparison of colour values (Uijttenboogaart, 1991).

SKIN COLOUR

Market studies in the United States in the early 1960s clearly showed pronounced regional differences in consumers' preferences for fresh whole broilers based solely on skin colour (Raskopf *et al.*, 1961; Courtenay and Branson, 1962; Davis, 1963; Heffner *et al.*, 1964). These studies showed that consumers generally prefer broiler skin colours ranging from white to pale yellow to deeply pigmented based on traditional regional supplies. Marion and Peterson (1987) showed that skin colour still influenced consumers' attitudes towards fresh poultry. Thus consumers tend to favour skin colours which were traditionally available and which were based on local feeding practices as well as genetic stock. In modern markets, consumers still tend to favour their traditional market forms. In the Eastern United States, deeply pigmented birds are the most desired; in the Southeastern US, moderately pigmented birds are preferred; in the Northwestern US, pale skin colour is preferred; in the United Kingdom, consumers prefer a white, non-pigmented skin. Similar differences in colour preferences exist all over the world, and are based primarily on historical and regional supplies.

Because of its market impact, much is known about the factors affecting skin pigmentation. As early as 1915, researchers recognized the principal pigment involved in the coloration of egg yolks and tissues of poultry (Palmer, 1915). Pigmentation, or the deposition of pigments in the skin of the bird, depends on the genetic capability of the bird, dietary pigments, health of the bird and processing. A review of the many factors affecting poultry carotenoid pigmentation was published by Fletcher (1989) and the current state of the art for pigmenting poultry products has been published in symposium form (Sunde, 1992; Hencken, 1992; Hamilton, 1992; Fletcher, 1992; Williams, 1992).

The skin colour of broilers is dependent on the genetic capability of the bird to produce melanin pigments in the dermal or epidermal melanophores and the genetic ability to absorb and then deposit carotenoid pigments in the epidermis (Table 6.1). In most commercial strains melanin production has long been eliminated through selection. With the exception of the Cornish breed, English Class birds lack this genetic ability to deposit carotenoid pigments in the skin thus these birds have a white appearance regardless of diet or other factors. Those birds that have the genetic disposition to deposit the carotenoid pigments in the skin must have them supplied in the diet. For this reason, numerous studies have been conducted to evaluate the skin pigmenting properties of a variety of both natural and synthetic sources. Disease, particularly coccidiosis, has been shown to have dramatic negative effects on pigmentation. Flock health is critical to uniform pigment absorption and deposition. Since the carotenoid pigments are deposited in the epidermis, care must also be exercised in processing not to remove this layer by over-scalding or damaging the skin during picking.

Table 6.1. Combinations of possible skin colour due to dietary xanthophyll being deposited in the epidermis or melanin being produced by the malanophores in either the dermis or epidermis.

Skin colour	Dermis	Epidermis
White	None	None
Yellow	None	Xanthophyll
Black	Melanin	Melanin
Blue (Slate)	Melanin	None
Green	Melanin	Xanthophyll

With the increase in further processing and changing markets, the relative importance of skin colour has decreased in recent years. The predominance of skinless raw products as well as further processing has reduced demand for whole birds and skin-on parts. The increased trend for further processing, which includes numerous breaded or coated products, has also resulted in a requirement by further processors to remove the epidermis during scalding so as to increase coating adherence during further processing and cooking. Thus even in areas which may prefer a yellow skinned bird, further processing demands for removing the epidermis has resulted in decreased economic incentives to maintain high carotenoid levels in the feed.

MEAT COLOUR

Colour of raw poultry meat is critical for consumer selection whereas colour of the cooked meat is critical for final evaluation. Colours which differ from the expected pale tan to pink raw meat or from the tan to grey cooked meat will result in consumer rejection of the product. This is especially true with the appearance of pinkness in fully cooked meat; a major defect in poultry meat products. A recent survey indicated that approximately 7% of skinless-boneless breast fillets, packaged four fillets to a pack, had one or more fillets which were noticeably different from the other three fillets (Fletcher, 1995 unpublished results). In a survey of five commercial broiler processing plants, breast meat colours were found to range with lightness values (L^*) from 43.1 to 48.8 with a strong negative correlation with muscle pH (Fletcher, 1995). These results indicate that significant variations in breast meat colour exist and are present at the retail level.

Mugler and Cunningham (1972) reviewed many of the factors affecting poultry meat colour. Such factors as bird sex, age, strain, processing procedures, chemical exposure, cooking temperature, irradiation and freezing conditions were all shown to affect poultry meat colour. In recent years additional factors have also been identified as affecting poultry meat colour. Froning (1995) presented the most recent review on many of these factors affecting poultry meat colour. Maga (1994) reviewed the primary factors influencing pink discoloration in cooked white meat.

Stress immediately before and during slaughter affects meat colour. Ante-mortem temperature stress and excitement just prior to slaughter have been shown to affect turkey meat colour (Froning *et al.*, 1978; Babji *et al.*, 1982; Ngoka and Froning, 1982). Walker and Fletcher (1993) reported that adrenaline injections just prior to slaughter, to simulate severe ante-mortem stress, resulted in darker breast meat due in part to both a higher muscle pH and increased haemoglobin content of the meat. Electrical stunning at high currents (greater than 100 mA) were shown to increase blood spots in broiler chicken breast meat (Veerkamp, 1987). However, other than for haemorrhaging effects on meat appearance, comparisons of low and high current stunning appears to show little direct effect on broiler breast meat colour (Papinaho and Fletcher, 1995; Craig and Fletcher, 1997). Gas stunning or gas killing has been shown to affect breast meat colour. Raj *et al.* (1990) reported that broiler breast muscles from birds killed with argon were less dark than those killed conventionally or with carbon dioxide. Fleming *et al.* (1991a) found that stunning with carbon dioxide resulted in significantly less red breast and thigh meat compared to electrically stunned turkeys. Maki and Froning (1987) showed that electrical stimulation resulted in redder raw breast meat but lighter cooked breast meat than non-stimulated controls. Froning and Uijttenboogaart (1988) reported that post-mortem electrical stimulation resulted in darker broiler breast meat. However, Owens and Sams (1997) reported no effects of electrical stunning on turkey breast meat colour.

The effect of chilling and leaching of haem pigments on poultry meat colour is not clear. Fleming *et al.* (1991b) reported no effect of immersion versus air chilling on broiler breast or thigh muscle colour or haem content. However, Boulianne and King (1995) attributed pale boneless broiler breast fillets to loss of heme pigments during storage in ice slush tanks. Yang and Chen (1993) found that lightness and redness values of ground breast and thigh meat decrease with storage.

The major contributing factors to poultry meat colour are myoglobin content, the chemical state and reactions of the myoglobin, and meat pH. Myoglobin content has been shown to be primarily related to species, muscle and age of the animal. The chemical state and reactions of myoglobin with other compounds greatly influence meat colour. Muscle pH, which has been shown to be primarily related to the biochemical state of the muscle at time of slaughter and following rigor mortis development, affects both the light reflectance properties of the meat as well as the chemical reactions of the myoglobin. It is the relationship between myoglobin content, and its reactions, as ameliorated by muscle pH that most contribute to meat colour and the occurrence of meat colour defects.

The relationship of animal species, muscle type and animal age on meat myoglobin content and visual colour was presented by Miller (1994). White meat from 8-week-old poultry had the lowest myoglobin content (0.01 mg myoglobin g^{-1} meat) compared to 26-week-old male poultry white meat (0.10 mg g^{-1}), young turkey white meat (0.12 mg g^{-1}), 8-week poultry dark meat (0.40 mg g^{-1}), 26-week male poultry dark meat (1.50 mg g^{-1}), 24-week male turkey dark meat (1.50 mg g^{-1}) and compared to 5-month-old pork (0.30 mg g^{-1}), young lamb (2.50 mg g^{-1}), dark meat fish species (5.3–24.4 mg g^{-1}), white meat fish species (0.30–1.0 mg g^{-1}), 3-year-old beef (4.60 mg g^{-1}), and old beef (16–20 mg g^{-1}).

Because of the importance of both fresh and processed meat colour, the biochemistry of the haem pigments and their reactions that affect meat colour are extremely well documented in the general meat science literature. Bodwell and McClain (1978) present a comprehensive coverage of the myoglobin reactions associated with fresh meat colour and cooking. The various ionic and covalent complexes of both the ferrous and ferric state of the haem with oxygen and other compounds to form the basic meat colour variations from the purplish red of deoxygenated myoglobin to the bright red of oxymyoglobin to the brown/grey of metmyoglobin are well established. Bard and Townsend (1978) discuss numerous haem reactions involved in meat curing. The reactions with various nitrogen compounds and heat to form stable nitrosyl haemochrome complexes to produce the desirable pink colour of cured red meats or the undesirable pinkness of some poultry products. A series of research reports by Ahn and Maurer (1990a,b,c) presented a comprehensive coverage of the complex haem reactions that affect turkey breast meat colour. This series of papers clearly illustrates the complexity of the numerous potential compounds and their effects on turkey meat colour. Their work also illustrated the pronounced effect of muscle pH on the formation of these complexes.

Muscle pH and meat colour are highly correlated. Higher muscle pH is associated with darker meat whereas lower muscle pH values are associated with lighter meat. In the extremes, high pH meat is often characterized as being dark, firm and dry (DFD) and the lighter meat as being pale, soft and exudative (PSE). The effect of pH on meat colour is complex. One effect, as noted earlier, is that many of the haem-associated reactions are pH dependent. In addition, muscle pH affects the water binding nature of the proteins and therefore directly affects the physical structure of the meat and its light reflecting properties (Briskey, 1964). Also, pH affects enzymatic activity of the mitochondrial system thereby altering the oxygen availability for haem reactivity (Ashmore et al., 1972; Cornforth and Egbert, 1985).

Muscle pH has been associated with numerous other meat quality attributes including tenderness, water-holding capacity, cook loss, juiciness and microbial stability (shelf-life). Allen et al. (1997, 1998) showed that variations in breast meat colour, presumably due primarily to pH effects, significantly affect breast meat shelf-life, odour development, moisture pick-up during marination, drip loss, water-holding capacity and cook loss.

VISUAL DEFECTS

Visual defects are those factors that can dramatically affect the appearance of the carcass or meat but may not be directly associated with the pigments, physical or chemical property of the skin or meat. The most important visual defects are those associated with bruising and haemorrhages. The discoloration

Table 6.2. Summary of poultry colour defects.

Defect	Description	Possible causes
Bruises and haemorrhages	Classic bruises, pin-point blood spots in meat, blood accumulation along bones and in joints	Physical trauma, nutrient deficiencies, mycotoxins, stunning
Over-scalding	Incomplete removal of epidermis, cooked discoloration on surface of meat	Too high scalding temperature, too long time in scalder
Surface drying	Mottled appearance of skin or meat due to surface dehydration	Incomplete removal of epidermis, (skin), exposed meat, poor packaging, freezing (freezer burn)
Haem reactions	Normal colour ranges from raw pink meat, tan to brown raw meat, grey to brown cooked meat, pink cooked meat, cured meat colour	Oxidative or redox state of the myoglobin, myoglobin complexing with nitrites/nitrates or other compounds such as carbon monoxide
Dark meat	Darker than normal appearing meat, possible mottling	High muscle pH due to ante-mortem depletion of muscle glycogen
Light meat	Pale breast meat	Low muscle pH (PSE-like condition)
Dark bones	Dark brown to black bones	Freezing, blood accumulation around bone

of muscle tissue due to bruising or due to the accumulation of blood in the tissue due to haemorrhages negatively affect product appearance. If severe enough, bruises and haemorrhages can result in product condemnation or product rejection by the consumer.

Bruising is due to physical trauma (without laceration) resulting in capillary rupture and haemorrhaging (escape of blood from the circulatory system) of blood into the surrounding tissue. Initially a bruise will impart a red discoloration to the damaged tissues but will begin to darken to a blue–black discoloration and finally to green and possibly yellow as the haem compounds degrade. Haemorrhaging refers directly to any capillary or blood vessel rupture resulting in blood pooling in the meat or below the skin. Therefore, bruises are due to ageing of capillary haemorrhaging in the tissue due to physical trauma whereas haemorrhages refers simply to any blood accumulation.

Because bruises are a major source of condemnation and downgrading (Bilgili, 1990) efforts to reduce or control their incidence have been identified. Factors identified which affect bruising include breed/strain, sex, housing density, feathering, bird size and age, season, light intensity, litter conditions, housing ventilation, disease, mycotoxins, vitamins, stress, holding conditions, unloading, hanging, stunning, killing and picking. Tung *et al.* (1971) reported that feed aflatoxins can result in capillary fragility and increased incidences of haemorrhages. Wu *et al.* (1994) found that corn containing *Fusarium moniliforme* resulted in significantly darker and more red turkey breast meat. As presented earlier, electrical stunning has been implicated in contributing to increased haemorrhaging and blood spotting in meat. However, it is often difficult to completely separate haemorrhaging from meat colour issues.

A summary of visual defects is presented in Table 6.2. In addition to bruises and haemorrhaging, processing errors in live bird handling, scalding, and packaging can result in several visual defects as previously described.

REFERENCES

Ahn, D.U. and Maurer, A.J. (1990a) Poultry meat color; kinds of heme pigments and concentrations of the ligands. *Poultry Science* 69, 157–165.

Ahn, D.U. and Maurer, A.J. (1990b) Poultry meat color, Heme-complex-forming ligands and color of cooked turkey breast meat. *Poultry Science* 69, 1769–1774.

Ahn, D.U. and Maurer, A.J. (1990c) Poultry meat color, pH and the heme-complex forming reaction. *Poultry Science* 69, 2040–2050.

Allen, C.D., Russell, S.M. and Fletcher, D.L. (1997) The relationship of broiler breast meat color and pH to shelf-life and odor development. *Poultry Science* 76, 1042–1046.

Allen, C.D., Fletcher, D.L., Northcutt, J.K. and Russell, S.M. (1998) The relationship of broiler breast color to meat quality and shelf-life. *Poultry Science* 77, 361–366.

The American Heritage College Dictionary (1993) Houghton Mifflin Company, Boston.

Ashmore, C.R., Parker, W. and Doerr, L. (1972) Respiration of mitochondria isolated from dark-cutting beef, postmortem changes. *Journal of Animal Science* 34, 46–48.

Babji, A.S., Froning, G.W. and Ngoka, D.A. (1982) The effect of preslaughter environmental temperature in the presence of electrolyte treatment on turkey meat quality. *Poultry Science* 61, 2385–2389

Bard, J. and Townsend, W.E. (1978) Cured meats. In: Price, J.F. and Schweigert, B.S. (eds) *The Science of Meat and Meat Products.* Food and Nutrition Press, Inc., Connecticut, pp. 452–483.

Bilgili, S.F. (1990) Broiler quality, grades are posted. *Broiler Industry* 53(1), 32–40.

Bird, H.R. (1943) Increasing yellow pigmentation in shanks of chickens. *Poultry Science* 22, 205.

Bodwell, C.E. and McClain, P.E. (1978) Chemistry of animal tissues. In: Price, J.F. and Schweigert, B.S. (eds) *The Science of Meat and Meat Products.* Food and Nutrition Press, Inc., Connecticut, pp. 78–207.

Boulianne, M. and King, A.J. (1995) Biochemical and color characteristics of skinless boneless pale chicken breast. *Poultry Science* 74, 1693–1698.

Briskey, E.J. (1964) Etiological status and associated studies of pale, soft, exudative porcine musculature. *Advances in Food Research* 13, 89–178.

Brown, W.L. (1930) Some effects of pimento pepper on poultry. *Georgia Experimental Station Bulletin,* no. 160.

Cornforth, D.P. and Egbert, W.R. (1985) Effect of rotenone and pH on the color of pre-rigor muscle. *Journal of Food Science* 50, 34–35, 44.

Courtenay, H.V. and Branson, R.E. (1962) Consumers image of broilers. *Texas Agricultural Experiment Station, Bulletin* 989.

Craig, E.W. and Fletcher, D.L. (1997) A comparison of high current and low voltage electrical stunning systems on broiler breast rigor development and meat quality. *Poultry Science* 76, 1178–1181.

Culton, T.G. and Bird, H.R. (1941) Effect of certain protein supplements in inhibiting pigment deposition in growing chicks. *Poultry Science* 20, 432.

Daniëls, H.P., Fris, C., Veerkamp, C.H., De Vries, A.W. and Wijnker, P. (1989) *Standard Methods Classification Broiler Carcasses.* Published by Commodity Board for Poultry and Eggs, The Netherlands.

Dansky, L.M. (1971) A role for alfalfa in high efficiency broiler rations. *Poultry Science* 50, 1569.

Davies, R.E., Jones, M.L. and Yacowitz, H. (1969) Direct instrumental measurement of skin colour in broilers. *Poultry Science* 48, 1800.

Davis, B.H. (1963) How do consumers react to broiler pigmentation. *Broiler Business,* July.

Day, E.J. and Williams, W.P. Jr (1958) A study of certain factors that influence pigmentation in broilers. *Poultry Science* 37, 1373.

Fleming, H. P., Blumer, T.N. and Craig, H.B. (1960) Quantitative estimations of myoglobin and hemoglobin in beef muscle extracts. *Journal of Animal Science* 19, 1164–1171.

Fleming, B.K., Froning, G.W., Beck, M.M. and Sosnicki, A.A. (1991a) The effect of carbon dioxide as a preslaughter stunning method for turkeys. *Poultry Science* 70, 2201–2206.

Fleming, B.K., Froning, G.W. and Yang, T.S. (1991b). Heme pigment levels in chicken broilers chilled in ice slush and air. *Poultry Science* 70, 2197–2200.

Fletcher, D.L. (1988) Methods of determining broiler skin pigmentation. *Proceedings of the National Pigmentation Symposium,* p. 37.

Fletcher, D.L. (1989) Factors influencing pigmentation in poultry. *CRC Critical Reviews in Poultry Biology* 2(2), 149–170.

Fletcher, D.L. (1992) Methodology for achieving pigment specifications. *Poultry Science* 71, 733–743.

Fletcher, D.L. (1995) Relationship of breast meat color variation to muscle pH and texture. *Poultry Science* 74 (Suppl. 1), 120.

Francis, F.J. and Clydesdale, F.M. (1975) *Food Colorimetry: Theory and Applications.* AVI Publishing Inc., Westport, Connecticut, p. v.

Froning, G.W. (1995) Color of poultry meat. *Poultry and Avian Biology Reviews* 6(1), 83–93.

Froning, G.W. and Uijttenboogaart, T.G. (1988) Effect of post-mortem electrical stimulation on color, texture, pH, and cooking loss of hot and cold deboned chicken broiler breast meat. *Poultry Science* 67, 1536–1544.

Froning, G.W., Daddario, J. and Hartung, T.E. (1968) Color and myoglobin concentration in turkey meat as affected by age, sex, and strain. *Poultry Science* 47, 1827–1835.

Froning, G.W., Babji, A.S. and Mather, F.B. (1978) The effect of preslaughter temperature, stress, struggle and anesthetization on color and textural characteristics of turkey muscle. *Poultry Science* 57, 630–633.

Fry, J.L., Ahmed, E.M., Herrick, G.M. and Harms, R.H. (1969) A reflectance method of determining skin and shank pigmentation. *Poultry Science* 48, 1127.

Ginger, I.D., Wilson, G.D. and Schweigert, B.S. (1954) Biochemistry of myoglobin quantitative determination in beef and pork muscle chemical studies with purified metmyoglobin. *Journal of Agricultural and Food Chemistry* 2, 1037–1040.

Hamilton, P.B. (1992) The use of high-performance liquid chromatography for studying pigmentation. *Poultry Science* 71, 718–724.

Harms, R.H., Ahmed, E.H. and Fry, J.L. (1971) Broiler pigmentation – factors affecting it and problems in its measurement *Proceedings of the Maryland Nutrition Conference*, p. 81.

Heffner, J., Roy, E.P., Davis, B.H. and Hilton, W.B. (1964) Consumer preference for broiler pigmentation in New Orleans, *Louisiana, Bulletin 586,* Louisiana Agricultural Experiment Station.

Heiman, V. and Carver, J.S. (1935) The yolk color index. *The U.S. Egg and Poultry Magazine,* August.

Heiman, V. and Tighe, L.W. (1943) Observations on the shank pigmentation of chicks. *Poultry Science* 22, 102.

Hencken, H. (1992) Chemical and physiological behavior of feed carotenoids and their effects on pigmentation. *Poultry Science* 71, 711–717.

Hinton, C.F., Fry, J.L. and Harms, R.H. (1973) Subjective and colorimetric evaluation of the xanthophyll utilization of natural and synthetic pigments in broiler diets. *Poultry Science* 52, 2169.

Janky, D.M. (1986) The use of the Minolta Reflectance Chroma Meter II for pigmentation evaluation of broiler shanks. *Poultry Science* 65, 491.

Maga, J.A. (1994) Pink discoloration in cooked white meat. *Food Reviews International* 10(3), 273–286.

Maki, A. and Froning, G.W. (1987) Effect of post-mortem electrical stimulation on quality of turkey meat. *Poultry Science* 66, 1155–1157.

Marion, J.E. and Peterson, R.A. (1987) Composition, pigmentation, and yield by parts of different brands of broilers in grocery stores. *Poultry Science* 66, 1174–1179.

Marusich, W.L. (1970) Collaborative ANRC broiler pigmentation standard study – final report. *Feedstuffs* 42(10), 30.

Miller, R.K. (1994) Quality characteristics. In: Kinsman, D.M., Kotula, A.W. and Breidenstein, B.C. (eds) *Muscle Foods; Meat, Poultry, and Seafood Technology.* Chapman & Hall, New York, pp. 296–332.

Mugler , D.J. and Cunningham, F.E. (1972) Factors affecting poultry meat color – a review. *World's Poultry Science Journal* 28(4), 400–406.

Ngoka, D.A. and Froning, G.W. (1982) Effect of free struggle and preslaughter excitement on color of turkey breast muscles. *Poultry Science* 61, 2291–2293.

Owens, C.M. and Sams, A.R. (1997) Muscle metabolism and meat quality of pectoralis from turkeys treated with postmortem electrical stimulation. *Poultry Science* 76, 1047–1051.

Palmer, L.S. (1915) Xanthophyll, the principal natural yellow pigment of the egg yolk, body fat, and blood serum of the hen. The physiological relation of the pigment to the xanthophyll of plants. *Journal of Biological Chemistry* 23, 261–279.

Papinaho, P.A. and Fletcher, D.L. (1995) Effect of stunning amperage on broiler breast muscle rigor development and meat quality. *Poultry Science* 74, 1527–1532.

Parker, S.L., Gossman, S.S. and Lippincott, W.A. (1925) Studies on egg quality, I, Introductory note on variations in yolk color. *Poultry Science* 5, 131.

Potter, L.M., Bunnell, R.H., Matterson, L.D. and Singsen, E.P. (1956) The effect of antioxidants and a vitamin B_{12} concentrate on the utilization of carotenoid pigments by the chicks. *Poultry Science* 35, 452.

Raj, M. A.B., Grey, T.C., Audsely, A.R. and Gregory, N.G. (1990) Effect of electrical and gaseous stunning on the carcass and meat quality of broilers. *British Poultry Science* 31, 725–733.

Raskopf, B.D., Kidd, I.H. and Goff, O.E. (1961) Effects of diets containing milo on broilers. *Tennessee Agricultural Experimental Station Bulletin* no. 324.

Ringrose, R.C., Norris, L.C. and Heuser, G.F. (1939), The value of corn gluten meal for feeding poultry. *Cornell Agricultural Experimental Station Bulletin* no. 725.

Saffle, R.L. (1973) Quantitative determinaton of combined hemoglobin and myoglobin in various poultry meats. *Journal of Food Science* 38, 968–970.

Scholtyssek, V.S. (1977) Ein technisches verfahren zur bestimmung der pigmentierung von broilern einschlieslich zweier anwendungsbeispiele. *Archives Geflugelkunde* 41, 37.

Stone, H.A., Collins, W.M. and Urban, W.E. Jr (1971) Evaluation of carotenoid concentration in chicken tissue. *Poultry Science* 50, 675.

Sunde, M.L. (1992) Introduction to the symposium; the scientific way to pigment poultry products. *Poultry Science* 71, 709–710.

Tung, H.T., Smith, J.W. and Hamilton, P.B. (1971) Aflatoxicosis and bruising in the chicken. *Poultry Science* 50, 795–800.

Twining, P.V. Jr, Bossard, E.H., Lund, P.G. and Thomas, O.P. (1971) Relative availability of xanthophylls from ingredients based on plasma levels and skin measurements, *Proceedings of the Maryland Nutrition Conference* p. 90.

Twining, P.V. Jr, Quarles, C.L. and Schwartz, J.H. (1986) The evaluation of the Minolta Croma Meter for reading shank pigmentation of live broilers. *Poultry Science* 65 (Suppl. 1), 196.

Uijttenboogaart, T.G. (1991) Colour of fresh and cooked poultry meat. *Workshop on Welfare, Hygiene, and Quality Aspects of Poultry Processing.* University of Bristol, October, pp. 16–17.

Veerkamp, C.H. (1987) Stunning and killing broilers. *Proc. 8th European Symposium on Poultry Meat Quality,* Budapest, Hungary, pp. 121–126.

Vuilleumier, J.P. (1969) The 'Roche Yolk Color Fan' – an instrument for measuring yolk color. *Poultry Science* 48, 767.

Waldroup, P.W. and Johnson, Z.B. (1974) Lack of repeatability among persons using the Roche color fan to assess the shank color of broilers. *Poultry Science* 53, 437.

Walker, J.M. and Fletcher, D.L. (1993) Effect of ante-mortem epinephrine injections on broiler breast meat color, pH, and heme concentration. *Poultry Science* 72 (Suppl. 1), 138.

Williams, W.D. (1992) Origin and impact of color on consumer preference for food. *Poultry Science* 71, 744–746.

Wu, W., Jerome, D. and Nagaraj, R. (1994) Increased redness in turkey breast muscle induced by Fusarial culture materials. *Poultry Science* 73, 331–335.

Yacowitz, H., Davies, R.E. and Jones, M.L. (1978) Direct instrumental measurement of skin color in broilers. *Poultry Science* 57, 443.

Yang, C.C. and Chen, T.C. (1993) Effects of refrigerated storage, pH adjustment, and marinade on color of raw and microwave cooked chicken meat. *Poultry Science* 72, 355–362.

PART II
Production and harvesting factors affecting meat quality

CHAPTER 7
Live production factors influencing yield and quality of poultry meat

E.T. Moran, Jr
Poultry Science Department, Auburn University, AL 36849-5416, USA

INTRODUCTION

Poultry meat originates with the live bird. Throughout live production many factors influence its ultimate value for the consumer. These factors may be simplistically categorized as age of the bird at marketing, sex, genetic background, nutrition received and environment. Product value represents a combination of amount and quality relative to cost. Measurements of quality differ with the progression from live bird to carcass and consumer. The following is an overview of facets in live production as they influence yield of poultry meat and quality characteristics. This information overwhelmingly relates to the broiler chicken because of its world dominance in all respects.

AGE AND SEX

Growth that occurs with age is accurately represented by the Gompertz function (Knizetova *et al.*, 1991). Most broilers and turkeys are marketed at the inflection point which is a transition from an increasing to decreasing rate of growth that occurs from juvenile to adolescent development. Females have an inflection point a few days in advance of males. The sum of all changes that occur during the interim influence carcass and meat characteristics and are of particular importance.

Growth of skeleton, muscles and fat depots are continually being altered. The gastrointestinal system decreases as the need to support rapid growth diminishes; in turn, yield of the carcass after processing improves (Moran, 1977). Muscle growth continues at the inflection point as skeletal development diminishes and an increase in overall meat yield occurs. The breast musculature is a dominant contributor in this respect and defects to this part that result in downgrading are important to carcass quality. Bruising increases with age and weight of the bird due to handling in preparation for slaughter, particularly that creating extensive muscular damage (Mayes, 1980b). The relative incidence of breast blisters parallels bruising (Mayes, 1980a). Males generally suffer from both defects more than females.

Growth of the body's muscles may not remain proportional to one another with change in age. Breast and thigh muscles differ in emphasis with development. Breast musculature is negligible at hatch, then extraordinary growth occurs for 2 weeks which subsequently diminishes. Thigh muscles are well developed at hatch, whereupon their growth is moderate until 2 weeks and similar to breast thereafter (Iwamoto et al., 1993). Presumably, advanced thigh development relates to the need for emergence and posthatch mobility.

Muscle growth through juvenile development can be attributed to progressive increases in fibre length and diameter. The pectoralis major is the overwhelming contributor to breast meat and its fibres are exclusively the fast-glycolytic (IIB) type (Smith and Fletcher, 1988). Many muscles contribute to thigh meat, each of which can differ in the proportions of slow-oxidative (I), fast-oxidative glycolytic (IIA) and fast-glycolytic (IIB) fibres (Iwamoto et al., 1993).

Fibre contribution to the thigh muscles may change with age. A decrease in the proportion of type IIB in some muscles is more than recovered by an expansion in diameter to make them a major contributor with growth (Table 7.1). Breast having all type IIB fibres exhibits a particular advantage in growth over other muscles because of dominance in this respect.

Breast and thigh muscles also change in their composition with age, especially at the inflection point. Touraille et al. (1981) performed an array of measurements with experimental male chickens having an inflection point between 12 and 14 weeks of age. At these ages, lipid in pectoralis major and the composite of thigh muscles decreased (Table 7.2). Collagen associated with breast decreased in total; whereas, its solubility as a proportion of total collagen in thigh increased with myoglobin. Overall changes in sensory

Table 7.1. Growth of breast and thigh muscles by fibre type and size[1].

Age (weeks)	Weight (g)	Type II A		Type II B	
		%	Diameter (µm)	%	Diameter (µm)
Pectoralis major					
1	1.78	0	—	100	10.1
2	4.48	0	—	100	17.7
5	14.3	0	—	100	23.2
10	34.1	0	—	100	30.2
15	62.6	0	—	100	38.3
20	95.6	0	—	100	47.1
Iliotibialis					
1	0.32	21.5	9.4	78.6	9.3
2	0.73	34.3	11.8	65.7	14.2
5	2.58	36.6	20.7	63.4	25.6
10	6.99	35.9	29.5	64.1	38.7
15	11.9	39.1	31.5	60.9	40.1
20	18.6	39.1	40.3	60.9	49.0

[1]Selected data from Ono et al. (1993) using male New Hamphire chickens.

Table 7.2. Composition of breast and thigh muscles of broiler males from juvenile to preadolescent development[1].

Age (weeks)	Muscle 'as is'			% Dry matter	myoglobin (mg g⁻¹ DM)	Collagen		mg CP g⁻¹ 'as is'		Total lipid % 'as is'
	wt (g)	% Live wt	pH			mg g⁻¹ DM	% Soluble	Total	myofibre	
Total breast muscle[2]										
8	113	10.3	5.9	25.2	0.48	8.7	–	36.2	17.5	1.79
10	145	10.2	–	23.9	0.48	8.0	–	38.3	17.4	1.41
12	196	10.3	5.8	25.6	0.45	8.7	–	36.5	16.9	1.39
14	261	11.5	5.7	24.7	0.46	6.6	–	37.3	17.1	1.04
16	319	12.5	5.9	24.6	0.50	7.3	–	40.9	19.4	1.05
Total thigh muscle[2]										
8	105	9.5	6.2	25.4	1.12	16.1	32.2	31.2	16.6	5.20
10	131	9.2	–	23.9	1.39	16.5	30.0	31.9	18.7	4.40
12	184	9.6	6.2	24.5	1.63	16.1	27.8	33.0	17.6	4.53
14	224	9.9	6.0	23.6	1.57	16.7	–	31.6	–	3.70
16	276	10.8	6.1	25.6	1.53	17.4	26.5	34.4	19.7	3.58

[1] Selected data from Touraille *et al.* (1981) using experimental chicken males.
[2] Breast muscle was the pectoralis major, whereas, the thigh muscles were all represented.

evaluations with age favour tenderness when young, and flavour after the approximate inflection point in growth (Touraille *et al.*, 1981; Scholtyssek and Sailer, 1986).

GENETICS

The amounts of meat and fat on the carcass together with live performance are desirable traits in meat bird genetics. Given that the inflection point represents a benchmark for transitions that influence carcass quality, then awareness of its occurrence would be important in any selection strategy. Knizetova *et al.* (1991) evaluated the Gompertz function for nine broiler lines and observed that the age of inflection varied between 48 and 56 days for cockerels and 48 and 53 days for females. Gous *et al.* (1992) found similar ages using six breeds of commercial broilers (45–50 days for cockerels and 45–53 days for females).

Concurrent selection to increase meat yield and decrease fatness is not antagonistic. Overall results from a symposium conducted by Leclercq and Whitehead (1988) supports the view that direct and/or indirect measurements of either trait may be used without adverse effect on the other. Such selection is known to be of advantage for improved feed conversion, decreased fatness and increased meat; but, a variety of results occurs to carcass appearance.

A large part of total body fat is in the skin, particularly in association with the main feather tracts. Apparently, these depots can act to minimize the effect and/or perception of traumas from handling prior to slaughter. A decrease of this fat layer along the pelvic back results in an accentuation of bruising (Table 7.3). Conversely, skin tears that occur with processing usually appear along feather tracts and a decrease in fatness also reduces their likelihood.

Genetic improvement in meat yield has focused on the breast because of its extensive contribution to the total and economic value. Either subjective scoring of its prominence relative to the keel (Vereijken, 1992) or direct measurement of depth (Migineishvili, 1991) have proven to be effective for selection in this respect. Accentuation of breast musculature appears to protect the associated skeleton from abuse. A comparison of several commercial source males differing in their percentage of pectoralis major correlate with the relief of breast blisters and to a lesser extent the incidence of broken clavicles (Table 7.4).

Selection for increased breast meat does not appear to be fully realized until the inflection point in growth. Acar *et al.* (1993) measured pectoralis major development between two commercial source broilers known to differ in this respect. Although the greatest proportion of muscle growth occurred in the first 2 weeks, strain difference did not maximize until the inflection point, which occurred at 7–8 weeks of age. Concentrations of DNA and RNA decreased with age and were identical between strains.

Table 7.3. Abdominal fat and appearance of defects associated with the chilled carcasses from diverse strains of commercial broilers and the influence of sex (7 weeks of age)[1].

Contrasts	Carcass[2] (g)	Abdominal fat (%)	Wings Dislocated (%)	Wings Broken (%)	Wings Bruise (%)	Breast Blister (%)	Breast Broken clavicle (%)	Back Bruise (%)	Back Skin tear (%)	Drum red hock (%)	Grade A (%)
Strain	*	***	NS	*	*	NS	NS	*	*	NS	*
A	1926^a	2.95^b	9.9	4.3^{ab}	20.7^a	2.4	22.0	14.7^{ab}	6.5^{ab}	5.6	46.6^{ab}
B	1863^b	2.75^c	13.2	7.4^a	13.6^{ab}	3.4	20.2	25.0^a	4.4^b	8.3	42.0^b
C	1869^b	3.15^a	12.2	1.2^b	9.9^b	0.8	14.5	12.5^b	9.1^a	6.1	56.5^a
D	1858^b	3.02^b	12.8	2.7^{ab}	11.3^b	2.0	23.4	13.2^{ab}	5.5^{ab}	6.4	56.2^{ab}
Sex	***	***	**	**	NS	**	**	NS	***	*	NS
M	2072	2.67	15.2	5.9	12.6	3.9	23.8	17.2	3.1	2.5	49.5
F	1686	3.27	8.8	1.9	15.1	0.4	16.8	15.5	9.7	10.6	51.0

Figures in any one column not having a common letter are statistically significant ($P < 0.05$).
[1]Data are presented as contrasts of strains and sex in the absence of significant interactions ($P > 0.05$). E.T. Moran, unpublished data.
[2]Carcass after 4 h static chilling in slush-ice without neck and giblets.

Table 7.4. Yield of pectoralis major and incidence of breast defects among commercial strains of broiler males at 7 weeks of age[1]. (Data from Moran, 1996b.)

Strain	Chilled carcass[2]		Pectoralis major		% Breast defects		Grade A (%)
	wt (g)	% of live wt	wt (g)	% of carcass	Blister	Broken clavicle	
A	2245[a]	69.0[a]	509[a]	23.3[a]	0.6[c]	23.4[c]	48.7[a]
B	1932[c]	64.8[c]	383[c]	19.8[c]	29.2[a]	48.5[a]	34.2[b]
C	2127[b]	66.4[b]	439[b]	20.9[b]	19.8[b]	32.7[b]	30.3[b]
D	2166[b]	67.1[b]	492[a]	22.7[a]	1.9[c]	32.7[b]	32.7[b]

Figures in any one column not having a common letter are statistically significant ($P < 0.05$).
[1]All birds were reared in pens on pine shaving litter, then processed 'on-line' using automated equipment typical of commercial plants.
[2]Carcass without neck, giblets, and abdominal fat on an absolute basis and relative to the full-fed live weight after 4 h of static immersion chilling in slush-ice.

Selection for whole body growth where all muscles benefit led to an increase in total myofibre number and cross-sectional area, but the proportions of fibre types is not perceptibly altered (Remignon *et al.*, 1994, 1995). Fast-glycolytic (type IIB) fibres expand their cross-sectional area more so than the other fibre types and the pectoralis major benefits to the largest extent (Table 7.5). Although such accentuation of type IIB tends to increase glycolytic metabolic influence associated with the meat, no significant alteration in pH, colour and drip loss occur (Remignon *et al.*, 1996).

Turkeys appear to respond to selection for growth and breast meat yield in a similar manner to broiler chickens. Swatland (1980) examined commercial strains having the same body weights but different amounts of breast meat. The pectoralis major from the low-yielding strain had myofibre cross-sectional areas 80–85% of those from the high-yielding strain.

Meat composition is a function of many issues. Given a potentially large

Table 7.5. Pectoralis major development and myofibre cross-sectional area between fast-growing (FGL) and slow-growing (SGL) lines of chickens[1]. (From Remignon *et al.*, 1995.)

Age (weeks)	Body weight (g)		P. major (g)		Myofibre[2] (μm^2)	
	FBL	SGL	FGL	SGL	FGL	SGL
0	36	31	—	—	20	23
1	84	43	—	—	62	27
3	285	119	8.9	3.0	244	165
5	670	230	24.6	7.0	537	301
11	1882	675	84.2	26.3	1256	664
55	3685	1883	181.2	82.8	2754	1946

[1]Chickens selected over 31 generations for fast or slow growth.
[2]All myofibres were classified as fast glycolytic IIB.

array of selection strategies that involve growth rate, breast meat yield, fatness and fecundity, variation in meat composition among commercial sources of meat birds is to be expected. Xiong *et al.* (1993) measured composition, pH and protein extractability on pectoralis major plus minor to represent breast meat and all muscles of the thigh on eight broiler sources. Although their results reveal considerable variation, its meaning for food manufacturing and consumer is elusive. Large differences in fatness are known to have minimal influence on sensory value (Chambers *et al.*, 1989).

NUTRITION

Feeds used in the commercial production of meat birds are usually formulated on the basis of minimum nutrient requirements. The National Research Council (1994) values are given for progressive intervals from start until marketing to accommodate alteration in growth. Such 'requirements' must be considered as no more than 'estimates' given their fixed nature through periods when extent and type of growth is constantly changing. Genetic differences further defy any one value being the 'requirement'. Hancock *et al.* (1995) characterized growth and compositional alterations with six commercial genotypes. Differences were sufficiently extensive to warrant separate nutrient requirements.

Although an inadequacy of any nutrient is bound to have repercussions on the amount of meat and perhaps quality, only a few are of consistent concern in practice. Feeds are invariably assembled on a least-cost basis using ingredient prices together with their nutrient contents. In most situations, attaining the requirements for a few nutrients is particularly expensive and calculated levels do not exceed the stated minimum. More often than not, these few nutrients are energy, protein and phosphorus.

Inadequacies of these few nutrients in a commercial context are usually submarginal to need rather than any blatant deficiency. Expression of these 'small' inadequacies is seldom obvious in terms of live performance, but repercussions become progressively important to yield and quality as product objective proceeds to carcass then further-processed parts. Breast musculature, which represents about one-third of all meat and nearly half the total edible protein, is particularly vulnerable in its skinless boneless form.

Energy levels employed in 'high performance' feeds require the use of added fat, which is the most expensive contributor in this respect. Reduction in energy, particularly with a decrease in either fat or its digestibility, is unlikely to have an adverse effect when the levels of all other nutrients are maintained. On the contrary, additional feed intake occurs in response to a reduction in feed energy level, in turn so does intake of associated nutrients. Moran (1997) replaced added dietary fat with corn in the diets of male broilers. Although feed conversion was adversely affected, body weight, carcass quality and skinless–boneless meat yield did not suffer. Consumption of additional protein in this manner fosters a reduction in fatness (Cornejo *et al.*, 1991).

Should reduction in dietary energy be accompanied by a commensurate decrease in other nutrients, particularly protein, then a feed 'dilution' occurs.

These dilutions necessitate increased feed intake which cannot readily be accommodated by the very young and early growth is impaired; however, subsequent adaptation enables recovery in all respects that becomes assured as marketing age is lengthened (Campbell *et al.*, 1988; Moran, 1996a).

Protein inadequacies affect the amount of meat more than its quality. Asghar *et al.* (1986a, b) provided 'submaintenance feeding' to growing broilers from 4 to 8 weeks of age that reduced yield of breast and thigh muscle weights by 30–35% of those fed *ad libitum*. Overall, sarcoplasmic protein was reduced to a small extent only in breast as were lysosomal, microsomal and soluble fractions. However, no single protein or fraction of proteins was distinct in this respect, other than collagen which tended to increase and alter its amino acid composition. In another study, Roth *et al.* (1990) increased dietary protein of broilers during ages corresponding to the inflection point in a manner that enabled additional breast meat formation. Measurement of amino acid retention by meat was of a consistent pattern with few alterations (Table 7.6).

Table 7.6. Effect of dietary protein supply on the amino acid retention in breast meat of broiler males between 5 and 8 weeks of age[1].

Amino acid	21.0 g day⁻¹		27.3 g day⁻¹		33.5 g day⁻¹	
	mg total	%	mg total	%	mg total	%
Essential						
Arginine	96[a]	7.6	133[b]	7.5	157[c]	7.6
Histidine	52[a]	4.2[A]	95[b]	5.4[B]	107[b]	5.1[B]
Isoleucine	60[a]	4.6[B]	83[b]	4.7[B]	86[b]	4.3[A]
Leucine	104[a]	8.2	145[b]	8.1	168[c]	8.2
Lysine	135[a]	10.6	190[b]	10.6	223[c]	10.8
Methionine	35[a]	2.8	53[b]	3.0	57[b]	2.8
Phenylalanine	48[a]	3.8	68[b]	3.7	83[c]	3.9
Threonine	67[a]	5.3[B]	91[b]	5.2[B]	100[b]	4.8[A]
Valine	61[a]	4.8[B]	83[b]	4.7[B]	85[b]	4.1[A]
Total	673[a]	53.0[A]	960[b]	54.0[b]	1089[c]	52.7[A]
Non-essential						
Alanine	66[a]	5.1[A]	97[b]	5.4[B]	121[c]	5.8[c]
Aspartic acid	128[a]	10.0[B]	164[b]	9.2[A]	214[c]	10.2[B]
Glutamic acid	193[a]	15.2[B]	247[b]	13.9[A]	305[c]	14.7[B]
Glycine	45[a]	3.4[A]	69[b]	3.9[B]	83[c]	3.9[B]
Proline	49[a]	3.9[B]	70[b]	4.0[B]	75[b]	3.6[A]
Serine	53[a]	4.3[AB]	78[b]	4.5[B]	86[b]	4.1[A]
Tyrosine	45[a]	3.6	64[b]	3.6	73[c]	3.5
Total	598[a]	47.0[B]	816[b]	46.0[A]	987[c]	47.3[B]
Crude protein[2]	1246[a]	102.0	1769[b]	100.3	2123[c]	98.6

[1]Selected data from Roth *et al.* (1990). Dietary protein came from conventional feedstuffs and was balanced with respect to amino acid proportions.
[2]Amino acids as 16 g N.
[a–c]in rows corresponds to multiple range test for mg total amino acid, whereas[A–B] relates to % (mg amino acid per 100 mg amino acids).

Protein inadequacies may be encountered in commercial practice in any one of three situations. Dietary protein is usually decreased in a progression of feeds from start to finish in a manner that satisfies need and economics. These feeds also decrease markedly in cost. Providing later feeds early in the progression is economically favourable but limits protein intake. Although little impact is apparent on live performance, carcass fatness increases (Saleh *et al.*, 1996) and breast meat recovery in further processing suffers (Table 7.7).

Failure to provide sufficient amounts of limiting essential amino acids also impairs meat formation. Lysine is of particular concern because of its very high proportions in muscle protein and its usual marginal levels in most feeds. Such inadequacies are likely to occur prior to marketing and result in additional carcass fat and decreased breast meat yield (Moran and Bilgili, 1989; Holsheimer and Rueskin, 1993). Although sulphur amino acid inadequacies are also common, their potential impact is less than lysine because relative muscle content is low whereas final feeds are seldom limiting in this respect (Moran, 1994).

There has recently been concern about the non-essential amino acids. The availability of lysine, methionine, tryptophan and threonine for commercial use often leads to a reduction in total crude protein. Even though 'requirements' for all the essential amino acids have been satisfied, increased fatness and reduced breast meat yields occur when there is extensive reduction in crude protein (Moran and Bushong, 1992). Marginal decreases in crude protein do not alter meat yield; but, additional fatness is obvious and an accentuation of carcass bruising is seen (Moran and Stilborn, 1996). Reduced fatness and relief of bruising by supplemental glutamic acid suggests a need for non-essential amino acids to fully realize connective tissue formation.

Table 7.7. Effect of abbreviating the feeding sequence of advocated nutrient levels on broiler males over a 7-week production period[1]. (From Moran, 1996b.)

	Live bird and processed carcass				
	Live gain (g)	F/G	% Carcass[2]	Abdominal fat (g)	% Grade A
Regimen[3]	NS	*	***	***	NS
NRC	3192	1.87	67.5	40	35.1
Abbrev.	3138	1.89	66.3	45	37.7

	Further processing yields (g)[4]				
	Wings	Drums	P. major	P. minor	Thigh meat
Regimen	NS	NS	**	*	NS
NRC	244	298	466	107	335
Abbrev.	241	297	450	103	325

[1]Represented by four different strain-crosses and four replicates.
[2]Carcass without neck, giblets, and abdominal fat; static slush-ice chilled for 4 h
[3]NRC regimen corresponded to three progressive feeds each meeting advocated nutrient levels through to 7 weeks of age (i.e. 0–3, 3–6 and 6–7 weeks). The abbreviated regimen reduced access to the first two feeds (i.e. 0–2, 2–5 and 5–7 weeks).
[4]Cone-deboned by processing plant personnel.

Phosphorus requirements necessitate the use of relatively expensive inorganic ingredients in most feeds. Contrary to submarginal protein, phosphorus inadequacies tend to improve live performance without adverse effects on either carcass fatness or skinless–boneless meat yield (Moran and Todd, 1994). Such inadequacies appear to 'weaken' the skeleton and advantage to live performance arises from a lack of ready mobility, in turn, decreasing energy expenditure. Absence of live performance 'sensitivity' to low phosphorus has occasionally been extended to omitting inorganic sources from the final feed as an economic measure to which there are no obvious repercussions on the whole carcass (Chen and Moran, 1994).

The consequence of low dietary phosphorus does not appear until further-processing, then an array of carcass defects which reduce quality are seen. Impaired mobility, on the one hand, is of advantage by reducing breast blisters and back bruising; however, increased skeletal vulnerability to the traumas of transportation and automated processing lead to additional broken bones (Table 7.8). Such breakages create bloodsplash, if occurring in the live bird, and bone chips which are a concealed consumer threat when they occur during processing.

ENVIRONMENT

The environmental influences on poultry meat may be either direct or indirect. Temperature and lighting are influential in large part by modulating feed intake; whereas, stocking density and flooring impose varying conditions to the body itself. No one environmental factor is 'unto itself', but each has the ability to modify expression of the others.

Temperature alters feed intake by influencing energy 'need.' Energy is needed to support productive activity and maintain daily functions. Optimal environmental temperatures enable growth to maximize while maintenance is minimal. Although body mechanisms exist to continue favourable operation with moderate departures from optimum, extensive change has an impact on the carcass. Smith and Teeter (1987) compared cold and hot environments with optimal, using broilers grown through juvenile development (Table 7.9). Ad libitum feed consumption increased by 25% when temperature was reduced to ca. 7°C and both meat and fat deposition decreased. Increasing the temperature to 35°C decreased feed intake by 10% and again both meat yield and fatness decreased.

High temperatures are the most difficult to accommodate in practice and repercussions are accentuated when dietary nutrient adequacy is compromised. Marginal protein and essential amino acids are particularly influential in increasing body fatness (Halvorson et al., 1991; Cahaner et al., 1995; Waibel et al., 1995). Likewise, the extent of feathering can influence the body's ability to either conserve or dissipate heat, which in turn alters expression of fatness (Hanzl and Somes, 1983: Ajang et al., 1993). Breast meat usually suffers more than other parts of the carcass when body weight is not fully realized (Howlinder and Rose, 1989; Smith, 1993); however, these adverse effects do not readily alter sensory value (Sonaiya et al., 1990).

Table 7.8. Effect of a chronic phosphorus inadequacy during rapid development followed by omission of inorganic phosphate from the final feed on broiler males further-processed at 7 weeks of age[1]. (Data from Chen and Moran, 1995.)

			Whole chilled carcass	
	Preslaughter	Abdominal	Carcass without abdom. fat	
Contrast	wt loss (g)	fat wt (g)	weight (g)	% preslaughter wt
3–6 weeks	NS	***	***	*
NRC	169	55	1909	67.8
Low AP	184	45	1769	67.2
6–7 weeks	*	NS	NS	NS
NRC	186	50	1852	67.5
w/o Ca P	167	50	1827	67.5

	Incidence of carcass defects (%)			
	Broken		Breast	Back
	Drumsticks	Clavicle	blister	bruised
3–6 weeks	NS[2]	NS	**	***
NRC	0.6	25.0	26.3	22.1
Low AP	2.8	25.3	17.0	13.6
6–7 weeks	*[2]	*	*	**
NRC	0.5	21.3	28.9	21.3
w/o Ca P	3.0	29.0	18.4	14.4

	Further-processed parts			
	% Skinless–boneless meat		Femur[3]	
	P. major	Thigh	kg Max. load	% Broken head
3–6 weeks	NS	NS	***	NS
NRC	20.5	15.5	31.4	9.3
Low AP	20.5	15.2	25.3	13.1
6–7 weeks	NS	NS	***	***
NRC	20.3	15.4	31.6	3.0
w/o Ca P	20.5	15.3	25.1	19.4

[1]All values are the least square means derived from 32 pens each providing 12 birds. Data are given as the contrasts of main factors because no significant interactions occurred ($P > 0.05$) except as footnoted.
[2]Interaction ($P < 0.05$): low 3–6 wk P + NRC = 0.5; low 3–6 wk P + w/o Ca P = 5.2; NRC + NRC = 0.4; NRC + w/o Ca P = 0.9.
[3]Femur obtained after cone deboning was evaluated for proximate epiphysis head breakage and shaft subjected to instron stress.

Lighting of short duration has been used to restrict feed intake, thereby relieving mortalities due to rapid development. Such restriction is most efficacious shortly after hatching when followed by extended lighting to enable compensatory recovery. Although final live body weight and ultimate

Table 7.9. Carcass responses of broilers to extremes in temperature imposed from 28 to 52 days within environmental chambers.[1] (Data from Smith and Teeter, 1987.)

Measurements at 52 days	Temperature (°C) (70% RH)		
	7.2	23.9	35
Feed intake 100 g^{-1} RW	11.8	9.4	8.5
Chilled carcass	803	1063	800
Abdominal fat	1.5	11.5	7.6
Breast[1]	156	203	138
Thigh[1]	111	152	113

[1]Whole parts as separated from the carcass.

feed conversion of light-restricted birds is similar to controls, the carcass and meat yield appear to suffer. Additional time lying down during the dark period accentuates incidence of breast blisters (Renden *et al.*, 1992a) and buttons (Newberry, 1992). Breast meat appears to be the last part of the body to realize recovery (Table 7.10).

Stocking density is most influential prior to marketing when live weight per unit pen area maximizes. At this time, bird-to-bird contact is the dominant factor determining meat quality; however, concurrent temperature and humidity increases together with deterioration in air quality also play a small role (Tegethoff and Hartung, 1996). Bird-to-bird contacts are likely to involve the claws and cause skin scratches (Elfadil *et al.*, 1996); however, decreased back bruising has also been observed by Bilgili *et al.* (1991) which was attributed to a reduction in overall flock activity. Toenail clipping alleviates scratching (Hargis *et al.*, 1989; Frankenhuis *et al.*, 1991) and their appearance can be improved by soft-scalding during processing rather than hard-scalding (Sams *et al.*, 1990).

Litter conditions can also affect meat bird quality with the extent of involvement being aggravated by high temperature, humidity and stocking density. There are many different sources of litter and problems with carcass quality with most are low compared to the use of alternate floorings (Andrews *et al.*, 1990). Breast blisters and buttons can be minimized by avoiding coarse and hard-packed litters (Newberry, 1993), whereas, ulcerative dermatitis results from contacts that have high microbial activity when moisture level is excessive (Martland, 1985; Weaver and Meijerhof, 1991). Additional microbial load of the litter does not perceptibly increase levels associated with the carcass after processing (Reiber *et al.*, 1990).

CONCLUSIONS

The yield and quality of poultry meat are readily influenced by several aspects of live production. Most marketing occurs at the inflection point as defined by the Gompertz function. Although the rate of skeletal development and myofibre lengthening decreases at this time, muscles with fast-glycolytic fibres

Table 7.10. Effect of restricted lighting of broiler males on yields of carcass and skinless boneless meats at progressively older market ages. (Data from Renden *et al.* (1992b.)

Lighting treatment[1]	Days of age			
	35	42	49	56
Live body weight (kg)				
$P<$	***	**	NS	NS
Continuous	1841	2313	2953	3456
Restricted	1784	2253	2901	3427
Feed conversion to date				
$P<$	*	*	*	NS
Continuous	1.59	1.70	1.77	1.80
Restricted	1.55	1.65	1.72	1.77
Chilled carcass (% live wt)				
$P<$	NS	NS	NS	NS
Continuous	74.9	73.7	74.6	80.1
Restricted	74.5	73.5	75.1	79.2
Pectoralis major (% carcass)				
$P<$	NS	NS	*	**
Continuous	17.1	17.3	17.7	17.7
Restricted	16.5	17.1	17.1	17.1
Skinless boneless thigh (% carcass)				
$P<$	*	***	NS	**
Continuous	16.0	16.2	16.3	15.8
Restricted	16.3	16.8	16.7	16.4

[1]Continuous lighting = 23 h light : 1 hour dark; restricted lighting = 6L : 18D, 0–14 days then 1L : 3D thereafter.

rapidly increase their cross-sectional area at this time compared to the slow-oxidative and fast-oxidative glycolytic types. Breast is exclusively represented by fast-glycolytic fibres and its meat is particularly responsive. The inflection point is also the hallmark for other changes which improve overall sensory value.

Genetic selection has increased the amount of meat and decreased carcass fatness. Breast meat has been the focus of attention and additional yield is largely due to expansion of myofibre cross-sectional area. Protein nutrition is particularly crucial to breast meat yield, whereas, submarginal phosphorus can weaken the skeleton and create an array of quality defects. High temperature and reduced duration lighting decrease feed intake and breast meat is acute in response. Increased stocking rate and poor litter impair carcass quality by creating an array of skin problems. Adverse effect on the functional and sensory properties of poultry meat because of most facets of live production are not usually serious.

REFERENCES

Acar, N., Moran, E.T., Jr and Mulvaney, D.R. (1993) Breast muscle development of commercial broilers from hatching to 12 weeks of age. *Poultry Science* 72, 317–225.

Ajang, O.A., Prijono, S. and Smith, W.K. (1993) Effect of dietary protein content on growth and body composition of fast and slow feathering broiler chickens. *British Poultry Science* 34, 73–91.

Andrews, L.D., Whiting, T.S. and Stamps, L. (1990) Performance and carcass quality of broilers grown on raised floorings and litter. *Poultry Science* 69, 1644–1651.

Asghar, A., Morita, J.-I., Samejima, K. and Yasui, T. (1986a) Variations of proteins in subcellular sarcoplasmic fractions of chicken red and white skeletal muscles influenced by under-nutrition. *Agricultural and Biological Chemistry* 50, 1913–1940.

Asghar, A., Morita, J.-I., Samejima, K. and Yasui, T. (1986b) Variation of proteins in myofibrils and connective tissue of chicken red and white skeletal muscles influenced by under-nutrition. *Agricultural and Biological Chemistry* 50, 1941–1949.

Bilgili, S.F., Revington, W.H., Moran, E.T., Jr and Bushong, R.D. (1991) The influence of diet and stocking density on carcass quality of broilers processed under soft-and hard-scald conditions. In: Ujittenboogaart, T.G. and Veerkamp, C.H. (eds) *Quality of Poultry Products I. Poultry Meat*. Spelterholt Center, Beekbergen, The Netherlands, pp. 263 271.

Cahaner, A., Pinchasov, Y., Nir, I. and Nitsan, Z. (1995) Effects of dietary protein under high ambient temperature on body weight, breast meat yield and abdominal fat deposition of broiler stocks differing in growth rate and fatness. *Poultry Science* 74, 968–975.

Campbell, G.L., Salmon, R.E. and Classen, H.L. (1988) Effect of nutrient density on broiler carcass composition as influenced by age. *Nutritional Reports International* 37, 973–981.

Chambers, J.R., Fortin, A., Mackie, D.A. and Larmond, E. (1989) Comparison of sensory properties of meat from broilers of modern stocks and experimental strains differing in growth and fatness. *Canadian Institute of Food Science and Technology Journal* 22, 353–358.

Chen, X. and Moran, E.T., Jr (1994) Response of broilers to omitting dicalcium phosphate from the withdrawal feed, live performance, carcass down-grading and further-processing yields. *Journal of Applied Poultry Research* 3, 74–79.

Chen, X. and Moran, E.T., Jr (1995) The withdrawal feed of broilers, carcass responses to dietary phosphorus. *Journal of Applied Poultry Research* 4, 69–82.

Cornejo, S., Lopez, A., Pokniak, J., Gonzalez, N. and Cordeiro, A. (1991) Effect of energy/protein ratio on productive performance and carcass composition of male broilers. *Journal of Veterinary Medicine Archives* 38, 126–133.

Elfadil, A.A., Vaillancourt, J.-P. and Meek, A.H. (1996) Impact of stocking density, breed and feathering on the prevalence of abdominal skin scratches in broiler chickens. *Avian Diseases* 40, 546–552.

Frankenhuis, M.T., Vertommen, M.H. and Hemminga, H. (1991) Influence of claw clipping, stocking density and feeding space on the incidence of scabby hips in broilers. *British Poultry Science* 32, 227–230.

Gous, R.M., Hancock, C.E. and Bradfield, G.D. (1992) A characterization of the potential growth rate of six breeds of commercial broiler. In: *Proceedings of the 19th World's Poultry Science Association Meeting*, Volume 2, Amsterdam, The Netherlands, pp. 189–192.

Halvorson, J.C., Waibel, P.E., Oju, E.M., Moll, S.L. and El Halawani, M.E. (1991) Effect of diet and population density on male turkeys under various environmental conditions. 2. Body composition and meat yield. *Poultry Science* 70, 935–940.

Hancock, C.E., Bradford, G.D., Emmans G.C. and Gous R.M. (1995) The evaluation of the growth parameters of six strains of commercial broiler chickens. *British Poultry Science* 36, 247–264.

Hanzl, C.J. and Somes, R.G., Jr (1983) The effect of naked neck gene, Na, on growth and carcass composition of broilers raised in two temperatures. *Poultry Science* 62, 934–941.

Hargis, B.M., Moore, R.W. and Sams, A.R. (1989) Toe scratches cause scabby hip syndrome. *Poultry Science* 68, 1148–1149.

Holsheimer, J.P. and Rueskin, E.W. (1993) Effect on performance, carcass composition, yield and financial return of dietary energy and lysine levels in starter and finisher diets fed to broilers. *Poultry Science* 72, 806–815.

Howlinder, M.A.R. and Rose, S.P. (1989) Rearing temperature and the meat yield of broilers. *British Poultry Science* 30, 61–67.

Iwamoto, H., Hara, Y., Gotoh, T.Y., Ono, Y. and Takahara, H. (1993) Different growth rates of male chicken skeletal muscles related to their histochemical properties. *British Poultry Science* 34, 925–938.

Knizetova, H., Hyanek, J., Knize, B. and Roubicek, J. (1991) Analysis of growth curves of fowl. I. Chickens. *British Poultry Science* 32, 1027–1038.

Leclercq, B. and Whitehead, C.C. (1988) *Leaness in Domestic Birds, Genetic, Hormonal and Metabolic Aspects.* Butterworth, London.

Martland, M.F. (1985) Ulcerative dermatitis in broiler chickens, the effects of wet litter. *Avian Pathology* 14, 353–364.

Mayes, F.J. (1980a) The incidence of breast-blister down-grading in broiler chickens. *British Poultry Science* 21, 497–504.

Mayes, F.J. (1980b) The incidence of bruising in broiler flocks. *British Poultry Science* 21, 505–509.

Migineishvili, A. (1991) Criterion of selection for higher broiler chicken breast yield. In: Ujittenboogaart, T.G. and Veerkamp, C.H. (eds) *Quality of Poultry Products I. Poultry Meat.* Spelterholt Center, Beekbergen, The Netherlands, pp. 235–241.

Moran, E.T., Jr (1977) Growth and meat yield in poultry. In: Boorman, K.N. and Wilson, B.J. (eds) *Growth and Poultry Meat Production.* British Poultry Science Ltd, Edinburgh, pp. 145–173.

Moran, E.T., Jr (1994) Response of boiler strains differing in body fat to inadequate methionine, live performance and processing yields. *Poultry Science* 73, 1116–1126.

Moran, E.T., Jr (1996a) Diet dilution by omitting added fat with broilers for further processing. *Journal of Applied Poultry Research* 5, 254–259.

Moran, E.T., Jr (1996b) Broiler feeding regimen and yield. In: *Proceedings of the Western Canada Nutrition Conference*, Edmonton, Canada, pp. 5–13.

Moran, E.T., Jr (1997) Response of broilers to added dietary fat and pellet quality. In: *Proceedings of the 11th European Symposium on Poultry Nutrition*, Faaborg, Denmark, pp. 7–10.

Moran, E.T., Jr and Bilgili, S.F. (1989) Processing losses, carcass quality and meat yield of broiler chickens receiving diets marginally deficient to adequate in lysine prior to marketing. *Poultry Science* 69, 702–710.

Moran, E.T., Jr and Bushong, R.D. (1992) Effects of reducing dietary crude protein to relieve litter nitrogen on broiler performance and meat yields upon further-processing the carcass. In: *Proceedings of the 19th World's Poultry Science Association Meeting*, Volume 3, Amsterdam, The Netherlands, pp. 466–470.

Moran, E.T., Jr and Stilborn, H.L. (1996) Effect of glutamic acid on boilers given submarginal CP and adequate essential amino acids using feeds high and low in potassium. *Poultry Science* 75, 120–129.

Moran, E.T., Jr and Todd, M.C. (1994) Continuous submarginal phosphorus with broilers and the effect of preslaughter transportation, carcass defects, further-processing yields and tibia–femur integrity. *Poultry Science* 73, 1448–1457.

National Research Council (1994) *Nutrient Requirements of Poultry*, 9th rev. edn. National Academy Press, Washington, DC.

Newberry, R.C. (1992) Influence of increasing photoperiod and toe clipping on breast buttons of turkeys. *Poultry Science* 71, 1471–1479.

Newberry, R.C. (1993) The role of temperature and litter type in the development of breast buttons in turkeys. *Poultry Science* 72, 467–474.

Ono, Y., Iwamoto, H. and Takahara, H. (1993) The relation between muscle growth and growth of different fiber types in the chicken. *Poultry Science* 72, 568–576.

Reiber, M.A., Hierholzer, R.E., Adams, M.H., Colberg, M. and Izat, A.L. (1990) Effect of litter condition on microbiological quality of freshly killed and processed broilers. *Poultry Science* 69, 2128–2133.

Remignon, H., Lefaucheur, L., Blum, J.C. and Ricard, F.H. (1994) Effects of divergent selection for body weight on three skeletal muscles characteristics in the chicken. *British Poultry Science* 35, 65–76.

Remignon, H., Gardahaut, M.-F., Marche, G. and Ricard, F.-H. (1995) Selection for rapid growth increases the number and size of muscle fibers without changing their typing in chickens. *Journal of Muscle Research and Cell Motility* 16, 95–102.

Remignon, H., Desrosiers, V. and Marche, G. (1996) Influence of increasing breast meat yield on muscle histology and meat quality in the chicken. *Reproduction and Nutritional Development* 36, 523–530.

Renden, J.A., Bilgili, S.F. and Kincaid, S.A. (1992a) Effects of photoschedule and strain cross on broiler performance and carcass yield. *Poultry Science* 71, 1417–1426.

Renden, J.A., Bilgili, S.F. and Kincaid, S.A. (1992b) Live performance and carcass yield of broiler strain crosses provided either sixteen or twenty-three hours of light per day. *Poultry Science* 7, 1427–1435.

Roth, F.X., Kirchgessner, M., Ristic, M. Kreuzer, M. and Manrus-Kukral, E. (1990) Amino acid pattern of the breast meat of broilers during an extended finishing period as affected by protein and energy intake. *Fleischwirtschaft* 70, 608–612.

Saleh, E.A., Watkins, S.E. and Waldroup, P.W. (1996) Changing time of feeding starter, grower and finisher diets for broilers. 1. Birds grown to 1 kg. *Journal of Applied Poultry Research* 5, 269–275.

Sams, A.R., Hargis, B.M., Hyatt, D.T. and Breger, C.R. (1990) Scalding conditions can improve the appearance of broilers with scabby-hip syndrome. *Poultry Science* 69, 1006–1008.

Scholtyssek, S. and Sailer, K. (1986) Differences in the taste of poultry meat. *Archives Geflugelkunde* 50, 49–54.

Smith, D.P. and Fletcher, D.L. (1988) Chicken breast muscle fiber type and diameter as influenced by age and intramuscular location. *Poultry Science* 67, 908–913.

Smith, M.O. (1993) Parts yield of broilers reared under cycling high temperatures. *Poultry Science* 72, 1146–1150.

Smith, M.O. and Teeter, R.G. (1987) Influence of feed intake and ambient temperature stress on the relative yield of broiler parts. *Nutritional Reports International* 35, 299–306.

Sonaiya, E.B., Ristic, M. and Klein, F.W. (1990) Effect of environmental temperatures, dietary energy, age and sex on broiler carcass portions and palatability. *British Poultry Science* 31, 121–128.

Swatland, H.J. (1980) A histological basis for differences in breast meat yield between two strains of white turkeys. *Journal of Agricultural Sciences, Cambridge* 94, 383–388.

Tegethoff, U. and Hartung, J. (1996) A field study on stocking density and air quality in broiler production and recommendations to avoid heat stress in summer. *Deutsche Tierärztliche Wochenschrift* 103, 87–91.

Touraille, C., Ricard, F.H., Kopp, J., Valin, C. and Leclercq, B. (1981) Chicken meat quality. 2. Changes with age of some physico-chemical and sensory characteristics of meat. *Archives Geflugelkunde* 45, 97–104.

Vereijken, A.L.J. (1992) Genetics of body conformation and breast meat yield in broilers. In: *Proceedings of the 19th World's Poultry Science Association Meeting*, Volume 2, Amsterdam, The Netherlands, pp. 98–100.

Waibel, P.C., Carlson, C.W., Liu, J.K., Brannon, J.A. and Noll, S.L. (1995) Replacing protein in corn–soybean turkey diets with methionine and lysine. *Poultry Science* 74, 1143–1158.

Weaver, W.D., Jr and Meijerhof, R. (1991) The effect of different levels of relative humidity and air movement on litter conditions, ammonia levels, growth and carcass quality for broiler chickens. *Poultry Science* 70, 746–755.

Xiong, Y.L., Cantor, A.H., Pescatore, A.J., Blanchard, S.P. and Straw, M.L. (1993) Variations in muscle chemical composition, pH and protein extractability among eight different broiler crosses. *Poultry Science* 72, 583–588.

CHAPTER 8
Nutritional effects on meat flavour and stability

M. Enser
Division of Food Animal Science, School of Veterinary Science, University of Bristol, Langford, Bristol BS40 5DU, UK

INTRODUCTION

The fatty acid composition of meat lipid is a major determinant of the flavour and shelf-life stability of fresh and cooked meats. In stored fresh meats lipid peroxidation leads to the development of rancid odours and flavours. In cooked meats this same process is more rapid, as a result of tissue disruption, and is exacerbated by reheating to give 'warmed-over flavour'. However, thermal activation of fatty acid peroxidation during cooking produces compounds which react with other components of the heated meat to produce the desirable characteristic flavours and odours of cooked meat.

Susceptibility of meat to oxidation depends on the degree of unsaturation of its fatty acids and the concentration of pro-oxidants such as iron compounds and antioxidants such as vitamins C and E and selenium-containing enzymes. In poultry, the fatty acid composition of the tissue lipids is markedly affected by dietary fatty acids, especially the feeding of the essential fatty acids linoleic and α-linolenic acids and the C_{20} and C_{22} polyunsaturated fatty acids (PUFA) in fish oils which are readily incorporated into neutral and phospholipids. Their innate instability can be counteracted in part by feeding increased amounts of tocopherols, particularly α-tocopherol (vitamin E). However, increasing the concentration of n-3 PUFA by feeding linseed or additional fish oil to improve the value of poultry in human nutrition puts considerable stress on the antioxidants. Furthermore, the change from n-6 to n-3 PUFA may result in a stronger, less acceptable flavour. Despite this there are few recent studies of the effect of high n-3 PUFA on flavour. Most investigations rely on chemical determination of oxidative stability despite the uncertain relationship of assays of malonaldehyde content (TBARS) with flavour assessed by taste panels or consumers. This chapter considers the factors governing the fatty acid composition of poultry meat and its modification by diet, particularly to increase the content of n-3 PUFA. Methods of assessing flavour and oxidative stability are assessed together with the ability of antioxidants to improve or maintain the oxidative stability of meat with increased concentrations of n-3 PUFA.

THE EFFECT OF DIETARY FATTY ACIDS ON TISSUE FATTY ACID COMPOSITION

Fatty acids fed to poultry are absorbed unchanged and deposited in tissues either directly or after metabolic conversion. Since birds are normally fed a diet containing added fat there is no standard control diet so that comparison can only be made between one dietary fat and another. An example of the effects of three dietary oils: corn oil, linseed oil and menhaden (fish) oil on the composition of the total lipids of the thigh muscles of broilers is shown in Table 8.1. These tissue compositions arise from an interaction of many factors which are outlined below.

Source of Fatty Acids: Exogenous or Endogenous

Birds can synthesize saturated and monounsaturated fatty acids and on a fat-free diet the major products are palmitic and oleic acids followed by stearic and palmitoleic acids (Bottino *et al.*, 1970). The amount of *de novo* synthesis depends on the availability of surplus energy which may be increased if protein intake is inadequate (reviewed by Fisher, 1984). Linoleic acid ($18:2$ *n*-6) and α-linolenic acid ($18:3$ *n*-3) are essential fatty acids and must be obtained from the feed hence the high concentrations in birds fed corn oil and linseed oil which are major sources of these two fatty acids respectively (Table 8.1). The bird can convert them into longer, more unsaturated fatty acids such as eicosapentaenoic (EPA, $20:5$ *n*-3) and docosahexaenoic acid (DHA, $22:6$ *n*-3) formed from α-linolenic acid. The latter two can also be supplied in the feed directly as fish oil (Table 8.1) or as a component of fish meal (Table 8.2). Dietary fatty acids, particularly linoleic acid, may decrease endogenous oleic acid synthesis by inhibiting the Δ^9 desaturase enzyme (Wahle, 1974). Most fatty acids are readily digested and absorbed when present in a mixed lipid but high concentrations of saturated fatty acids, particularly tristearin, may be poorly digested.

Table 8.1. The fatty acid composition (g kg^{-1}) of total fatty acids of thigh muscles from broilers fed dietary oils (50 g kg^{-1} feed). (Data from Chanmugam *et al.*, 1992.)

Fatty acid	Corn oil	Linseed oil	Menhaden oil
$14:0$	33	25	61
$16:0$	164	140	213
$16:1$	33	36	99
$18:0$	56	52	70
$18:1$ *n*-9	304	296	287
$18:2$ *n*-6	375	214	152
$18:3$ *n*-3	13	219	19
$20:4$ *n*-6	8	3	4.4
$20:5$ *n*-3	0.1	3.1	38
$22:5$ *n*-3	0.5	2.5	13
$22:6$ *n*-3	1.6	2.8	24

Table 8.2. Effect of dietary redfish meal on the PUFA composition, (g kg^{-1}) fatty acid, of muscles from female broilers. (Data from Ratnayake *et al.*, 1989.)

	\multicolumn{8}{c}{Redfish meal (g kg^{-1})}						
	\multicolumn{2}{c}{0}	\multicolumn{2}{c}{40}	\multicolumn{2}{c}{80}	\multicolumn{2}{c}{120}
Fatty acids	White	Dark	White	Dark	White	Dark	White	Dark
18 : 2 *n*-6	170	189	160	170	139	138	128	131
20 : 4 *n*-6	40	25	39	27	23	21	23	16
18 : 3 *n*-3	6	9	5	6	4	6	4	6
20 : 5 *n*-3	8	3	15	7	18	13	31	13
22 : 5 *n*-3	17	4	12	9	22	17	22	11
22 : 6 *n*-3	32	6	30	19	49	30	58	27

Metabolic Fate of Fatty Acids

Fatty acids absorbed from the gut may be deposited in tissue lipids, converted into other fatty acids which may, in turn, be deposited or be removed through oxidation to provide energy or by conversion into other compounds such as prostaglandins.

The net deposition of dietary fatty acids in chicken has been reported for fish oil (Opstvedt, 1973) and for mixtures of tallow and vegetable oils with increasing levels of linoleic and α-linolenic acids (Pinchasov and Nir, 1992). In the latter study the deposition of myristic and stearic acids decreased as their concentration in the feed decreased. However, the total quantity in the carcass relative to the amount fed increased. For palmitic acid the quantity deposited was a constant proportion of the quantity eaten and oleic acid behaved similarly. All of these fatty acids can be synthesized *de novo* and it would be wrong to assume that all of those deposited in the tissues were derived from the feed even when it contained 10% fat and the amount of body fat was only 88% of that consumed overall. The data clearly indicated synthesis of myristic and particularly stearic acid at low intakes with the ratio of the amount deposited over that consumed exceeding 1.0. The effect was much more pronounced for palmitoleic acid with deposition exceeding intake at all levels. These findings for stearic acid agree with earlier studies by Marion and Woodroof (1963) that a sevenfold increase in the stearic acid content of feed produced only a 37% increase in carcass stearic acid. This effect was independent of the other fatty acids in the feeds which varied from coconut oil, high in medium-chain fatty acids, safflower oil, high in linoleic acid or menhaden oil, rich in EPA and DHA.

In contrast to the saturated and monounsaturated fatty acids increases in intake were not matched by proportionate increases in deposition for linoleic and α-linolenic acid. The ratio of carcass content to intake was 0.6–0.8 for linoleic acid and about 0.35 for α-linolenic acid. This may be explained partly by high rates of oxidation, which increase with increasing unsaturation, and conversion into other fatty acids, although the latter process may be more important for α-linolenic acid. Whereas α-linolenic acid products may be

15–20% of the total n-3 PUFA in dark muscle of broilers, products from linoleic acid are only 4% of the total n-6 PUFA (Chanmugam et al., 1992). Opstvedt (1973) observed much lower carcass retention of linoleic and α-linolenic acid at 16% and 14%, respectively. The value for EPA was 5% and DHA was 9% in agreement with later reports of poor deposition of EPA compared with DHA in chicken tissues and eggs.

Type of Tissue Lipids

Tissue lipids consist of storage triacylglycerols and structural lipids, mainly phospholipids. The fat content and proportion of the two components varies according to the tissue. Adipose tissue contains 60–80% lipid of which 99% is triacylglycerol, whereas white muscle may contain 1% lipid, only half of which is triacylglycerol (Katz et al., 1966). The fatty acid composition of triacylglycerols tends to consist mainly of oleic, palmitic, linoleic, stearic and palmitoleic acids in decreasing amounts with very little C_{20} and C_{22} PUFA. Furthermore, they are of similar composition in muscle and adipose tissue and are readily altered by manipulation of dietary fatty acids (Lin et al., 1989). Whereas the tissue content of triacylglycerols is variable, the content of phospholipids is relatively fixed and their fatty acid composition is constrained by functional requirements. They tend to contain higher proportions of stearic acid and lower proportions of oleic and palmitic acids than the triacylglycerols but are characterized by containing significant amounts of C_{20} and C_{22} PUFA of both the n-6 and n-3 series. Since the phospholipid level is fixed an increase in one fatty acid, for example DHA, can only occur through the displacement of a similar fatty acid, usually arachidonic acid.

Although most diets are fed continuously from a relatively young age until slaughter, for example from seven days of age in broilers, changes in dietary lipid can result in rapid alterations of tissue fatty acid composition. In turkeys 50% of the total change may occur within two and a half weeks or less (Salmon and O'Neil, 1973; Hartfiel, 1995).

INCREASING THE *N*-3 PUFA CONTENT OF POULTRY MEAT

The manipulation of dietary fatty acids to increase n-3 PUFA in poultry has been reviewed by Hargis and Van Elswyck (1993) and Leskanich and Noble (1997). The aim of raising the concentrations of EPA and DHA can be achieved by feeding these fatty acids directly in fish oil, fish meal (Table 8.2) or marine algae or by feeding α-linolenic acid and relying on the bird to synthesize and deposit the longer chain fatty acids (Table 8.1). The deposition of α-linolenic acid itself in the tissues is also advantageous since it can lower the $18:2:18:3$ (n-6 : n-3) ratio in the human diet which should increase EPA and DHA synthesis in humans. A ratio of 5 or less is recommended for the human diet (British Nutrition Foundation, 1992; Department of Health, 1994). Potential sources of α-linolenic acid are rapeseed, soybean or linseed.

However, the α-linolenic acid content of the first two oils is usually less than 120 g kg^{-1} compared with 500 g kg^{-1} for linseed. With the poor deposition of α-linolenic acid high dietary fat levels are needed for effective deposition from rapeseed or soybean oil. A rapeseed oil diet containing 133 g kg^{-1} lipid with 86 g kg^{-1} α-linolenic fed to turkeys for 24 weeks only resulted in a 18:2 to 18:3 ratio approaching 5 (Salmon and O'Neil, 1973). The response of broilers to rapeseed oil was similar to that of turkeys. A feed with 100 g kg^{-1} lipid and containing 78 g kg^{-1} of α-linolenic acid fed for 56 days gave n-6 : n-3 ratios of 5.9, 5.0 and 3.7 for the breast meat, thigh meat and whole carcass, respectively (Ajuyah *et al.*, 1991). However, when the α-linolenic acid content of the feed was only 55 g kg^{-1} the ratios were 12.2, 9.1 and 5.0. At both levels of a-linolenic acid intake there were only small effects on tissue EPA and DHA contents. Soybean is a less desirable source of α-linolenic acid than rapeseed because of its high linoleic acid content. Soybean oil with 73 g kg^{-1} α-linolenic acid added to a soybean/wheat diet at 50 g kg^{-1} and fed to broilers for 56 days produced tissue levels of approximately 30 g kg^{-1} α-linolenic acid in the muscle lipid. However, the n-6 : n-3 ratio was about 12 and synthesis of EPA and DHA was not increased (Phetteplace and Watkins, 1989).

Linseed or linseed oil is much more effective in raising tissue levels of n-3 PUFA in broilers as expected from its high content of α-linolenic acid. However, three studies using 25–28 g kg^{-1} of α-linolenic acid in the feed have produced somewhat different results. Ajuyah *et al.* (1991) found breast muscle to contain 41 g α-linolenic kg^{-1} fatty acids whereas Ahn *et al.* (1995) found 108 g kg^{-1}. For DHA the proportions were reversed with the latter authors finding 24 g kg^{-1} compared with 48 g kg^{-1} (Table 8.3). A plausible explanation for these results is differences in the fat content of the muscles between the studies. As the fat content of the muscle falls the proportion of phospholipids in the total lipid rises, with an increase in the proportion of DHA which is present at much higher levels in phospholipids than in neutral lipids. On the other hand the proportion of α-linolenic acid falls because of its relatively low level in phospholipids (Lin *et al.*, 1989). The results of Lin *et al.* (1989) gave higher concentrations of α-linolenic than Ahn *et al.* (1995) for breast muscle which had a rather high fat content at 24 g kg^{-1}, partly because the birds were

Table 8.3. PUFA composition of breast muscle from broilers fed full-fat linseed (g kg^{-1} total fatty acids).

Fatty acid	Control 1	Linseed 1	Control 2	Linseed 2
18 : 3 n-3	12[a]	41[b]	12[c]	108[d]
20 : 5 n-3	8[a]	21[b]	3[c]	17[d]
22 : 5 n-3	20[a]	31[b]	6[c]	29[d]
22 : 6 n-3	25[a]	48[b]	7[c]	24[d]
18 : 2 n-6	184[a]	206[b]	179[c]	209[d]
20 : 4 n-6	80[a]	48[b]	32[c]	29[c]

Control 1 and Linseed 1 data from Ajuyah *et al.* (1991). Control 2 and Linseed 2 data from Ahn *et al.* (1995). Means within trials with different superscripts differ significantly, *P* < 0.05.

one week older at slaughter. Given the variation between studies and in the absence of data for the fat content of the muscles, calculation of the quantities of n-3 PUFA contributed to the human food supply are not justified. However, based on the control broilers in the studies, 26 g kg^{-1} dietary α-linolenic acid approximately doubles the tissue concentrations of EPA and DHA, whereas increases in α-linolenic acid vary from twofold to tenfold. The effect on the 18:2 to 18:3 ratio and the Σn-6:Σn-3 ratio of feeding linseed or its oil indicated a marked improvement in human nutritional value. At dietary levels of 26 g kg^{-1} α-linolenic acid the n-6:n-3 ratios were below 4.3 in both white and dark meat and the Σn-6:Σn-3 ratios were below 2, well within the recommended range for human nutrition. Compared with broilers, the meat of spent laying hens fed a wheat soybean feed was very low in n-3 PUFA, particularly EPA which was undetectable (Ajuyah et al., 1992). Continuous feeding of 36 g kg^{-1} α-linolenic acid was only partially effective in raising the levels of these fatty acids towards those in broilers indicating the drain on the synthetic systems imposed by the production of egg lipids.

The lipids of fish are rich in EPA and DHA although the proportions vary according to the species and season (Enser, 1991). Extracted oil may be added to the feed or be incorporated as a component of fish meal which has a residual lipid content of 80–100 g kg^{-1} (Opstvedt, 1985). Since the lipid in the meal contains a high proportion of phospholipid the proportion of long-chain n-3 PUFA are higher than in the oil from the same species. These factors make comparisons between the effects of feeding fish oil and fish meal difficult unless data for both the total fatty acid content and composition are provided. Ratnayake et al. (1989) (Table 8.2) fed redfish meal containing 109 g kg^{-1} lipid at a level of 120 g kg^{-1} of feed and obtained similar deposition of DHA to Chanmugam et al. (1992) who fed 50 g kg^{-1} of menhaden oil. Both feeds provided DHA at approximately 10 g kg^{-1} of the feed fatty acids and resulted in levels of approximately 60 g kg^{-1} and 25 g kg^{-1} in the lipids of white and red muscle, respectively. EPA, as expected, was deposited half as effectively as DHA but a threefold higher dietary level in the study by Chanmugam et al. (1992) resulted in a threefold higher tissue concentration than in the study by Ratnayake et al. (1989). Since in broilers dark muscle contains approximately twice as much lipid as white muscle both types of meat will provide similar quantities of EPA and DHA per 100 g serving of meat. In both studies tissue levels of docosapentaenoic acid (22:5 n-3) were much higher than expected from their dietary concentrations relative to DHA indicating more efficient deposition and probable synthesis from EPA by chain extension.

These and other studies (Hulan et al., 1988, 1989; Ajuyah et al., 1992; Phetteplace and Watkins, 1992; Scaife et al., 1994) confirm the ability of poultry to deposit significant amounts of DHA and EPA in edible parts of the carcass. Although the proportions of these fatty acids in skin are half to one-third those in dark muscle, the high fat content of skin, approximately 30 g kg^{-1}, means that it makes a significant contribution if consumed. Overall, a 100 g serving of chicken, from birds supplemented with fish oil that contributes 250–550 mg kg^{-1} of $C_{20} + C_{22}$ n-3 PUFA to the feed, will contain 100–200 mg of these fatty acids or from half to all the recommended daily intake. Levels of fish oil which yield that result will preclude the inclusion of excessive amounts of vegetable oils so that the *n*-6 to *n*-3 ratio will usually be below 5. However, additional linseed or linseed oil in the feed would lower the ratio further by supplying α-linolenic acid, although its contribution to EPA and DHA synthesis is very limited (Tables 8.1 and 8.3).

FLAVOUR AND ODOUR

Fatty acids contribute positively and negatively to flavour and odour characteristics of meat. Thermal oxidation of fatty acids during cooking produces reactive molecules, particularly aldehydes and ketones, which condense with Maillard products to form compounds that give the typical odour and flavour of cooked meats. The details of these reactions are discussed elsewhere in this volume. The types of fatty acids in the meat can alter the flavour and its acceptability. Although the effect of different dietary fatty acids in poultry has not been related to different positive effects on flavour, in cattle and sheep, grass feeding produces a stronger flavoured meat, preferred in the United Kingdom and New Zealand whereas feeding cereals produces a milder flavoured meat which is preferred in Spain and the USA. This difference produced by the type of feed is generally attributed to whether the main dietary fatty acid is α-linolenic which produces a strong flavour or linoleic acid which produces a mild flavour (Purchas *et al.*, 1979; Melton, 1990; Sanudo *et al.*, 1998). Poultry and pork normally have high levels of linoleic acid in their tissues and this partly contributes to their mild flavour.

The negative flavour effects of fatty acids are also related to their reaction with oxygen. At low temperatures the development of oxidative rancidity limits storage life. Excessive oxidation during cooking may lead to off odours and flavours and in stored cooked meat, particularly that which is reheated before serving, further oxidation leads to stale, cardboardy or warmed-over flavour. The susceptibility of meat to develop rancid odours and flavours depends on the fatty acids present. The more unsaturated the fatty acid, the greater its propensity to undergo peroxidation (Arakawa and Sagai, 1986) and it is well established that feeding high levels of fish oils containing EPA and DHA results in a fishy taint in the meat (Opstvedt, 1984). Other factors regulating lipid peroxidation are the levels of antioxidants and the accessibility of pro-oxidants to the fatty acids.

Before discussing the effects of fatty acids on meat flavour it is necessary to consider how we assess flavour. Clearly the ultimate test is whether the flavour is acceptable to the consumer. However, consumer studies are expensive and present many difficulties in interpretation of the results because of lack of consistency in cooking and consuming the meat. Trained taste panels make use of the high sensitivity of the human palate and integrating capacity of the brain. However, although they may detect differences between samples, the level of such differences that would be significant for consumers at large is usually not known since the control samples are usually specific to the experiment and do not represent the normal range of meat available to the consumer. Consumers presumably buy meat because they like it, which means that most meat is generally acceptable yet taste panel scores for overall liking are often at the 20% level for high quality control samples. For studies of meat deterioration due to lipid oxidation measurement of reaction products is often used in lieu of a taste panel. The most common method is to measure substances which react with thiobarbituric acid (TBA) to give an absorption peak around 532 nm; the TBARS or TBA test. The major reactant is malonic dialdehyde and results are expressed as mg malonic dialdehyde per kg of meat. However, the value obtained depends on the assay method with the distillation procedure of Tarladgis et al. (1960) giving values approximately twice as high as the extraction procedures used by others (Salih et al., 1987). The results from the two methods are highly correlated but only the distillation procedure has been related to panel-assessed odour with a value of 0.5–1.0 as the threshold for detectable rancidity in pork. Similar values were reported for chicken with panel scores of slight to no warmed-over flavour for TBA numbers of 0.5–1.0 (Igene et al., 1985). However, Ang and Lyon (1990) observed TBA numbers of 0.97 and 3.3 in white and dark chicken meat cooked to similar temperatures and assayed by the same method but the sensory scores for warmed-over flavour and rancidity were not different between the two types of tissue and were both low (Table 8.4). Although the TBA numbers increased almost linearly over 5 days storage of the meat at 2°C, sensory score changes occurred mainly in the first 2 days of storage. In ground turkey patties of mixed muscle types Younathan et al. (1980) detected no significant difference in odour scores for meat with TBA numbers of 5.9 and 11.3. There is clearly considerable difficulty in relating sensory and chemical measures of rancidity in cooked meat even when similar methods are used. This has been discussed by Lai et al. (1995) who observed some evidence for a threshold effect and that discrimination may be poor at high TBA numbers as observed by Ang and Lyon (1990). Thus, no TBA number or probably any other chemical measure of lipid oxidation can be related to meat flavour with certainty except for

Table 8.4. TBA numbers and sensory attributes of cooked broiler muscles stored at 2°C for 0 to 5 days. (Data from Ang and Lyon, 1990.)

Muscle	Storage time (days):	0	1	2	3	5
		TBA numbers (SD)				
Breast		0.97	4.06	7.27	8.37	11.43
		(0.25)	(0.48)	(0.20)	(0.54)	(0.51)
Thigh		3.30	6.13	7.83	8.76	12.57
		(0.63)	(0.28)	(0.46)	(2.25)	(0.84)
		Sensory scores (rancidity)				
Breast		4	34	37	53	57
Thigh		5	29	43	53	58

Sensory evaluation of line scale 1–100, weak–strong.

within-laboratory studies in which it has been standardized against taste panel assessments over the range within which the organoleptic response is approximately linear. However, TBA numbers offer a cheap and quick procedure to determine the relative stability of meat from different treatments.

The effects of increasing the concentration of *n*-3 PUFA in poultry meat on its oxidative stability have been reviewed by Hargis and Van Elswyck (1993) and Leskanich and Nobel (1997). Ajuyah *et al.* (1993a) observed significant increases in TBA numbers and rancid flavour scores for broilers fed 150 g kg^{-1} full-fat linseed compared with birds fed animal fat. The scores for rancid flavour of the fresh meat, 5–6 on a 15-point scale, indicate that such meat would be unacceptable (Table 8.5). Storage for 5 days at 4°C increased off-flavours to 8–9 (Table 8.5). The feed increased the level of α-linolenic acid in the triacylglycerols approximately tenfold (Table 8.6, Ajuyah *et al.*, 1993b). Increases in EPA, DPA and DHA in lecithin and ethanolamine phosphatides ranged from twofold to fourfold and were similar in white and dark meat. Thus the increased deposition of α-linolenic acid was proportional to the 12-fold higher level in the feed but increases in the longer-chain *n*-3 PUFA were less. Although in normal poultry meat the phospholipid PUFA oxidize most (Igene *et al.*, 1980; Pikul *et al.*, 1984), it is likely that the high content of α-linolenic acid would lead to its oxidation in the triacylglycerols, not only within the muscles but also in adipose tissue and skin. The findings of Ajuyah *et al.* (1993b) were confirmed by Ahn *et al.* (1995) using meat patties prepared from broilers fed 2.6% α-linolenic acid (see Table 8.2 for meat fatty acid composition). Although no organoleptic studies were carried out, the authors

Table 8.5. Dietary effects of full-fat flax seed on TBA numbers and rancid flavour of cooked fresh and stored, white and dark broiler meat. (Data from Ajuyah *et al.*, 1993a.)

Storage (days)	Broiler diet		
	Control	Flax seed	Flax seed + tocopherols
	TBA numbers, white meat		
0	1.4	3.3	0.8
5	6.3	8.4	4.7
	TBA numbers, dark meat		
0	1.2	4.7	1.9
5	7.7	9.9	12.7
	Rancid flavour, white meat		
0	3.7	5.4	2.3
5	2.3	9.2	5.4
	Rancid flavour, dark meat		
0	2.0	6.3	4.3
5	3.5	7.8	5.1

TBA numbers expressed as mg malonaldehyde per kg meat (Salih *et al.*, 1987).
Flavour score based on 15 cm line scale anchored as none (0) – strong (15).

Table 8.6. Effect of dietary full-fat flax seed on the *n*-3 PUFA composition (g kg⁻¹) of triacylglycerols, phosphatidylethanolamine and lecithin of broiler white and dark muscle. (Data from Ajuyah *et al.*, 1993b.)

Fatty acid	Broiler diet		
	Control	Flax seed	Flax seed + tocopherols
	Triacylglycerols white meat (dark meat)		
18 : 3	20 (15)	176 (185)	178 (217)
20 : 5	0 (0)	2 (3)	8 (5)
22 : 6	0 (0)	0 (1)	2 (3)
	Phosphatidylethanolamine		
18 : 3	6 (3)	0 (25)	28 (34)
20 : 5	0 (16)	27 (25)	49 (51)
22 : 6	42 (33)	103 (41)	11.2 (92)
	Lecithin		
18 : 3	0 (5)	6 (9)	10 (15)
20 : 5	0 (0)	13 (11)	22 (13)
22 : 6	8 (5)	13 (13)	14 (12)

considered the patties to be rancid within 3 h of cooking, based on an 'extraction' TBA number of 2–3. Allowing for differences in the TBA methods and cooking these two studies confirm the results of Lin *et al.* (1989). Raw white and dark muscle, obtained from broilers fed 55 g kg⁻¹ linseed oil for 7 weeks, which had been held at 4°C for 2 days, had TBA numbers (distillation method) of 0.64 and 1.4, respectively. After 3 days at 4°C the TBA number for the white meat had risen to 1.4, exceeding the threshold for detection of rancidity. Clearly dietary supplementation of broiler feed with 26 g kg⁻¹ α-linolenic acid may increase EPA and DHA one- to twofold, but the meat is unacceptable because of its increased susceptibility to oxidation. The levels of EPA and DHA obtained were below those of broilers fed 40 g kg⁻¹ redfish meal (Ratnayake *et al.*, 1989) and which produced acceptable meat which clearly indicates that the raised α-linolenic concentration was contributing to the oxidative instability.

   After considering the older and more recent literature, Leskanich and Noble (1997) suggested that fish meal and fish oil in broiler diets should not exceed 12% and 1% by weight, respectively, if fishy taints are to be avoided. These are similar to the levels recommended by Barlow and Pike (1977). However, such a conclusion should be treated with caution. Ratnayake *et al.* (1989) observed no effect of 120 g kg⁻¹ redfish meal on the flavour of freshly cooked broilers. Without quoting this paper, Poste (1990) reported that when the meat was held refrigerated at 4°C overnight, before tasting, a loss of chicken flavour and development of a fishy off-flavour occurred at 80 g kg⁻¹ fish meal. When the study was replicated using menhaden meal instead of redfish meal (O'Keefe *et al.*, 1995) peroxide values and hexanal levels in cooked meat stored at 4°C were considered too high for diets with 80 g kg⁻¹ and

120 g kg^{-1} fish meal, although there were no organoleptic assessments. These findings are contrary to those of Huang and Miller (1993) who found no negative flavour effects in freshly cooked, cooked and refrigerated, and frozen stored broilers fed fish oil (MaxEPA) at 10 g kg^{-1}. However, after 3 days at −3° to 0°C storage, TBARS increased significantly. There are several possible explanations for these differences in the findings of the two studies despite the similarities in fatty acid composition of the meat. The most likely is the difference in the levels of vitamin E added to the feed which was 20 IU kg^{-1} and 50 IU kg^{-1}, respectively. The discrimination by the trained taste panel used by Poste (1990) may also have been greater than the apparently untrained panel and less well controlled cooking in the Huang and Miller (1993) study. Overall, these results would indicate that the content of fish meal and fish oil in broiler diets should not exceed 50 g kg^{-1} and 5 g kg^{-1} (Opstvedt *et al.*, 1991) unless the oxidative stability of the meat can be increased by feeding vitamin E as discussed in the next section.

EFFECT OF ANTIOXIDANTS

α-Tocopherol (vitamin E) is the major antioxidant in meat post-mortem and its addition to poultry feeds to increase the oxidative stability of the meat has been established for many years (Marusich *et al.*, 1975) (Table 8.7). It is deposited in tissue membranes, intercalated with the phospholipid fatty acids, and within the lipid deposits in fat-cells. Its deposition from the feed is concentration and time dependent and, at equilibrium, concentrations vary between tissues (reviewed by Sheehy *et al.*, 1997). In broilers, equilibration in both thigh and breast meat takes approximately 5 weeks (Marusich *et al.*, 1975; Morrissey *et al.*, 1997). The efficiency of vitamin E deposition in turkey muscle is approximately one-quarter that of broilers (Marusich *et al.*, 1975), as a result of greater glucuronide synthesis in the liver and excretion via the bile (Sklan *et al.*, 1982). Equilibration in breast and leg muscle of turkeys given feed supplements of α-tocopheryl acetate at 300 mg kg^{-1} and 600 mg kg^{-1} required 13 weeks (Sheehy *et al.*, 1997). However, high level feeding for only 4 weeks before slaughter can have marked effects on the development of TBARS during refrigerated storage of carcasses (Table 8.7).

Table 8.7. Effect of dietary α-tocopherol on concentrations in hen turkey breast muscle and TBARS after storage (Marusich *et al.*, 1975).

Dietary α-tocopherol (IU kg^{-1})	Daily intake (IU)	Breast muscle (mg kg^{-1})	TBARS after storage at 1°C	
			4 days	7 days
50	11	1.05	0.71	1.64
150	30	1.30	0.63	0.81
250	57.6	1.85	0.44	0.62
450	88.9	2.05	0.30	0.39

The ability of supplementary dietary α-tocopherol to prevent the development of fishy taints in broilers and turkeys fed fish oils is well established (Opstvedt *et al.*, 1971; Crawford *et al.*, 1975). Many of the more recent studies aimed at raising the levels of *n*-3 PUFA have recognized the need to use supplemental vitamin E to prevent a decrease in the oxidative stability of the meat. Huang and Miller (1993) obtained meat with an acceptable shelf-life, both cooked and fresh frozen, and flavour when vitamin E was included, 250 IU kg^{-1}, in broiler feeds containing fish oil, 20 g kg^{-1}. This level of protection was similar to the study of Crawford *et al.* (1975) who added 200 IU vitamin E to turkey feed containing 20 g kg^{-1} tuna oil and assessed the flavour of freshly cooked muscle. Storage trials were not performed but, unlike the muscle, the flavour of skin was only normal at this vitamin E level when the tuna oil in the feed was decreased to 10 g kg^{-1}. Although this indication of lower oxidative stability in the turkey would be anticipated from the less efficient deposition of vitamin E, in terms of breast muscle *n*-3 PUFA the levels were similar for turkeys on 10 g kg^{-1} tuna oil and broilers given 20 g kg^{-1} MaxEPA. Meat from laying hens fed 35 g kg^{-1} of menhaden oil with mixed tocopherols at 367 mg kg^{-1} had similar TBARS after one month of frozen storage to chickens fed palm oil with or without supplemental vitamin E (Cherian *et al.*, 1996). The α-tocopherol content of the feed was 90 mg kg^{-1} compared with 37 mg kg^{-1} in the unsupplemented feed but levels in breast and thigh meat were less than a third of those in the Huang and Miller (1993) study using α-tocopheryl acetate, 50 mg kg^{-1} of feed. With muscle levels of *n*-3 PUFA similar in the two studies it is probable that more exacting studies of oxidation stability would have revealed decreased stability in the meat from the laying hens fed menhaden oil despite increased dietary vitamin E. The poor deposition of α-tocopherol in the laying hens compared with broilers, despite supplementation for four weeks, may result from secretion in the eggs or a slower rate of equilibration between feed and muscle in older birds. The use of free tocopherols rather than the acetate esters may have led to some loss through oxidation in the feed since the tissue α-tocopherol levels were somewhat higher when oils less susceptible to oxidation were fed. If the production of eggs with raised levels of *n*-3 PUFA becomes significant allowance will need to be made for the potentially low oxidative stability of the meat from the spent hens.

The use of supplemental dietary α-tocopherol to increase the stability of meat from birds fed linseed or linseed oil has been reported by Ajuyah *et al.* (1993a, b) and Ahn *et al.* (1995). In the earlier two studies the tocopherols were fed at 200 mg kg^{-1} of feed and consisted of mixed tocopherols, 80% of which were non-alpha forms. The addition of tocopherols to the feed resulted in a significant increase in the *n*-3 PUFA content of the raw white meat, particularly in the phosphatidylethanolamine fracture (Table 8.6). In the cooked meat the phosphatidylethanolamine of the dark meat also contained twice the proportion of *n*-3 PUFA when the linseed was supplemented with tocopherols. Since cooking did not affect the *n*-3 PUFA levels of the white meat significantly, it is likely that the main effect of the natural tocopherol mixture was to prevent loss of α-linolenic acid by oxidation in the feed.

However, these differences in n-3 PUFA, which were relatively small for total muscle lipid but resulted in this doubling in the phosphatidylethanolamine faction, must be taken into account when considering the ability of α-tocopherol to delay oxidative changes, particularly because of the involvement of this phospholipid in oxidative changes during the storage and cooking of meat (Keller and Kinsella, 1973; Igene and Pearson, 1979). The tocopherol supplement significantly lowered the high TBA numbers of the freshly cooked meat from birds fed linseed although they remained above the level in control birds for dark meat. After storage of the cooked white meat for 5 days the effect of the tocopherols remained. However, in the cooked dark meat the TBA number was higher in meat from the birds fed the linseed and tocopherol than in those fed linseed alone, presumably because of the higher n-3 PUFA in the former group. The lower effectiveness of the tocopherols in the dark meat, despite their higher concentrations compared with those in white meat, could result from the higher iron content or higher phospholipid levels compared with the white meat and both factors could contribute to the higher TBA numbers in brown meat.

In a subsequent similar study (Ahn *et al.*, 1995) the findings were reversed with the tocopherol supplement failing to protect the white meat, both raw and cooked, from the oxidative instability induced by feeding 2.6% α-linolenic acid as linseed. On the other hand the tocopherols halved the TBA numbers of the dark meat from birds fed linseed but levels generally were significantly higher than in the control meat both before and after storage. The only significant difference between this and the previous study appears to be the use of comminuted muscle rather than whole meat but that cannot account for the differences in the findings. The lack of an effect of dietary tocopherols on the stability of the breast meat is particularly unexpected in that feeding tocopherols did not increase the deposition of n-3 PUFA as it did in the first study. The tocopherol concentrations were higher in the leg meat, as expected, but the increments due to feeding were proportionately similar in white and dark meat. In both these studies the failure of 200 mg kg^{-1} of tocopherols to protect the meat from oxidation stems in part from the low α-tocopherol content which is the most effective component (Jensen *et al.*, 1995) and the use of free tocopherols which may be oxidized in the feed. Overall, these studies do not provide a clear answer to the effectiveness and levels of dietary α-tocopherol needed to protect high n-3 poultry meat from oxidative instability produced by feeding α-linolenic acid. The fish oil studies suggest adequate protection is possible, particularly if a sensible approach is taken to the overall aims; to lower the n-6 : n-3 ratio to less than 4 and to double the concentration of EPA and DHA (British Nutrition Foundation, 1992; Department of Health, 1994). For broilers this would require approximately 5 g kg^{-1} fish oil or 50 g kg^{-1} fish meal, together with 10 g kg^{-1} α-linolenic acid or 50 g kg^{-1} whole linseed. Supplementation with α-tocopherol would need to be 200 mg kg^{-1}. If it is economically possible to decrease the dietary concentration of linoleic acid less α-linolenic acid would be required to lower the n-6 : n-3 ratio.

Recent studies have demonstrated that other dietary antioxidants are ineffective in protecting stored poultry meat from peroxidation. King *et al.* (1995) found no protective effects in either raw or cooked meat after feeding β-carotene or L-ascorbic acid (Table 8.8) and the lack of effect of dietary vitamin C was confirmed by Lauridsen *et al.* (1997). Vitamin A did not reduce the TBARS in an induced oxidation test of thigh muscle from broilers fed 1.03 and 10.3 mg retinyl acetate kg⁻¹ feed for 5 weeks. Nor did the high level depress tissue tocopherol concentrations (Bartov *et al.*, 1997). De Vore *et al.* (1983) reported that supplementing a corn/soybean diet with selenium, 0.31 mg kg⁻¹, increased glutathione peroxidase activity and lowered the TBA numbers in meat stored at 4°C for 4 days (Table 8.9). The feed contained a calculated vitamin E content of 14.1 IU kg⁻¹ and tissue levels were not determined. However, the most likely explanation of the effect of selenium is an increase in tissue vitamin E due to a sparing effect of the glutathione peroxidase *in vivo*. Additional evidence for such an effect comes from a reported decrease in drip loss in chicken fed supplementary selenomethionine (Anon, 1996; Edens *et al.*, 1996). High membrane concentrations of vitamin E inhibit phospholipase A_2 post-mortem so that the levels of non-esterified fatty acids, which denature the membranes and increase fluid loss, are decreased. Although the relationship between dietary amounts of selenium and vitamin on the oxidative stability of poultry meat need to be examined, these reported effects of additional selenium will probably disappear at higher dietary levels of vitamin E.

Table 8.8. Effect of dietary α-tocopherol, β-carotene and ascorbic acid as antioxidants in broiler meat (King *et al.*, 1995).

Treatment	Content (mg per 100 g meat)			TBARS* (mg kg⁻¹)
	α-Tocopherol	β-Carotene	L-Ascorbic	
Control	3.8[b]	< 0.005		0.67[b]
α-Tocopherol	13.3[a]	< 0.005	–	0.25[a]
β-Carotene	2.7[b]	< 0.005	–	0.78[c]
L-Ascorbic acid	3.5[b]	< 0.005	33.7	0.66[b]

[a–c]Means within columns with different superscripts are significantly different ($P < 0.05$).
*Raw leg meat after grinding.

Table 8.9. Effect of dietary selenium on glutathione peroxidase activity and TBARS in chicken meat. (From DeVore *et al.*, 1983.)

Feed	Peroxidase activity		TBA number	
	Basal	+ Se	Basal	+ Se
Breast	1.9 ± 0.4[c]	4.0 ± 1.1[d]	1.0 ± 0.47[a]	0.4 ± 0.12[b]
Leg	2.4 ±1.3[c]	9.7 ± 1.9[e]	1.0 ± 0.44[a]	0.3 ± 0.12[b]

[a–e]Means within assays with different superscripts are significantly different, $P < 0.05$.

CONCLUSION

Nutritional effects on the flavour of poultry meat are mainly negative and stem from feeding excessive quantities of *n*-3 PUFA derived from fish or linseed. The high susceptibility of these fatty acids to peroxidation results in a rapid production of off-odours and flavours that reduce the shelf-life of both raw and cooked meat. Increasing the quantity of vitamin E in the feed can help to reverse the oxidative instability produced by these fatty acids. It seems probable, from the studies reported, that poultry meat can be modified successfully to meet nutritional guidelines with regard to the *n*-6 : *n*-3 PUFA ratio and the concentration of EPA and DHA. Such modification would require supplementation with sources of α-linolenic acid and EPA and DHA because of the inefficient synthesis of the latter two from α-linolenic acid. Supranutritional levels of vitamin E in excess of 100 mg kg^{-1} would be required and the testing for stability of such meat should be carried out on material known to be highly susceptible to oxidation such as frozen comminuted products and refrigerated cooked meat. Organoleptic assessment of the modified meat is the preferred method to determine effects on flavour and when cost necessitates the use of other methods such as the TBA test, these should be evaluated against a taste panel to give practically useful results.

REFERENCES

Ahn, D.U., Wolfe, F.H. and Sim, J.S. (1995) Dietary α-linolenic acid and mixed tocopherols and packaging influences on lipid stability in broiler chicken breast and leg muscle. *Journal of Food Science* 60, 1013–1018.

Ajuyah, A.O., Lee, K.H., Hardin, R.T. and Sim, J.S. (1991) Changes in the yield and the fatty acid composition of whole carcass and selected meat portions of broiler chickens fed full-fat oil seeds. *Poultry Science* 70, 2304–2314.

Ajuyah, A.O., Hardin, R.T., Cheung, K. and Sim, J.S. (1992) Yield, lipid, cholesterol and fatty acid composition of spent hens fed full-fat oil seeds and fish meal diets. *Journal of Food Science* 57, 338–341.

Ajuyah, A.O., Fenton, T.W., Hardin, R.T. and Sim, J.S. (1993a) Measuring lipid oxidation volatiles in meat. *Journal of Food Science* 58, 270–273, 277.

Ajuyah, A.O., Hardin, R.T. and Sim, J.S. (1993b) Effect of dietary full fat flaxseed with and without antioxidant on the fatty acid composition of major lipid classes of chicken meats. *Poultry Science* 72, 125–136.

Ang, C.Y.W. and Lyon, B.G. (1990) Evaluations of warmed-over flavour during chill storage of cooked broiler breast, thigh and skin by chemical, instrumental and sensory methods. *Journal of Food Science* 55, 644–648, 673.

Anon. (1996) Drip loss decrease with organic selenium. *Poultry International* 35, 82.

Arakawa, K. and Sagai, M. (1986) Species differences in lipid peroxide levels in lung tissue and investigation of their determining factors. *Lipids* 21, 769–775.

Barlow, S.M. and Pike, I.H. (1977) The role of fat in fish meal in pig and poultry nutrition. *Technical Bulletin no 4,* International Association of Fish Meal Manufacturers, Potters Bar, UK.

Bartov, I., Sklan, D. and Friedman, A. (1997) Effect of vitamin A on the oxidative stability of broiler meat during storage: lack of interaction with vitamin E. *British Poultry Science* 38, 255–257.

Bottino, N.R., Anderson, R.E. and Reiser, R. (1970) Animal endogenous triglycerides: 2. Rat and chicken adipose tissue. *Lipids* 5, 165–170.

British Nutrition Foundation (1992) Unsaturated fatty acids: nutritional and physiological significance. *Report of the British Nutrition Foundations Task Force.* Chapman & Hall, London.

Chanmugam, P., Boudreau, M., Boutte, T., Park, R.S., Hebert, J., Berio, L. and Hwang, D.H. (1992) Incorporation of different types of *n*-3 fatty acids into tissue lipids of poultry. *Poultry Science* 71, 516–521.

Cherian, G., Wolfe, F.W. and Sin, J.S. (1996) Dietary oils with added tocopherols: effects on egg or tissue tocopherols, fatty acids and oxidative stability. *Poultry Science* 75, 423–431.

Crawford, L., Kretsch, M.J., Peterson, D.W. and Lilyblade, A.L. (1975) The remedial and preventative effect of dietary α-tocopherol on the development of fishy flavour in turkey meat. *Journal of Food Science* 40, 751–755.

Department of Health (1994) Nutritional aspects of cardiovascular disease. *Report on Health and Social Subjects no 46.* HMSO, London.

De Vore, V.R., Colnago, G.L., Jensen L.S. and Greene, B.F. (1983) Thiobarbituric acid values and glutathione peroxidase activity in meat from chickens fed a selenium supplemented diet. *Journal of Food Science* 48, 300–301.

Edens, F.W., Carter, T.A. and Sefton, A.E. (1996) Influence of dietary selenium sources on post mortem drip from breast muscle of broilers grown on different litters. *Poultry Science* 75, 60.

Enser, M. (1991) Animal carcass fats and fish oils. In: Rossell, J.B. and Prichard, J.L.R. (eds). *Analysis of Oilseeds, Fats and Fatty Foods.* Elsevier Applied Science, London, pp. 329–394.

Fisher, C. (1984) Fat deposition in broilers. In: Wiseman, J. (ed.) *Fats in Animal Nutrition.* Butterworths, London, pp. 437–470.

Hargis, P.S. and van Elswyck, M.E. (1993) Manipulating the fatty acid composition of poultry meat and eggs for the health conscious consumer. *Worlds Poultry Science Journal* 49, 251–264.

Hartfiel, W. (1995) Schlachtkörper von Geflügel. Auswirkungen des futterfettes auf die qualität. *Fleischwirtschaft* 75, 90–92.

Huang, Y.X. and Miller, E.L. (1993) The effect of dietary oils and α-tocopherol on the *n*-3 fatty acid content and oxidative stability of broiler meat. In: Wood, J.D. and Lawrence, T.L.J. (eds) *Safety and Quality of Food from Animals.* British Society of Animal Production, Penicuik, UK, pp. 108–111.

Hulan, H.W., Ackman, R.G., Ratnayake, W.M.N. and Proudfoot, F.G. (1988) Omega-3 fatty acid levels and performance of broiler chickens fed redfish meal or redfish oil. *Canadian Journal of Animal Science* 68, 533–547.

Hulan, H.W., Ackman, R.G., Ratnayake, W.M.N. and Proudfood, F.G. (1989) Omega-3 fatty acid levels and general performance of commercial broilers fed practical levels of redfish meal. *Poultry Science* 68, 153–162.

Igene, J.O. and Pearson, A.M. (1979) Role of phospholipids and triglycerides in warmed-over flavour development in meat model systems. *Journal of Food Science* 44, 1285–1290.

Igene, J.O., Pearson, A.M., Dugan, L.R. and Price, J.F. (1980) Role of triglycerides and phospholipids on development of rancidity in model meat systems during frozen storage. *Food Chemistry* 5, 263–276.

Igene, J.O., Yamauchi, K., Pearson, A.M., Gray, J.I. and Aust, S.D. (1985) Evaluation of 2-thiobarbituric acid reactive substances (TBRS) in relation to warmed-over flavour development in cooked chicken. *Journal of Agricultural and Food Chemistry* 33, 364–367.

Jensen, O., Skibsted, L.H., Jacobsen, K. and Bertelsen, G. (1995) Supplmentation of broiler diets with all-rac-α- or a mixture of natural source RRR-α-γ-δ-tocopherol acetate. 2. Effect on the oxidative stability of raw and precooked broiler meat products. *Poultry Science* 74, 2048–2056.

Katz, M.A., Dugan, L.R. and Dawson, L.E. (1966) Fatty acids in neutral lipids and phospholipids from chicken tissues. *Journal of Food Science* 31, 717–720.

Keller, J.D. and Kinsella, J.E. (1973) Phospholipid changes and lipid oxidation during cooking and frozen storage of raw ground beef. *Journal of Food Science* 38, 1200–1204.

King, A.J., Uijttenboogaart, T.G. and de Vries, A.W. (1995) α-tocopherol, β carotene and ascorbic acid as antioxidants in stored poultry muscle. *Journal of Food Science* 60, 1009–1012.

Lai, S.-M., Gray, J.I., Booren, A.M., Crackel, R.L. and Gill, J.L. (1995) Assessment of off-flavour development on restructured chicken nuggets using hexanal and TBARS measurements and sensory evaluation. *Journal of the Science of Food and Agriculture* 67, 447–452.

Lauridsen, C., Jensen, C., Jacobsen, K., Engberg, R.M., Anderson, J.O., Jensen, S.K., Sorensen, P., Henckel, P., Skibsted, L.H. and Bertelsen, G. (1997) The influence of vitamin C on the antioxidative status of chickens *in vivo*, at slaughter and on the oxidative stability of broiler meat products. *Acta Agriculturae Scandinavica A* 47, 187–196.

Leskanich, C.O. and Noble, R.C. (1997) Manipulation of the *n*-3 polyunsaturated fatty acid composition of avian eggs and meat. *Worlds Poultry Science Journal* 53, 155–183.

Lin, C.F., Gray, J.I., Asghar, A., Buckley, D.J., Booren, A.F. and Flegel, C.J. (1989) Effects of dietary oils and α-tocopherol supplementation on lipid composition and stability of broiler meat. *Journal of Food Science* 54, 1457–1460, 1484.

Marion, J.E. and Woodroof, J.G. (1963) The fatty acid composition of breast, thigh and skin tissues of chicken broilers as influenced by dietary fats. *Poultry Science* 42, 1202–1207.

Marusich, W.L., De Ritter, E., Ogrinz, E.F., Keating, J., Mitrovich, M. and Bunnell, R.H. (1975) Effect of supplemental vitamin E in control of rancidity in poultry meat. *Poultry Science* 54, 831–844.

Melton, S.L. (1990) Effects of feeds on flavour of red meat: a review. *Journal of Animal Science* 68, 4421–4435.

Miller, D. and Robisch, P. (1969) Comparative effect of herring, menhaden and safflower oils on broiler tissues fatty acid composition and flavour. *Poultry Science* 48, 2146–2157.

Morrissey, P.A., Brandon, S., Buckley, D.J., Sheehy, P.J.A. and Frigg, M. (1997) Tissue content of α-tocopherol and oxidative stability of broilers receiving dietary α-tocopherol acetate supplement for various periods pre-slaughter. *British Poultry Science* 38, 84–88.

O'Keefe, S.F., Proudfood, F.G. and Ackman, R.G. (1995) Lipid oxidation in meats of omega-3 fatty acid-enriched broiler chickens. *Food Research International* 28, 417–424.

Opstvedt, J. (1973) Influence of residual lipids on the nutritive value of fish meal, V. Digestive and deposition of marine fatty acids in chicken. *Acta Agriculturae Scandinavica* 23, 200–208.

Opstvedt, J. (1984) Fish fats. In: Wiseman, J. (ed.) *Fats in Amimal Nutrition*. Butterworths, London, pp. 53–82.

Opstvedt, J. (1985) Fish lipids in animal nutrition. *Technical Bulletin No 22,* International Fishmeal and Oil Manufacturers Association, St Albans, UK.

Opstvedt, J., Nygard, E. and Olson, S. (1971) Influence of residual lipids on the nutritive value of fish meal. III. Antioxidant stabilised and solvent extracted fish meal in diets for broiler chickens with different levels of added vitamin E and 1, 2-dihydroxy-6-ethoxy, 2, 2, 4-trimethylquinoline. *Acta Agriculturae Scandinavica* 21, 125–143.

Opstvedt, J., Miller, E.L. and Pike, I.H. (1991) Complementary effect of fish meal with soyabean meal replacers in broiler diets. *Technical Bulletin no. 26.* International Association of Fish Meal Manufacturers, Potters Bar, UK.

Phetteplace, H.W. and Watkins, B.A. (1989) Effects of various n-3 lipid sources on fatty acid compositions in chicken tissues. *Journal of Food Composition and Analysis 2,* 104–117.

Phetteplace, H.W. and Watkins, B.A. (1992) Influence of dietary n-6 and n-3 polyunsaturates on lipids in chickens divergently selected for body weight. *Poultry Science* 71, 1513–1519.

Pikul, J., Leszczynski, D.E. and Kummerow, F.A. (1984) Relative role of phospholipids, triacylglycerols and cholesterol esters on malonaldehyde formation in fat extracted from chicken meat. *Journal of Food Science* 49, 704–708.

Pinchasov, Y. and Nir, I. (1992) Effect of dietary polyunsaturated fatty acid concentration on performance, fat deposition and carcass fatty acid composition in broiler chickens. *Poultry Science* 71, 1504–1512.

Poste, L.M. (1990) A sensory perspective of effect of feeds on flavour in meats: poultry meats. *Journal of Animal Science* 68, 4414–4420.

Purchas, R.W., Obrien, L.H. and Pendleton, C.M. (1979) Some effects of nutrition and castration on meat production from male Suffolk cross (Border Leicester–Romney cross) lambs. *New Zealand Journal of Agricultural Research* 22, 375–383.

Ratnayake, W.M.N., Ackman, R.G. and Hulan, H.W. (1989) Effect of redfish meal enriched diets on the taste and n-3 PUFA of 42 day old broiler chicken. *Journal of the Science of Food and Agriculture* 49, 59–74.

Salih, A.M., Smith, D.M., Price, J.F. and Dawson, L.E. (1987) Modified extraction 2-thiobarbituric acid method for measuring lipid oxidation in poultry. *Poultry Science* 66, 1483–1488.

Salmon, R.E. and O'Neil, J.B. (1973) The effect of the level and source and of a change of source of dietary fat on the fatty acid composition of the depot fat and the thigh and breast meat of turkeys as related to age. *Poultry Science* 52, 302–314.

Sanudo, C., Nute, G.R., Campo, M., Maria, G., Baker, A., Sierra, I., Enser, M. and Wood, J.D. (1998) Assessment of commercial lamb meat quality by British and Spanish taste panels. *Meat Science* 48, 91–100.

Scaife, J.R., Moyo, J., Galbraith, H., Michie, W. and Campbell, V. (1994) Effect of different dietary supplemental fats and oils on the tissue fatty acid composition and growth of female broilers. *British Poultry Science* 35, 107–118.

Sheehy, P.J.A., Morrissey, P.A., Buckley, D.J. and Wen, J. (1997) Effects of vitamins in the feed on meat quality in farm animals: vitamin E. In: Garnworthy, P.C. and Wiseman, J. (eds) *Recent Advances in Animal Nutrition, 1997.* Nottingham University Press, Nottingham, UK., pp. 1–27.

Sklan, D., Bartov, I. and Hurwitz, S. (1982) Tocopherol absorption and metabolism in the chick and turkey. *Journal of Nutrition* 112, 1394–1400.

Tarladgis, B.G., Watts, B.M., Younathan, M.T. and Dugan, L. (1960) A distillation method for the quantitative determination of malonaldehyde in rancid foods. *Journal of the American Oil Chemists Society* 37, 44–48.

Wahle, K.W.J. (1974) Desaturation of long-chain fatty acids by tissue preparations of the sheep, rat and chicken. *Comparative Biochemistry and Physiology* 48B, 87–105.

Yau, J.C., Denton, J.H., Bailey, C.A. and Sams, A.R. (1991) Customising the fatty acid content of broiler tissues. *Poultry Science* 70, 167–172.

Younathan M.T., Marjan, Z.M. and Arshad, F.B. (1980) Oxidative rancidity in stored ground turkey and beef. *Journal of Food Science* 45, 274–275, 278.

CHAPTER 9
The influence of ante-mortem handling on poultry meat quality

P.D. Warriss, L.J. Wilkins and T.G. Knowles
Division of Food Animal Science, School of Veterinary Science, University of Bristol, Langford, Bristol BS40 5DU, UK

INTRODUCTION

There is considerable potential for ensuring good quality poultry carcasses and lean meat in the period between leaving the production unit and slaughter. In the UK, about 700 million broilers, 35 million turkeys and 40 million culled hens are killed annually. Because of the large number of individuals processed, even small effects on each bird may be economically very significant to the industry as a whole. The increase in further processing of carcasses has drawn attention to meat quality by exposing defects that previously may have gone unrecognized.

The effects of handling include loss of potential meat yield, depreciation of the value of the meat through haemorrhage, bruising and broken bones and undesirable colour and water-holding capacity. Effects are likely to be greater where the handling time between farm and processing plant is longer. In the UK this time can be prolonged (Table 9.1). It is also likely that the effects that variation in handling during this period and at slaughter can have on quality are larger than those attributable to variation in husbandry factors during rearing.

PROBLEMS OF ANTE-MORTEM HANDLING

Broilers are mostly reared on litter in environmentally controlled sheds housing up to 30,000 birds. They are 'harvested' at 6–7 weeks of age. Harvesting consists of manual catching of the birds and placing them in transport crates (cooping) or the drawers of 'modules' which are then stacked

Table 9.1. Marketing times for poultry in the UK.

Species	Average marketing time (h)	Maximum recorded time (h)	Reference
Broiler	3.6	12.8	Warriss *et al.* (1990)
Turkey	2.2–4.5	10.2	Warriss and Brown (1996)

Poultry Meat Science (eds R.I. Richardson and G.C. Mead)

on a vehicle for transport to the processing plant. One vehicle may carry 5000 to 6000 birds. Most hens are still housed in battery cages and removal from these is more difficult than catching broilers. Older designs of cage especially do not allow easy access. Catching hens from 'alternative' systems, such as percheries, is also difficult because of the large amount of furniture and structure associated with perches and nest boxes which prevent easy access. Handling of broilers and hens is usually by the legs and operatives may carry up to five birds, each held by one leg, in each hand. The potential for trauma is therefore considerable. In particular, it may lead to dislocation of the femur at the hip joint. Development and adoption of mechanization of broiler harvesting has seen little progress in the UK despite prototype machines being in existence for some time. A major constraint is the nature of the accommodation which often does not allow either easy access or unhindered movement within the broiler shed.

Close environmental control in the crates or modules on the vehicle is difficult, mainly because on most vehicles ventilation is passive and is impeded by the close stacking of adjacent crates. Birds on the inside of a load may suffer hyperthermia whereas those on the outside may experience hypothermia. In cold conditions side curtains may be used to protect these outermost birds. Nevertheless, the high probability of thermal stress being suffered by at least some birds in transit has been well documented (Webster *et al.*, 1993; Kettlewell *et al.*, 1993).

Often, problems of carcass and meat quality are associated with marketing processes and conditions which are stressful to the live bird. There is much evidence that the harvesting, transport and handling of poultry is stressful (Duncan, 1989). Transport of broilers (Cashman *et al.*, 1989) and culled hens (Mills and Nicol, 1990) results in fear based on tonic immobility measurements. Handling and crating of broilers (Kannan and Mench, 1996) and transportation (Freeman *et al.*, 1984; Mitchell *et al.*, 1992) are associated with physiological and biochemical changes indicating that the birds find the processes stressful.

MORTALITY IN TRANSIT

Birds dead on arrival (DOA) at the plant represent complete loss of economic value. The average frequency of DOA broilers has ranged up to 0.5% in various European studies (Knowles and Broom, 1990; Warriss and Knowles, 1993); the mortality rate for culled (end of lay) hens is generally higher and more variable. Occasional, very high mortalities have been reported. Swarbrick (1986) cites a case of 26% of a load of culled hens dead on arrival and Warriss *et al.* (1992) recorded a case of 15% of broilers dead in one load. These are undoubtedly exceptional but illustrate the potential for distress to be caused to birds in transit by inadequate control of environmental conditions and the consequent economic loss. In the UK, an average morality rate of about 0.2% (Warriss *et al.*, 1992; Yogaratnam, 1995) would correspond to complete loss of about 1.2 to 1.4 million broilers a year. A rate of 0.42% (Bayliss, 1986) corresponds to a figure of 2.9 million birds.

Reduced mortality will result from closer control of environmental conditions during transit and more careful bird handling to reduce trauma. Particularly when hot weather is expected, it is important to reduce stocking density in the crates or module drawers to control the build-up of heat and humidity. This is illustrated by data from Warriss *et al.* (1992). Mortality was reduced from 0.22% to 0.16% between March and August in one UK plant, despite the increasing ambient temperature, by reducing stocking density progressively from on average 17.3 to 15.8 birds per transport crate. Birds thermoregulate in confined conditions largely by panting. At high humidities the effectiveness of panting is reduced or nullified and hot, humid conditions therefore limit the bird's ability to lose body heat (Kettlewell and Turner, 1985). The importance of reducing trauma in controlling mortality is demonstrated by the findings of Gregory and Austin (1992). They found that 35% of broilers dead on arrival at the six plants they studied died from the effects of trauma.

Mortality is higher in consignments of broilers transported further (Warriss *et al.*, 1992). For journeys lasting less than 4 h the prevalence of dead birds was 0.156%. For longer journeys (up to 9 h) it was 0.283%, an increase of about 80%. Warriss and Knowles (1993) estimated that limiting journeys to 4 h in the UK would save more than a quarter of a million birds annually.

WEIGHT LOSS DURING MARKETING

Birds do not have access to food or water during transport and, additionally, these may have been withdrawn several hours before crating. Prolonged food and/or water withdrawal periods lead to loss of live weight and loss of potential carcass yield. With longer withdrawal times the rate of loss may also increase. The actual loss varies with the holding conditions, particularly temperature and ventilation. The information presented in Fig. 9.1 shows the wide range of reported losses. Some of the variation is possibly attributable to whether both feed and water, or just feed, is withdrawn. However, our own observations suggest that deprivation of food reduces water consumption to very low levels at ambient temperatures of about 20°C and therefore this distinction may not be important in practice. Temperature is important as illustrated by the results of Chen *et al.* (1983) (Table 9.2). This is obviously a reflection of the effect of temperature on metabolic rate, as explained by Veerkamp (1986). Veerkamp showed that a broiler producing heat at a rate of 5 W $kg^{0.75}$ would lose 0.22% of its body weight per hour assuming an energy value for animal tissue of 7500 J g^{-1}. He pointed out that this figure corresponded to equivalent experimentally determined minimum values and to the average of literature data. Heat production decreases with increasing environmental temperature by about 1.5 W 10°C^{-1} rise so at higher temperatures birds will tend to lose less weight. However, at very high temperatures and low humidities more moisture will be lost by evaporation during panting.

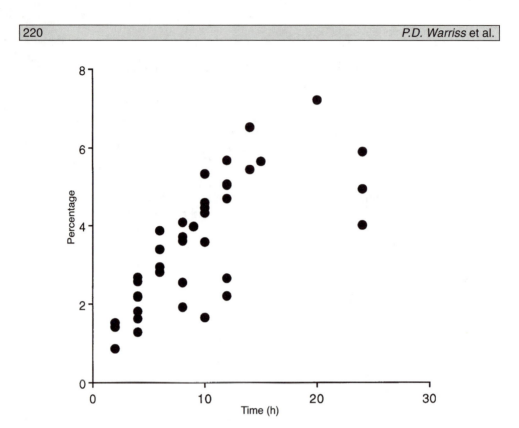

Fig. 9.1. Variation in the percentage live weight loss from broilers after food and water withdrawal. Data from Wabeck (1972), Fletcher and Rahn (1982) and Benibo and Farr (1985).

Table 9.2. Rates of live weight loss measured over 12 to 24 h of food/water withdrawal.

Reference	Rate of loss (% h^{-1})
Wabeck (1972)	0.18–0.24
Fletcher and Rahn (1982)	0.39–0.42
Chen *et al.* (1983)	0.22 at 10°C
	0.51 at 32.2°C
Benibo and Farr (1985)	0.35–0.39
Veerkamp (1986)	0.24
Warriss *et al.* (1988)	0.23

With very prolonged food deprivation, carcass yield may also be reduced (Wabeck, 1972; Chen *et al.*, 1983) although the size of the reduction is poorly defined. Food deprivation will also reduce liver yield. Birds fasted for 10 h had livers weighing 7% less than birds deprived of food for less than 1 h (Warriss *et al.*, 1993).

IMPLICATIONS OF FOOD WITHDRAWAL FOR CARCASS HYGIENE

A potentially important hygiene problem is the accidental contamination of the carcass at slaughter and evisceration by gut contents, particularly by faecal material, and especially the spread of pathogens such as *Salmonella* and *Campylobacter*. To reduce the danger, food is normally withdrawn some time before crating for transport. This reduces the pressure on the intestines and minimizes leakage of contents if the gut is accidentally broken. Various fasting periods from 4 to 10 h have been advocated (Anon., 1965; Wabeck, 1972). However, even prolonged food withdrawal will probably not completely prevent defaecation occurring during ante-mortem handling and there is therefore also the potential for faecal contamination of the outsides of live birds during crating and transport. Several factors make this more likely. Stress may increase defaecation. Because floor shavings are not used in crates, excreta are not absorbed and will be easily spread to other birds. In crates with perforated floors this will also occur between crates, birds being contaminated with the droppings of those in crates above. Dirty crates can obviously therefore become sources of contamination and effective cleaning and sterilization of crates between use is essential. Birds may become systemically infected very rapidly (≤2 h) after exposure (Humphrey *et al.*, 1993), particularly if fed.

As well as influencing the chances of live bird and carcass contamination with faecal material, food withdrawal may also affect the actual microbiological flora. There is evidence that, paradoxically, with longer food withdrawal times, the prevalence of *Salmonella* spp. in the crop of laying hens increases. Humphrey *et al.* (1993) found that the frequency of recovery of *Salmonella* spp. in the 24 h after their inoculation into the crops of birds either fasted or allowed feed *ad libitum* for the previous 24 h was significantly greater from the fasted birds. However, although starvation increased the survival of *Salmonella enteritidis* in the crop, the speed with which the lower parts of the gut were colonized decreased. The increased survival was attributed to the reduction in the population of normally resident lactobacilli in the crop by fasting. These normally compete with the salmonellae and also produce lactic acid which decreases the pH of the crop contents. Starvation leads to an increase in pH of these contents.

The crop and caeca are regarded as major sources of *Salmonella* contamination. Hargis *et al.* (1995) found that 52% of crops and 15% of caeca from broiler flocks known to be *Salmonella*-positive were contaminated with salmonellae when examined at slaughter. Also, crops were 86-fold more likely than caeca to rupture during processing. The crop in particular may therefore be a very important source of *Salmonella* contamination in processing plants.

Longer feed withdrawal (up to 24 h) was associated with a higher prevalence of birds testing positive for *Campylobacter jejuni* in cloacal swabs before slaughter and caecal swabs after slaughter (Willis *et al.*, 1996). Withholding water as well as feed increased the frequency of *Campylobacter*-positive birds. The conclusion was that any feed withdrawal time would lead to a higher potential for caecal contamination of the carcass with *C. jejuni*.

BRUISING AND CARCASS DAMAGE

Bruising is the presence of blood in tissues caused by trauma. Bruises and haemorrhages are unsightly and downgrade the value of the meat. They are mostly not detectable in the live bird and become visible only during the primary processing after feather removal. As a consequence, haemorrhagic conditions are sometimes erroneously attributed to the stunning and slaughter operations when they may have been inflicted at an earlier stage to the live bird. For instance, the presence of red wingtips, which may be influenced by the stunning procedure, has also been shown to be associated with severe flapping ante-mortem (Gregory and Austin, 1992). Similarly, bruising in turkeys in the area covering the rostral end of the keel bone has been attributed to the electrical stunner whereas investigations showed that the birds were arriving at the processing plant already bruised and that the bruise was being inflicted when the birds impacted with the front lip of the transport module. The prevalence of such bruising could be reduced by increasing the size of the module.

Estimates of the levels of bruising vary widely. Mayes (1980) recorded 2.63% in one processing plant in Northern Ireland. Griffiths and Nairn (1984) concluded that bruising occurred in 3.5–8.0% of all birds processed in four Australian plants whereas Taylor and Helbacka (1968) reported an average bruising level of about 20% in the USA. Most bruises occur on the breast, followed by the legs and wings, then the backs and thighs. Some variation is attributable to strain differences (Taylor and Helbacka, 1968), although this has been thought unlikely by other authors (Griffiths and Nairn, 1984), and seasonal effects. Well-muscled birds, which are heavy for their age, and females, have been claimed to be more susceptible. The importance of careful handling is illustrated by differences in bruising prevalence attributable to different catching teams (Taylor and Helbacka, 1968). Wilson and Brunson (1968) recorded more haemorrhaging in the thighs of broilers which had been handled more. Birds handled by one leg showed a higher frequency and severity of haemorrhaging in the thigh of that leg and the authors concluded that the problem was caused mainly by live bird handling during loading and processing, and by struggling on the shackles before slaughter. Certainly, the general view is that most bruising occurs during the last 12–24 h before slaughter (Hamdy *et al.*, 1961; Barbut *et al.*, 1990).

Turkeys appear to be very prone to carcass damage during handling, especially modern strains which are bigger but younger at slaughter (Barbut *et al.*, 1990). These authors showed the benefits of better designed, new transport cages over older equipment which allowed trapping of wings and legs by cage doors, greater cage heights (43 vs. 33 cm), and careful unloading procedures. Toenail trimming and spur clipping have been reported to reduce skin scratches whereas increased transport times increased half-wing trim and drumstick bruising (McEwen and Barbut, 1992).

LEAN MEAT pH, COLOUR AND WATER-HOLDING CAPACITY

The pH of muscle during life is about 7.2. After death, the muscle acidifies to values of 6 or less through the accumulation of lactic acid. The lactic acid derives from the postmortem breakdown of glycogen by glycolysis, in the process liberating energy in the form of adenosine triphosphate (ATP). The ATP serves to keep the muscle extensible. When it is used up the muscle enters the state of rigor mortis and becomes inextensible. Preslaughter handling can deplete muscle glycogen stores and affect the rate at which they are broken down after death, thus influencing the rate and extent of acidification.

The pattern of acidification may affect the colour and water-holding capacity (WHC) of the meat. At rigor the extent of contraction of the muscle will determine the textural qualities of the meat after cooking. Preslaughter handling may therefore potentially influence several important quality characteristics of the lean meat, either through influencing acidification, or rigor development. Unfortunately, the exact effects of different ante-mortem handling treatments are poorly understood for poultry (Uijtenboogaart, 1996).

FACTORS INFLUENCING GLYCOGEN DEPLETION

Glycogen reserves can be depleted by prolonged food withdrawal (fasting) and the stress of transport. In broiler chickens killed at various times up to 36 h after food (but not water) withdrawal, liver glycogen was reduced to negligible amounts (< 1 mg g^{-1}) within 6 h of deprivation (Warriss *et al.*, 1988). Glycogen in the 'red' biceps femoris (BF) muscle of the leg was also reduced but that in the 'white' pectoralis superficialis (PS) muscle of the breast was not. There was a corresponding elevation of the ultimate pH (pHu) in the BF but not in the PS (Fig. 9.2).

Warriss *et al.* (1993) transported broilers for 2, 4 or 6 h after they had been subjected to food withdrawal times of < 1 h or 10 h. The longer fast reduced liver glycogen by 40% but did not affect that in the PS. However, pHu in the BF was elevated, implying ante-mortem glycogen depletion. Transport progressively reduced liver glycogen concentration and increased pHu in the BF, again implying glycogen depletion. Recently we have confirmed this effect of transport in reducing liver and BF glycogen concentrations (unpublished observations) using commercially transported (for between about 2 and 3 h) broilers. In this study we also investigated the effects of keeping birds in lairage at the processing plant before slaughter. Liver glycogen was depleted with holding times longer than about 2 h. Glycogen in the PS was unaffected, that in the BF was not progressively reduced but pHu in the PS was elevated (5.84 vs. 5.78, $P < 0.01$) after 1 h in lairage.

An interesting observation from this work was that body temperature also rose progressively with longer holding so that birds killed after 4 h in lairage were 0.6°C warmer ($P < 0.001$) than birds killed immediately on arrival at the plant (Fig. 9.3). This could imply that birds were unable to thermoregulate

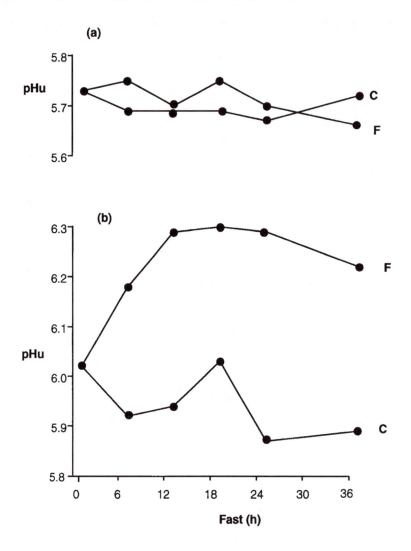

Fig. 9.2. Ultimate pH in the (a) pectoralis superficialis and (b) biceps femoris muscles of broiler chickens deprived of food for up to 36 h (F) compared with that in muscles from birds with *ad libitum* access to food (C). From Warriss *et al.* (1988).

effectively under the holding conditions in lairage, possibly because of inadequate ventilation of the holding crates. Higher body temperatures might have implications for meat quality. Holm and Fletcher (1997) held broilers at 7, 18 or 29°C for 12 h prior to slaughter. Breast fillets from birds held at 29°C had lower ultimate pH and cooking loss, and higher shear value than those from birds held at the lower temperatures.

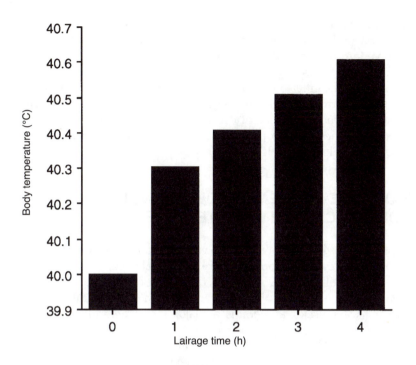

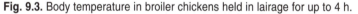

Fig. 9.3. Body temperature in broiler chickens held in lairage for up to 4 h.

PALENESS IN POULTRY MEAT

Ante-mortem glycogen depletion will tend to elevate muscle pHu. Particularly in redder muscles, such as those in the leg, this will potentially produce darker meat. Too pale meat, especially in the breast muscles which have low levels of the pigment myoglobin, has also been identified in poultry.

It has even been suggested that some poultry breast meat can exhibit properties similar to that of PSE (pale, soft, exudative) pork (Santé *et al.*, 1991). Sosnicki (1993) has described the evidence for the occurrence of PSE-like meat in turkeys. The problem is caused by a combination of the extreme muscular development of the birds, large size and a predominantly anaerobic metabolism of the breast muscles coupled with a poor response to ante-mortem stress leading to a rapid pH fall and rigor onset when the muscle temperature is still high (> 35°C). Sosnicki (1993) suggested that exposure to heat or cold stress ante-mortem, or the stress associated with transport, could cause local ischaemia in the breast muscle so promoting glycolytic metabolism and rapid pH fall. Farm-slaughtered birds, not subjected to the stresses of transport, had higher muscle pH than birds transported for 12 h to processing plants.

In Canada, Barbut (1996) has used Lightness (L*) values in the pectoral muscle to estimate the prevalence of PSE in turkeys. Between 18 and 34% of birds from eight flocks had L* values >50 and exhibited the characteristics of PSE meat. The problem of too pale breast meat also occurs in broiler chickens

(Boulianne and King, 1995) although it is unclear whether the aetiology is similar or whether part, at least, of the paleness is caused by leaching of myoglobin into the water used for chilling the meat.

The haemoglobin content of muscle, derived from residual blood, may contribute significantly to colour. This is known to be variable as a result of adrenergic control of the microvasculature, and indeed, the complex relationship of muscle vascularity to resultant haem pigment concentration has been hypothesized as a possible factor responsible for variation in breast muscle colour (Fletcher, 1991).

EFFECTS OF ANTE-MORTEM HANDLING ON pH, WATER-HOLDING CAPACITY AND TEXTURE

Poultry meat is generally tender. However, because the texture of poultry, particularly turkeys, does appear to vary considerably between individual birds (Klose and Scholtyssek, 1967), some effort has been devoted to trying to elucidate the mechanisms behind the variation. In general, the state of contraction of muscles at rigor is a major factor determining tenderness. Highly contracted muscles can be more tender if cooked in the prerigor state (Klose *et al.*, 1970). However, under normal conditions of cooking postrigor, greater contraction is likely to be associated with tougher meat.

Contraction of muscles immediately post-mortem will be controlled by the availability of ATP. If glycogen reserves have been depleted ante-mortem then regeneration of ATP may be affected. Complete depletion would severely limit ATP regeneration and inhibit contraction, leading to tender meat. If only some depletion takes place, enough glycogen may remain to allow continuing production of ATP and greater contraction. This will lead to tougher meat. Additionally, glycogen depletion will be associated with reduced acidification which may have implications for the normal processes of conditioning. Water-holding capacity is also affected by pH. The interaction between events ante-mortem and post-mortem processing probably contributes to the variation seen in final meat quality and the difficulty in defining exactly the influences of ante-mortem stressors.

To assess the effects of stress some workers have used anaesthetized groups of control birds. Froning *et al.* (1978) compared anaesthetized turkeys with birds subjected to cold or heat stress for up to 1 h preslaughter. These treatments did not affect pHu or WHC in the PS but heat stress made the meat tougher and darker. Allowing the birds to struggle freely at slaughter reduced pHu and also led to darker and tougher meat.

Ngoka *et al.* (1982) also examined the effect of anaesthesia on turkeys and, additionally, the influences of a 15 h fast or holding in lairage for 24 h to allow the birds to recover from the stresses associated with transport. Anaesthesia, compared with free struggle, increased initial pH and WHC, and decreased shear force and redness (aL) value. Feed withdrawal for 15 h increased pHu and WHC, and also reduced shear force. Birds killed immediately on arrival at the processing plant had higher WHC, redness (aL) value and lower shear force values.

Based on comparison with birds reared in the laboratory, Wood and Richards (1975a) could find no effect of 'normal' commercial handling of broilers on pH or shear value. However, heat and cold stress preslaughter did affect the rate of post-mortem glycolysis.

To overcome the difficulties of controlling preslaughter factors, in order to investigate their effects, some workers have used ante-mortem adrenaline (epinephrine) injections to simulate naturally occurring stress. Wood and Richards (1975b) injected adrenaline into broilers. Glycogen in the PS muscle was almost completely depleted within 8–12 h of treatment. The pHu was elevated from 6.04 in untreated controls to 6.77 after 8 h, 6.88 after 12 h and 6.11 after 24 h. Adrenaline also resulted in significantly tougher meat which seemed to be related to differences in the contractile properties of the muscles. A problem with this approach is that injected adrenaline may not accurately mimic normally occurring stress. Adrenaline seems to deplete glycogen from PS muscle (and possibly all muscles) whereas natural stressors may have an effect only in 'red' muscles. A similar effect occurs in red meat species.

CONCLUSIONS

Four major aspects of poultry meat quality can be influenced by ante-mortem handling. Yield may be reduced by death of birds in transit and by 'shrinkage' caused by prolonged food withdrawal preslaughter and transport stress. Food withdrawal times may also have implications for hygiene by influencing gut fill and the character of the microbial populations, particularly of pathogens, in the crop and caeca. Haemorrhages and bruising can also reduce yield if trimming of tissue is necessary. Even if this is not required, damage downgrades the appearance of the product. Lastly, ante-mortem handling may affect lean meat quality characteristics such as colour, water-holding capacity and texture. Various stressors have been shown to deplete muscle glycogen and potentially to lead to elevated ultimate pH and changes in water-holding capacity. It is less clear how the normal stresses associated with handling and transport affect cooked meat texture. There is some evidence that these stresses can also lead to PSE-like meat characteristics in susceptible birds, especially in the breast muscles of turkeys.

REFERENCES

Anon. (1965) *Table Chickens*, MAFF, Bulletin No 168, HMSO, London, p. 41.

Barbut, S. (1996) Estimates and detection of the PSE problem in young turkey breast meat. *Canadian Journal of Animal Science* 76, 455–457.

Barbut, S., McEwen, S.A. and Julian, R.J. (1990) Turkey downgrading: effect of truck, cage location and unloading. *Poultry Science* 69, 1410–1413.

Bayliss, P.A. (1986) A study of factors influencing mortality of broilers during transit to the processing plant. MSc Thesis, University of Bristol, Bristol, UK.

Benibo, B.S. and Farr, A.J. (1985) The effects of feed and water withdrawal and holding shed treatment on broiler yield parameters. *Poultry Science* 64, 920–924.

Boulianne, M. and King, A.J. (1995) Biochemical and color characteristics of skinless boneless pale chicken breast. *Poultry Science* 74, 1693–1698.

Cashman, P.J., Nicol, C.J. and Jones, R.B. (1989) Effects of transportation on the tonic immobility fear reactions of broilers. *British Poultry Science* 30, 211–221.

Chen, T.C., Schultz, C.D., Reece, R.N., Lott, B.D. and McNaughton, J.L. (1983) The effect of extended holding time, temperature and dietary energy on yields of broilers. *Poultry Science* 62, 1566–1571.

Duncan, I.J.H. (1989) The assessment of welfare during the handling and transport of broilers. In: *Proceedings of the 3rd European Symposium on Poultry Welfare,* Tours, France, pp. 93–107.

Fletcher, D.L. (1991) Ante mortem factors related to meat quality. In: Uijtenboogaart, T.G. and Verkamp, C.H. (eds) *Proceedings of the 10th European Symposium on the Quality of Poultry Meat,* pp. 11–19.

Fletcher, D.L. and Rahn, A.P. (1982) The effect of environmentally modified and conventional housing types on broiler shrinkage. *Poultry Science* 61, 67–74.

Freeman, B.M., Kettlewell, P.J., Manning, A.C.C. and Berry, P.S. (1984) Stress of transportation for broilers. *Veterinary Record* 114, 286–287.

Froning, G.W., Babji, A.S. and Mather, F.B. (1978) The effect of preslaughter temperature, stress, struggle and anethetization on color and textural characteristics of turkey muscle. *Poultry Science* 57, 630–633.

Gregory, N.G. and Austin, S.D. (1992) Causes of trauma in broilers arriving dead at poultry processing plants. *Veterinary Record* 131, 501–503.

Griffiths, G.L. and Nairn, M.E. (1984) Carcass downgrading of broiler chickens. *British Poultry Science* 25, 441–446.

Hamdy, M.K., May, K.N. and Powers, J.J. (1961) Some physical and physiological factors affecting poultry bruises. *Poultry Science* 40, 790–795.

Hargis, B.M., Caldwell, D.J., Brewer, R.L., Corrier, D.E. and DeLoach, J.R. (1995) Evaluation of the chicken crop as a source of *Salmonella* contamination for broiler carcasses. *Poultry Science* 74, 1548–1552.

Holm, C.G.P. and Fletcher, D.L. (1997) Antemortem holding temperatures and broiler breast meat quality. *Journal of Applied Poultry Research* 6, 180–184.

Humphrey, T.J., Baskerville, A., Whitehead, A., Rowe, B. and Henley, A. (1993) Influence of feeding patterns on the artificial infection of laying hens with *Salmonella enteritidis* phage type 4. *Veterinary Record* 132, 407–409.

Kannan, G. and Mench, J.A. (1996) Influence of different handling methods and crating periods on plasma corticosterone concentrations in broilers. *British Poultry Science* 37, 21–31.

Kettlewell, P. and Turner, M.J.B. (1985) A review of broiler chicken catching and transportation systems. *Journal of Agricultural Engineering Research* 31, 93–114.

Kettlewell, P., Mitchell, M. and Meehan, A. (1993) The distribution of thermal loads within poultry transport vehicles. *Agricultural Engineer* 48, 26–30.

Klose, A.A. and Scholtyssek, S. (1967) Sources of variability in turkey tenderness. *Poultry Science* 46, 936–938.

Klose, A.A., Luyet, B.J. and Menz, L.J. (1970) Effect of contraction on tenderness of poultry muscle cooked in the prerigor state. *Journal of Food Science* 35, 577–581.

Knowles, T.G. and Broom, D.M. (1990) The handling and transport of broilers and spent hens. *Applied Animal Behavioural Science* 28, 75–91.

Mayes, F.J. (1980) The incidence of bruising in broiler flocks. *British Poultry Science* 21, 505–509.

McEwen, S.A. and Barbut, S. (1992) Survey of turkey downgrading at slaughter: carcass defects and associations with transport, toe-nail trimming and type of bird. *Poultry Science* 71, 1107–1115.

Mills, D.S. and Nicol, C.J. (1990) Tonic immobility in spent hens after catching and transport. *Veterinary Record* 126, 210–212.

Mitchell, M.A., Kettlewell, P.J. and Maxwell, M.H. (1992) Indicators of physiological stress in broiler chickens during road transportation. *Animal Welfare* 1, 91–103.

Ngoka, D.A., Froning, G.W., Lowry, S.R. and Babji, A.S. (1982) Effects of sex, age, preslaughter factors, and holding conditions on the quality characteristics and chemical composition of turkey breast muscles. *Poultry Science* 61, 1996–2003.

Santé, V., Bielicki, G., Renerre, M. and Lacourt, A. (1991) Post mortem evolution in the *Pectoralis superficialis* muscle from two turkey breeds: relationship between pH and colour changes. *Proceedings of the 37th International Congress of Meat Science and Technology*, Kulmbach, paper 3, 36, pp. 456–468.

Sosnicki, A.A. (1993) PSE in turkey. *Meat Focus International,* February, pp. 75–78.

Swarbrick, O. (1986) The welfare during transport of broilers, old hens and replacement pullets. In: Gibson, T.E. (ed.) *The Welfare of Animals in Transit.* British Veterinary Association Animal Welfare Association, London, pp. 82–97.

Taylor, M.H. and Helbacka, N.V.L. (1968) Field studies of bruised poultry. *Poultry Science* 47, 1166–1169.

Uijtenboogaart, T.G. (1996) Poultry handling, slaughter and primary processing. In: Taylor, S.A., Raimundo, A., Severini, M. and Smulders, F.J.M. (eds) *Meat Quality and Meat Packaging*, ECCEAMST, Utrecht, The Netherlands, pp. 125–136.

Veerkamp, C.N. (1986) Preslaughter conditions for poultry – good handling gives better yield. *Poultry-Misset*, April, pp. 30–33.

Wabeck, C.J. (1972) Feed and water withdrawal time relationship to processing yield and potential faecal contamination of broilers. *Poultry Science* 51, 1119–1121.

Warriss, P.D., and Brown, S.N. (1996) The time spent by turkeys in transit to processing plants. *Veterinary Record* 139, 72–73.

Warriss, P.D. and Knowles, T.G. (1993) Welfare aspects of broiler transport in the United Kingdom. In: Collins, E. and Boon, C. (eds) *Proceedings of the Fourth International Symposium of the American Society of Agricultural Engineering: 'Livestock Environment'*, American Society of Agricultural Engineers, St Joseph, Michigan, USA. pp. 547–551.

Warriss, P.D., Kestin, S.C., Brown, S.N. and Bevis, E.A. (1988) Depletion of glycogen reserves in fasting broiler chickens. *British Poultry Science* 29, 149–154.

Warriss, P.D., Bevis, E.A. and Brown, S.N. (1990) Time spent by broiler chickens in transit to processing plants. *Veterinary Record* 127, 617–619.

Warriss, P.D., Bevis, E.A., Brown, S.N. and Edwards, J.E. (1992) Longer journeys to processing plants are associated with higher mortality in broiler chickens. *British Poultry Science* 33, 201–206.

Warriss, P.D., Kestin, S.C., Brown, S.N., Knowles, T.G., Wilkins, L.J., Edwards, J.E., Austin, S.D. and Nicol, C.J. (1993) The depletion of glycogen stores and indices of dehydration in transported broilers. *British Veterinary Journal* 149, 391–398.

Webster, A.J.F., Tuddenham, A., Saville, C.A. and Scott, G.B. (1993) Thermal stress on chickens in transit. *British Poultry Science* 34, 267–277.

Willis, W.L., Murray, C. and Raczkowski, C.W. (1996) The influence of feed and water withdrawal on *Campylobacter jejuni* detection and yield of broilers. *Journal of Applied Poultry Research* 5, 210–214.

Wilson, J.G. and Brunson, C.C. (1968) The effects of handling and slaughter method on the incidence of haemorrhagic thighs in broilers. *Poultry Science* 47, 1315–1318.

Wood, D.F. and Richards, J.F. (1975a) Effect of some antemortem stressors on postmortem aspects of chicken broiler pectoralis muscle. *Poultry Science* 54, 528–531.

Wood, D.F. and Richards, J.F. (1975b) Effect of preslaughter epinephrine injection on postmortem aspects of chicken broiler pectoralis muscle. *Poultry Science* 54, 520–527.

Yogaratnam, V. (1995) Analysis of the causes of high rates of carcase rejection at a poultry processing plant. *Veterinary Record* 137, 215–217.

CHAPTER 10
Effects of stunning and slaughter methods on carcass and meat quality

A.B.M. Raj

Division of Food Animal Science, School of Veterinary Science, University of Bristol, Langford, Bristol BS40 5DU, UK

PRODUCTION AND CONSUMPTION IN EUROPE

Chicken and turkey meat production and consumption have been increasing steadily in Europe (Table 10.1). Poultry meat is leaner and is less expensive than red meats and carcass portioning and deboning have given the consumer more choice (white breast and darker thigh or drumstick meat) and opportunity to purchase preferred quantity. In addition, developments in further processing of poultry meat has given them varieties of products with different taste and texture (whole, flaked or ground meat).

IMPORTANCE OF CARCASS AND MEAT QUALITY

Consumer awareness of quality has also improved considerably over recent years and the appearance of carcass or meat has become more important in

Table 10.1. Broiler chicken and turkey meat production and per capita consumption in European Union (12 Member States) (Sources: Foreign Agricultural Service, Commodity and Marketing Programs, Dairy, Livestock and Poultry Division).

	Year		
	1995	1996(p)	1997(f)
Production (1000 metric tonnes in ready-to-cook equivalents)			
Broiler	5280	5460	5530
Turkey	1561	1625	1668
Per capita consumption (kg)			
Broiler	14.8	15.4	15.6
Turkey	3.6	3.7	3.8

p = preliminary; f = forecast.

© CAB *International* 1999.
Poultry Meat Science (eds R.I. Richardson and G.C. Mead)

determining consumer acceptability and retail price. In general, carcass and meat quality problems can originate from various factors starting from catching on the farm to the evisceration process in the processing plant (Gregory and Wilkins, 1990a). However, immersion or convection chilling, in comparison with air chilling, can mask the appearance defects (Moran and Bilgili, 1995). In the USA, immersion chilling of broiler carcass is commonly used irrespective of whether the meat is sold fresh or frozen. By contrast, in Europe, all the fresh broiler meat should be air chilled and only frozen carcasses can be immersion chilled, and therefore, carcass appearance is more important in this continent. Turkey carcasses however can be immersion chilled in Europe.

Some of the carcass and meat quality defects are listed in Table 10.2 and the commercial significance of these defects varies according to market outlet. However, the prevalence of appearance defects can lead to downgrading and loss of value of fresh carcasses. Other conditions, such as haemorrhagic wing veins, may warrant trimming and loss of valuable portions. The broken pectoral bones (mainly furculum) come away with the breast fillets when the carcasses are prepared as portions and haemorrhages appear as dark spots when the fillets are cooked. These are undesirable from the consumer's point of view. Therefore, the fillets will have to be examined, bone fragments removed and haemorrhagic areas in the breast fillets trimmed prior to packaging. These procedures involve additional man-power, costs and loss in valuable meat. Broken coracoid bones frequently cause haemorrhaging in breast muscles due to either rupture of blood vessels adjacent to the bone or splinters damaging the muscle. Residual blood retained in the breast meat, occurring due to poor bleed out, might be squeezed out during retail packaging and this may appear either as a lump of clot or serum smear over the meat. In addition, engorged blood vessels may appear as dark streaks in cooked meats. These could be visually less appealing to the consumer.

Table 10.2. Carcass and meat quality defects leading to downgrading or trimming.

Carcass appearance defects:
Red wingtips
Red pygostyles
Red feather tracts
Engorged wing veins
Haemorrhagic wing veins
Haemorrhage in shoulders
Claw damage and torn skin
Haemorrhage in the muscles:
Breast
Leg
Dislocated or broken bones:
Pectoral bones
Wing bones
Leg bones

In Europe, the average loss in quantity of fresh poultry meat is estimated to be 1–3%, although some processing plants report up to 6% trimming loss in breast meat alone. At 1% loss, it can be estimated that 54,600 tonnes of prime broiler meat was lost during the year 1996. In December 1996, the producer price (pound sterling (£) equivalent) was 56 p kg^{-1} in the Netherlands, the lowest cost producer in Europe, and at this producer price, the actual loss for the year 1996 can be estimated at over £30 million. If the retail price of fresh turkey meat is considered to be £3 kg^{-1} and the minimal loss due to trimming happens to be 1%, then it is estimated that the European turkey industry had lost about £50 million worth of prime meat in the year 1996. Although the trimmings and downgraded portions or carcasses would have been sold at a reduced price, this certainly shows the importance of carcass and meat quality. To address the concerns of poultry processors and retailers, scientists around the world are relentlessly pursuing research and development.

BACKGROUND

In order to understand how stunning methods can affect carcass and meat quality, one needs to consider some of the anatomical features and physiological responses to stunning. Breast muscles, pectoralis major (pectoralis superficialis) and pectoralis minor (supracoracoidius), are the most valuable portions in a poultry carcass. The pectoralis minor muscle originates from the keel bone and inserts on the dorsal side of the humerus bone. The articular surface of the shoulder joint is formed by the scapula and coracoid bones, and they act as fulcrum to the supracoracoidius tendon of the pectoralis minor muscle. The main function of this muscle is therefore elevation and rotation of the humerus (elevation of wings or upwards stroke during flight). The pectoralis major muscle extends mainly from the clavicle (furculum) and the coracoclavicular membrane, and to a lesser extent from the keel of the sternum, to the pectoral crest of the humerus bone. The main function of this muscle is the depression of the humerus (depression of wings or downwards stroke during flight). Both chickens and turkeys are capable of fast flapping flights in which the thrust is produced solely during depression of the wings. Therefore, in these birds, the pectoralis major muscles are larger than the pectoralis minor muscles. Both the muscles are composed of predominantly (> 90%) fast twitch glycolytic fibres (Wiskus *et al.*, 1976; Chiang *et al.*, 1995). The activity of white fibre adenosine triphosphatase (ATPase) is faster than the red fibre ATPase. This has two implications, firstly, the muscles have the capacity to undergo rapid pH fall or rigor development post mortem. Secondly, in fast-twitch fibres, the development of tension in response to neural stimulation takes 7.5 ms compared with 100 ms for the slow-twitch red fibres (Ganong, 1993). When the stimulation rates are faster than the time course of fibre relaxation, a summation of contractions (tetanus) will occur and it has been reported that in this situation forces up to four times that found in twitch contraction can develop in muscles (Wilson, 1972). Due to the antagonistic functions of the pectoralis major and minor muscles, there is also likely to be a combination of shortening and stretching known as eccentric contraction (Warren *et al.*, 1993), resulting in damage to cell membranes (Cassens *et al.*, 1963) and supercontraction of muscle fibres (Leet *et al.*, 1977). From a meat quality point of view, these can lead to haemorrhaging in breast muscles and dislocation or fracture in pectoral bones. Because of the anatomical dispositions, there can be broken furculum and coracoid bones due to the contraction of pectoralis major and minor muscles, respectively. Similarly, haemorrhaging can also occur in leg muscles with antagonistic functions (abductor and adductor). However, leg bone breakage due to muscle contraction is uncommon.

Under stunning and slaughter situations, muscle contractions can occur due to:

1. stimulation of the central nervous system or removal of suppression of higher centres on brainstem and spinal cord;
2. stimulation of spinal motor neurones;
3. direct stimulation of muscle.

These three effects can occur concurrently during waterbath electrical stunning of poultry, in which the current flows from an electrified bath through the birds to a shackle line, the earth. The release of brainstem and spinal cord from the inhibition of higher centres can occur under gas stunning situations (Raj *et al.*, 1992a). However, the rate of induction of anaesthesia with gas mixtures, and thus the rate of removal of inhibition of higher centres, determines the severity of convulsions (wing flapping) occurring during gas stunning. For example, rapid induction of unconsciousness induced with either 90% argon in air or a high concentration (> 60%) of carbon dioxide in air results in severe convulsions. By contrast, gradual induction of unconsciousness with either 75–80% argon in air or 25–30% carbon dioxide in air produces very few convulsions. From the bird welfare point of view, slow induction of unconsciousness with gas mixtures can be aversive, and therefore, not recommended.

During electrical stunning, the contractile response of the muscles varies according to peak-to-peak voltage, wave form and frequency of current applied. Although the effects of these have not been elucidated in poultry, a rat model has been used to demonstrate the effects of transcranial, nerve or direct muscle electrical stimulation on the contractile responses in muscle (Simmons, 1995). In this model, a peak force of contraction is developed in muscle during the application of different voltages and frequencies, a common pattern of response seen in all three stimulation pathways. However, the peak contraction force was maintained throughout the period of stimulation with 50 Hz, whereas at higher frequencies, the peak force fell swiftly to a substantially reduced level for the rest of the period of stimulation. In all three stimulation pathways, the mean force of contraction reduced as the current frequency increased. In addition, when a multiple bird electrical waterbath stunner is supplied with a constant voltage source, the current that flows through each bird can vary according to the impedance offered, and therefore, some birds receive less and others receive more than the necessary currents

(Sparrey *et al.*, 1993). This could account for the highly variable carcass and meat quality seen under commercial electrical waterbath stunning conditions. The Silsoe Research Institute in the UK has developed a constant current stunner which will control the current flow through individual birds in a waterbath stunner and, when used commercially, can improve the situation.

STUNNING METHODS

The conventional method of poultry processing involves uncrating and shackling live birds and then electrically stunning them using a multiple bird waterbath stunner prior to neck cutting. The concept, mode of operation and recent developments in electrical waterbath stunners have been described by Bilgili (1992) and Sparrey *et al.* (1992, 1993). It should be noted that the amount of current (amperage) received by individual birds, rather than the voltage supplied to a waterbath stunner, determines the effectiveness of the stun and the carcass and meat quality.

In Europe, certain minimum RMS (root mean square) currents have been recommended by the Commission, however, they are yet to be made law (Table 10.3). Nonetheless, stunning poultry under commercial condition is a statutory requirement and the minimum current applied varies from 80 to 120 mA per broiler applied for a minimum of 4 s. In the USA, there is no statutory requirement to stun poultry; however, the majority of poultry processors voluntarily implement electrical stunning using 5–6 mA per broiler for a minimum of 10 s (Heath *et al.*, 1994).

It is very likely that various wave forms and frequencies of electric currents used commercially could have different effects on the birds. However, while using a 50 Hz sinusoidal alternating current in a waterbath stunner, these minimum currents will induce cardiac arrest in about 90% of birds (Gregory and Wilkins, 1989a, 1990b). There are two reasons for selecting cardiac arrest as a criterion for setting the minimum currents. First, it is the only method which produces rapid brain death following stunning, at least in chickens (Gregory and Wotton, 1986). Secondly, induction of cardiac arrest at stunning eliminates the chances of resumption of consciousness in birds due to delayed or inappropriate neck cutting. However, some scientists argue, on bird welfare grounds, that these current levels do not abolish brain responsiveness (somatosensory evoked potentials) immediately after stunning, and therefore, the recommended currents should be not less than 120 mA per

Table 10.3. Minimum RMS (root mean square) electric current (per bird) recommended in Europe for stunning chickens and turkeys.

	Waterbath stunning	Head-only stunning
Chickens	100 mA	240 mA
Turkeys	150 mA	400 mA
Minimum duration	4 s	3 s

chicken and 250 mA per turkey (Gregory and Wotton, 1990, 1991).

Alternatively, novel methods of killing poultry using gas mixtures (controlled atmosphere stunning) have been approved in the UK, under The Welfare of Animals (during Slaughter or Killing) Regulations (1995), for killing chickens and turkeys in their transport containers (HMSO, 1995). They are:

1. anoxia induced with 90% argon or other inert gases in air (leaving 8% residual nitrogen and 2% residual oxygen from air);
2. a mixture of 30% carbon dioxide and 60% argon or other inert gases in air (leaving 8% residual nitrogen and 2% residual oxygen from air).

There is no doubt that killing poultry in transport containers using gas mixtures will enable shackling to be performed on relaxed carcasses and this would eliminate the live bird handling at the processing plants.

These two gas mixtures have been selected on the basis of the following.

1. The induction of unconsciousness with anoxia is smooth and the birds, given a free choice, spontaneously enter this atmosphere and are killed.
2. The induction of unconsciousness with the carbon dioxide–argon mixture is rapid and the majority of birds, given a free choice, enter this atmosphere and are killed.
3. Birds find an atmosphere containing a high concentration of carbon dioxide aversive, and given a free choice, the majority of birds avoid it (Raj *et al.*, 1992a; Raj and Gregory, 1994; Raj, 1996).

BLOOD LOSS

It is known that, in comparison with mammals, poultry have unusually long blood clotting times. This is because they rely on tissue thromboplastin for homeostasis rather than on the generation of plasma thromboplastin as in mammals (Bigland, 1964). Therefore, any differences seen in the rate of bleed-out or total blood loss can be attributed to a combination of factors, such as, whether the birds have been killed or just stunned (resulting in relaxed carcasses with fibrillated hearts or birds with non-fibrillated hearts showing tremors during bleeding, respectively), the delay between killing and neck cutting, blood vessels cut and the bleed-out time permitted before scalding. A poor bleed-out can increase the prevalence of some of the carcass downgrading conditions. Nevertheless, in the UK, bleed out times of 90 s for chickens and 180 s for turkeys must be provided following electrical stunning. In the USA, a minimum of 90 s bleed out time has been recommended for chickens (Kuenzel *et al.*, 1978). In Europe, it is a common practice to cut the necks of poultry at the back of their heads severing a vertebral artery, or cut unilaterally on the ventral side of the necks severing one carotid artery and one jugular vein. By contrast, in the USA, a complete ventral neck cut, severing both carotid arteries and both jugular veins in the neck, is commonly practised. The bleed-out times are generally based on the fact that, if the birds were just stunned and had their necks cut, brain death should occur through exsanguination before they enter the scald tank. Therefore, duration of unconsciousness with a stunning procedure must be longer than the sum of the time taken to perform neck cutting and the time to onset of brain death through blood loss (Gregory and Wotton, 1986). Prevalence of red skin conditions has been reported to be due to an acute inflammatory reaction occurring in live birds entering the scald tank (Griffiths, 1985).

In the past, at least in Europe, poultry have been stunned using 50–60 Hz sine wave alternating current. Alternating current frequencies of up to 100 Hz can be more effective in inducing fibrillation of hearts (cardiac arrest) than higher frequencies of AC or DC. However, as described earlier, stunning with low frequency currents can lead to muscle contractions, and consequently, haemorrhaging in breast muscles. Therefore, the poultry industry in Europe, as in the USA, has opted to use high frequency (> 300 Hz) AC or DC.

Reports concerning blood loss in broilers following electrical stunning are conflicting. For example, Griffiths *et al.* (1985) found that neither bleed-out nor the residual blood in the carcass meat varied significantly between the birds which were stunned or killed with an electric current. Gregory and Wilkins (1989b) examined blood loss using seven different neck cutting methods in broilers and found that the total bleed-out after 2.25 min of neck cutting was similar in all the treatments. Dickens and Lyon (1993) also found that the total blood loss was very similar in chickens stunned with either 50 V AC or 200 V AC. By contrast, Veerkamp and de Vries (1983) found that blood loss at 285 s after neck cutting decreased as the stunning voltage increased from 75 to 200 V. Craig and Fletcher (1997) reported that, after 150 s bleed-out time, broilers stunned with 125 mA (50 Hz sine wave AC) lost on average 0.3% less blood than those stunned with 5–6 mA (500 Hz square wave pulsed DC). It is possible that, in birds which suffer cardiac arrest at stunning, the wings begin to relax very soon and hang lower than the shoulder joints which can result in pooling of blood in the wing veins. On the other hand, in birds which have non-fibrillated hearts, the wings are held stiffly against the breast muscle, and this, in association with the tremors can improve the drainage from the wing veins. These differences are apparent in the initial rate of bleed-out, however, the total blood loss is very similar (Raj and Johnson, 1997). In the case of turkeys, when compared with 50 Hz AC, high frequency electrical stunning results in a faster rate of bleed-out and higher total blood loss (Mouchoniere *et al.*, 1998). Nevertheless, irrespective of the stunning current parameters, cutting all the major blood vessels in the neck should become mandatory under commercial conditions.

Under the gas or controlled atmosphere killing of poultry in their transport containers, birds would leave the unit in large numbers. These crates will have to be emptied and carcasses shackled prior to neck cutting. Therefore, it is very likely that the time between end of killing and neck cutting is to be longer than the corresponding time under the electrical stunning systems. In addition to this delay in neck cutting, physiological effects of gases can also affect the bleed-out. For example, Kotula *et al.* (1957) and Kotula and Helbacka (1966) found that the birds stunned with carbon dioxide in air retained a higher percentage of blood in the internal organs. It has been suggested that, in laboratory models, anoxia or carbon dioxide combined with anoxia causes arterial dilatation and vasoconstriction, respectively (Shorr *et al.*, 1945; Messina *et al.*, 1992). However, Poole and Fletcher (1995) found that killing of broilers with either carbon dioxide, nitrogen or argon resulted in a very similar total blood loss. Raj and Gregory (1991a) found no significant difference in total blood loss in broilers stunned with either 45% carbon dioxide in air, 90% argon in air or an electric current.

More recently, the effect of delayed neck cutting on total blood loss was investigated in broilers and turkeys (Table 10.4). In broilers, electrical stunning with 1500 Hz AC resulted in carcasses with non-fibrillated hearts, and in these birds, when neck cutting was performed in less than 20 s the cumulative blood loss at 100 s was about 2 g kg^{-1} live weight more than that recorded for broilers which had fibrillated hearts and had their necks cut at 1 min after stunning

Table 10.4. Effect of stunning/killing methods, time to neck cutting and blood vessels cut on the average blood loss (after Raj and Gregory, 1991a; Raj *et al.*, 1994; Raj and Johnson, 1997).

Treatment	Time to neck cut	Method of cutting[a]	Average blood loss (g kg^{-1} live weight) Broilers (100 s)	Turkeys (170 s)
90% Argon	< 50 s	U	27.6	22.9
	1 min	V	31.0	—
		U	29.8	—
	3 min	V	26.5	—
		U	29.8	—
	5 min	V	30.0	—
		U	29.7	24.5
	10 min	U	—	22.0
Carbon dioxide –argon mixture	< 50 s	U	—	25.8
	1 min	V	30.0	—
		U	28.7	—
	3 min	V	26.1	—
		U	28.1	—
	5 min	V	26.0	—
		U	25.0	24.9
	10 min	U	—	25.2
Electrical 50 Hz	< 50 s	U	29.0	25.0
	1 min	V	34.2	—
		U	29.7	—
	3 min	V	26.0	—
		U	28.4	—
	5 min	V	29.1	—
		U	24.8	—
Electrical 1500 Hz	20 s	V	36.1	—

V = ventral cut aimed at severing both carotid arteries and both jugular veins.
U = Unilateral cut aimed at severing one carotid artery and one jugular vein.

with the 50 Hz sine wave AC. When compared with the high frequency electrical stunning, killing broilers with argon or carbon dioxide–argon mixture and delays of up to 5 min in neck cutting resulted in about 6–9 g kg^{-1} live weight less bleed-out. However, at corresponding neck cutting intervals, there were no significant differences between broilers killed with either gas mixtures or a 50 Hz sine wave AC. In the case of turkeys also the total blood loss was very similar in birds that were killed with either an electric current or a gas mixture (Raj *et al.*, 1994). Therefore, it appears that, in birds killed with either an electric current or gas mixtures, bleeding occurs through gravitational force and therefore all the major vessels in the neck should be cut as soon as possible to maximize the bleed-out.

Inadequate bleeding, particularly in turkeys, frequently results in retention of blood in the vessels of pectoral muscles and legs. It is possible that in large turkeys, when the wings hang low, they cause flexion resulting in narrowing of the pectoral trunk leading to impaired drainage. Inappropriate shackle size, in particular those causing abduction or adduction of legs could have a similar effect on the blood vessels in the leg. Therefore, it is suggested that extrinsic factors which can impede drainage of blood should also be considered when determining the effect of stunning methods on bleed-out.

RIGOR DEVELOPMENT

As mentioned previously, the nature of muscle contractions induced by the stunning procedure could vary according to stimulation parameters and this can influence the rate of onset of rigor. However, the direct effect of electrical stunning parameters, such as peak voltage, amperage and frequency of current and stunning duration, on the rate of rigor development is unclear. For example, Papinaho and Fletcher (1995a) found that, in comparison with 50 mA, stunning broiler chickens with 100–200 mA per bird resulted in higher mean pH values at 15 min post-mortem. Schutt-Abraham *et al.* (1983) found no significant differences in the pH at 15 min between groups of broilers stunned with currents ranging from 55 to 110 mA per bird. Craig and Fletcher (1997) compared broiler chickens stunned with either 125 mA delivered using 110 V, 50 Hz sine wave AC or 5–6 mA delivered using 11 V, 500 Hz pulsed square wave DC. In that study, the birds stunned with high current had a higher mean pH value at 15 min than those stunned with the low current (6.67 vs. 6.47). Poole and Fletcher (1995), although using the same currents, found that the breast muscles of broilers stunned with the high current reached a pH of below 6.0 at 5 h when compared with 3 h in broilers stunned with the low current. However, it is not certain whether these differences were solely due to the amount (mA) of current applied to birds or the frequency of current applied to birds. For example, high frequency (300–1000 Hz) electrical stunning of turkeys results in wing flapping during bleeding and this has been found to accelerate the pH fall early post-mortem.

There are conflicting reports on the effect of electrical stunning duration on the rate of rigor development. For example, Papinaho and Fletcher (1995b) reported that the duration of 5, 10, 20 or 40 s of electrical stunning with 100 V AC had no effect on the broiler breast muscle pH at 15 min post-mortem. By contrast, Young and Buhr (1997) stunned broilers with 50 V AC for either 0, 2, 4, 6, 8 or 10 s and found that the breast muscle pH measured after 1 h post-mortem increased with the duration of electrical stunning. However, it should be noted that, in these studies, there are differences in live bird handling, application of stunning, carcass chilling and pH measurement.

Papinaho *et al.* (1995) reported that, when broilers were restrained during electrical stunning or had their breast muscles denervated surgically prior to stunning, there was no significant effect of current (50 or 125 mA per bird) on the mean pH at 15 min post-mortem. Therefore, these authors concluded that the muscular activity occurring peri-mortem rather than the stunning current *per se* is responsible for any differences seen in the rate of rigor development. However, it should be noted that, in the denervated breast muscles, the effect of stimulation of the central nervous system and the spinal motor neurones has been removed, and therefore, the effect of electrical stunning on the denervated muscles would have been a consequence of direct stimulation of muscles only.

Wing flapping occurring during gas or controlled atmosphere stunning can accelerate the rate of pH fall early post-mortem depending on the physiological properties of the gas used in the stunning atmosphere. For example, in comparison with 45% carbon dioxide in air, stunning of broiler chickens with 90% argon in air resulted in significantly lower breast muscle pH at 20 min post-mortem (6.37 vs. 5.91; Raj *et al.*, 1990b). This is possibly due to:

1. argon induced anoxia at the cellular level triggering the break down of ATP, and thus, anaerobic glycolysis;
2. glycolysis being accelerated by the wing flapping occurring under the anoxic conditions.

Together, these effects appear to result in rigor development (pH < 6.0) within 20 min post-mortem in broilers (Raj *et al.*, 1990b, 1991) and turkeys (Raj, 1994a). In these studies, anoxia was induced in chickens and turkeys by exposing them very rapidly (less than 20 s) to < 2% oxygen in argon, whereas, Poole and Fletcher (1995) did not find rapid rigor development in broilers stunned with argon or nitrogen when anoxia was induced gradually (in about 1 min). In that study, although broilers exposed to anoxia showed severe wing flapping, the times to onset and duration of convulsions were found to be different. This implies that the rate of induction of anoxia at the cellular level may also have an effect on the rate of rigor development.

In contrast with the effect of true anoxia induced with argon, addition of carbon dioxide to argon (hypercapnic anoxia) appears to retard the rate of rigor development. For example, when 10%, 20% or 30% carbon dioxide was added to argon, leaving 5% residual oxygen in all the mixtures, it was found that the mean pH values in the breast muscles at 20 min post-mortem were 6.38, 6.60 and 6.61, respectively (Raj *et al.*, 1992b). A more recent study showed that stunning of broilers with a mixture of 30% carbon dioxide and 60% argon, leaving a residual oxygen of 2%, resulted in a mean breast muscle pH of 6.4 and 6.1 at 2 and 4 h post-mortem, respectively (Raj *et al.*, 1997). Poole and Fletcher (Georgia, 1997, personal communication) also found that broilers stunned with 30% carbon dioxide and 60% argon reached a pH of below 6.0 at 5 h post-mortem. These results show that, in comparison with the pure anoxia induced by argon, carbon dioxide gas inhibits the rate of rigor development. Sams and Dzuik (1995) reported that electrical stimulation (applied after bleed-out) of broilers killed with carbon dioxide (> 70%) failed to breakdown ATP or glycogen, as determined using R-value (adenosine to inosine compounds ratio) and pH at 1 h post-mortem. Based on these, the authors concluded that carbon dioxide killing negated the acceleration of rigor development induced by the electrical stimulation treatment. The exact mechanism by which carbon dioxide retards the rate of rigor development in poultry is not known. However, there is some evidence to suggest that the acidosis induced by carbon dioxide gas reduced the twitch force and the ATP cost per twitch by 50% in skinned cat skeletal muscle fibres when 10 s trains of twitches (2 s at 1 Hz) were induced (Harkema *et al.*, 1997). In addition, carbon dioxide acidosis can cause:

1. activation of potassium channels;
2. inhibition of calcium channels;
3. increases in intramitochondrial potential for ATP synthesis;
4. inhibition of the release of glycolytic enzymes either directly or through inactivation of the sarcoplasmic reticulum.

Theoretically, points **1** and **2** will induce muscle relaxation, and **3** and **4** will sustain ATP and glycogen reserves in muscles. Further research should clarify these effects in poultry. However, the relaxation of frog skeletal muscle was slower when intracellular pH was lowered, independent of other metabolites, with carbon dioxide, and the relaxation was prolonged when the tetanus duration was longer (Curtin, 1988). On the other hand, at low temperatures (12–20°C), a decreased tetanus tension and enhanced tension relaxation of rat skeletal muscle have been reported during carbon dioxide-induced acidosis (Ranatunga, 1987).

CARCASS APPEARANCE DEFECTS

The inevitable live bird handling is a universal welfare problem associated with the conventional electrical stunning systems. Wing flapping prior to stunning can lead to a higher prevalence of red wingtips in carcasses (Gregory *et al.*, 1989). Tipping of live birds from transport modules, hanging on tight shackles, and prestun electric shocks received at the entrance to waterbath stunners can cause wing flapping.

The effects of stunning current using 50 Hz sine wave AC on the prevalence of carcass and meat quality defects have been reported by Gregory and Wilkins (1989a; 1990b) for broilers and turkeys (Tables 10.5 and 10.6). These studies have shown that the prevalence of carcass downgrading

Table 10.5. Effect of stunning current (50 Hz sine wave AC) on the prevalence of carcass and meat quality defects in broilers (laboratory study) (after Gregory and Wilkins, 1989a).

	Average stunning current (mA)						
	45	85	121	141	161	181	220
Percentage of carcasses with:							
Appearance defects:							
Red wingtips	7	8	15	16	8	9	9
Haemorrhagic wing veins	4	7	11	16	12	8	9
Haemorrhagic shoulder	12	—	22	23	14	18	13
Haemorrhage in breast muscle	15	10	17	25	23	28	19

Table 10.6. Effect of stunning current (50 Hz sine wave AC) on the prevalence of carcass and meat quality defects in turkeys (laboratory study) (after Gregory and Wilkins, 1990b).

	Average stunning current (mA)		
	75	150	250
Percentage of carcasses with:			
Appearance defects:			
Red wingtips	0	1	1
Haemorrhagic wings	3	5	8
Shoulder haemorrhage	6	9	5
Haemorrhage in breast muscle	6	8	20
Broken furculum	6	4	5
Broken coracoid	10	3	6

conditions tend to be relatively high when a stunning current of 121–161 mA per broiler is applied. In the case of turkeys, the prevalence of haemorrhagic wings alone increased when the stunning current was raised from 75 to 250 mA per bird. The prevalence of carcass downgrading conditions was similar in broilers when the frequency of current was varied from 50, 250 or 350 Hz delivered with a pulsed square wave DC (Table 10.7). Gas or controlled atmosphere killing, in comparison with the waterbath electrical stunning, reduced the prevalence of some of the carcass downgrading conditions in broilers (Table 10.8) and turkeys (Table 10.9). However, Raj *et al.* (1990b) showed that the prevalence of carcass downgrading conditions are low in manually plucked broiler carcasses which implies that the severity of plucking could contribute to the occurrence of carcass downgrading conditions. For example, any residual blood in the superficial vessels will be massaged by the plucker fingers and exacerbate the conditions.

Table 10.7. Effect of stunning frequency (unipolar square wave (pulsed) DC current) on the prevalence of carcass and meat quality defects in broilers (laboratory study) (after Gregory *et al.*, 1991).

	Stunning frequency		
	50	250	350
Average current (mA) per bird	112	111	109
Percentage of carcasses with:			
Red wingtips	2	2	5
Wing haemorrhage	7	6	4
Engorged wing veins	2	2	0
Shoulder haemorrhage	7	5	9
Breast muscle haemorrhage	24	23	23
Broken coracoid	26	28	23
Broken furculum	25	18	24
Broken scapula	33	40	34

Table 10.8. Effect of stunning method on the prevalence of carcass and meat quality defects in broilers (after Raj *et al.*, 1992b, 1997).

	Laboratory study		Commercial study	
	30% CO_2 and 50% argon	Electrical[a]	30% CO_2 and 60% argon	Electrical[a]
Number of birds used	98	50	100	100
Prevalence (%) of carcass downgrading conditions:				
Appearance defects:				
Red wingtips	21	28	19	23
Wing vein haemorrhage	3	4	23	30
Shoulder haemorrhage	10	8	12	5
Wing vein engorgement	5	2	1	17
Red pygostyle	2	4	25	33
Breast muscle haemorrhaging	3	32	5	77
Prevalence of dislocations/broken bones:				
Carcasses (%) with dislocations and/or fractures				
Dislocations	15	6	NR	NR
Fractures	20	24	NR	NR
Wing bones				
Humerus	10	4	NR	NR
Radius	7	0	NR	NR
Ulna	7	0	NR	NR
Pectoral bones				
Coracoid	0	8	0	50
Furculum	8	24	24	35
Scapula	NR	NR	1	34

[a] Laboratory study: 120 mA per bird, 50 Hz full sine wave AC; commercial study: 80 mA per bird; 50 Hz clipped (half) sine wave AC.
NR = not recorded.

Table 10.9. Effect of stunning methods on the prevalence of carcass and meat quality defects in turkeys (commercial study) (after Raj, 1994b).

	Anoxia (90% argon in air)	30% CO$_2$ and 60% argon in air	Electrical[a] (150 mA per bird)
Turkey hens			
Carcasses (%) with			
Red wingtips	3.1	1.7	9.9
Wing haemorrhage	9.3	7.6	16.5
Shoulder haemorrhage	0.4	0.3	1.2
Haemorrhage in breast	0.8	2.7	62.5
16-week-old stags			
Carcasses (%) with			
Red wingtips	3.0	NR	2.1
Wing haemorrhage	6.6	NR	17.0
Shoulder haemorrhage	3.0	NR	2.1
Haemorrhage in breast	3.1	NR	85.1
22-week-old stags			
Carcasses (%) with			
Red wingtips	1.6	0.5	3.2
Wing haemorrhage	7.3	5.1	19.3
Shoulder haemorrhage	0.7	0.5	1.8
Haemorrhage in breast	4.0	1.4	59.2

[a] 50 Hz full sine wave AC.
NR = not recorded.

Haemorrhaging in Muscles

Breast muscle haemorrhaging occurred to a similar extent when stunning currents between 45 and 220 mA per broiler were applied using 50 Hz sine wave AC (Table 10.5). However, in the case of turkeys, the prevalence of breast muscle haemorrhaging increased significantly when the stunning current was raised to 250 mA per bird (Table 10.6). The frequency of stunning currents of 50, 250 to 350 Hz delivered with a pulsed square wave DC had a very similar effect on the incidence of breast muscle haemorrhaging (Table 10.7). It has been suggested that the tetanic muscle contractions occurring during electrical stunning are responsible for the higher incidence of haemorrhaging in breast muscles and broken pectoral bones (Raj *et al.*, 1992b). The prevalence of these conditions is higher in broilers stunned with a clipped sine wave than those stunned with an unclipped sine wave 50 Hz AC (Gregory *et al.*, 1995). It has been suggested that the severity of muscular contractions induced at stunning could be related to the peak voltage applied to the bird, and that the peak voltage required to deliver a preset stunning current is likely to be higher with a clipped than with an unclipped sine wave. In addition to the peak voltage, the stimulation response of muscles could also vary according to the frequency of stunning currents.

Hillebrand *et al.* (1996) found that the overall prevalence of haemorrhaging in breast muscles was very similar in broilers stunned on shackles using either head-only using tongs (25 V, 200 Hz) or whole-body using a waterbath stunner (100 V, 200 Hz). However, waterbath stunning resulted in haemorrhages in the middle of pectoralis major and minor muscles, whereas head-only stunning resulted in haemorrhages in the distal end of the muscles and in the shoulder joints. The shoulder haemorrhages were attributed to the wing flapping which occurred during the epileptic phase following head-only electrical stunning while the birds were hanging on shackles.

Wing flapping occurring while the birds are in transport containers during exposure to gas mixtures does not appear to result in haemorrhaging either in the shoulder or in the breast muscles of broiler chickens (Table 10.8) and turkeys (Table 10.9). It appears that wing flapping occurring on shackles is potentially more damaging to the breast muscles than that occurring in transport containers. However, in contrast with the tetanic muscle contractions occurring during waterbath electrical stunning, the clonic convulsions (wing flapping) occurring during gas or controlled atmosphere stunning are twitch contractions and they appear to be less detrimental to carcass and meat quality. This is probably because wing flapping occurring during controlled atmosphere stunning is very similar to that of flight and the breast muscles are capable of coping with it, irrespective of the severity, over a short duration.

Although haemorrhages occurring in leg muscles of birds stunned using waterbath electrical stunners are mainly attributed to the shackling procedure (Wilson and Brunson, 1968), electrical stunning *per se* can increase the prevalence of haemorrhaging in leg muscles (Walker *et al.*, 1993). Head-only, in comparison with waterbath, electrical stunning on shackles results in lower incidence of this condition (Hillebrand *et al.*, 1996).

Broken Bones

The prevalence of birds with one or more broken pectoral bones increased from 25% to 39% as the stunning current was raised from 74 to 269 mA per broiler using a 50 Hz sine wave AC (Gregory and Wilkins, 1989a). However, in the case of turkeys, the prevalence of broken pectoral bones is not found to be related to the amount of stunning current, and between 75 and 250 mA per turkey, the incidence appears to be very similar (Gregory and Wilkins, 1990b). The number of broken bones occurring in electrically stunned birds which are processed under commercial conditions (Table 10.8) appears to be significantly more due to the variations in the current flow through the individual bird. Stunning current frequencies of 50, 250 or 350 Hz applied with a pulsed square wave DC resulted in a similar prevalence of broken bones in broilers when the average current was 109–112 mA per bird (Gregory *et al.*, 1991).

By contrast, gas or controlled-atmosphere stunning of broilers in transport containers results in a smaller number of carcasses with broken pectoral bones and reduces the number of broken pectoral bones per carcass (Raj *et al.*, 1990a). It is likely that, under the batch stunning of chickens in transport containers using gas mixtures, the cushioning effect provided by the birds against each other reduces the incidence of broken bones which can otherwise occur due to wing flapping. Therefore, the stocking density in a crate could determine the incidence of dislocated or broken wing bones in gas stunned birds.

BREAST MEAT COLOUR

Colour of poultry meat, including the effect of electrical and carbon dioxide stunning methods, has been recently reviewed by Froning (1995). The effects of stunning broilers with either argon or carbon dioxide–argon mixture, in comparison with electrical stunning, is presented in Table 10.10. It appears that, excluding haemorrhagic areas, stunning methods do not adversely affect the colour of breast meat.

COOKING LOSS

Stunning methods do not appear to have a significant effect on cooking loss. For example, Raj *et al.* (1990b) found that stunning broilers with either an electric current, 90% argon in air, or 45% carbon dioxide in air did not significantly affect percentage cooking loss measured in the whole carcasses (on average 260, 261 and 262 g kg^{-1}, respectively). In the same study, it was also found that hand plucked carcasses lost significantly less weight during cooking than those that were mechanically plucked (249 and 272 g kg^{-1}). In another study, it was found that stunning broilers with either a mixture of 30% carbon dioxide and 60% argon in air or an electric current did not affect the cooking loss, however, regardless of the stunning method, breast muscles filleted early post-mortem (2, 3, 4 or 5 h) lost more weight during cooking than those filleted at 24 h post-

Table 10.10. Effect of stunning methods on the colour of broiler breast meat (after Raj *et al.*, 1990b, 1997).

| CIE colour parameters | Laboratory study | | Commercial study | |
	Anoxia (90% argon in air)	Electrical[a]	30% CO$_2$ and 60% argon in air	Electrical[a]
L*	52.16	54.02	54.3	55.5
a*	2.00	1.80	3.4	2.9
b*	−0.63	−0.23	4.0	4.0

[a] Laboratory study: 120 mA per bird, 50 Hz sine wave AC; commercial study: 80 mA per bird, 50 Hz clipped sine wave AC.

mortem (16 vs. 14%; Raj *et al.*, 1997). Therefore, it appears that the severity of plucking and filleting time, rather than stunning method, can significantly increase the cooking loss in broilers. However, this does not agree with the results of Papinaho *et al.* (1996) who reported that, in electrically stunned broilers, the percentage cooking loss was not significantly affected by the breast muscle filleting time (on average 20%). The difference between these two studies could be attributed to the differences in cooking methods.

Electrical stunning of turkeys resulted in slightly higher cooking loss than stunning with either 90% argon in air or a mixture of 30% carbon dioxide and 60% argon in air (Raj, 1994a). However, in that study, the effect of bird type was more significant than the effect of stunning methods. For example, large toms had a significantly higher cooking loss (37%) than the medium size toms (32%) and hens (30%). In the same study, interactions were found between bird type and filleting time, stunning method and filleting time, and bird type, stunning method and filleting time. However, the differences in the percentage cooking loss due to these interactions were found to be smaller than the effects of bird type.

OBJECTIVE TEXTURE

Poultry breast meat texture is an important eating quality criterion, though consumers' preferences vary widely. The major factors affecting texture are:

1. rate of rigor development;
2. rate of carcass chilling;
3. filleting time.

Stunning methods can affect texture mainly by altering the time course of rigor development and the extent of muscle contraction and relaxation occurring during early post-mortem. The rate of chilling can change the severity of muscle tension development and the time course of relaxation early post-mortem. Separation of breast muscles from carcasses, before the completion of rigor, would remove the restraint offered by the skeleton and this could result in irreversible rigor and/or cold shortening to produce tough meat. In addition, since pectoralis major and p. minor muscles have opposite functions, cutting of supracoracoideus tendon at the humeral insertion soon after evisceration results in contraction in both the muscles and toughening of cooked meat (Cason *et al.*, 1997).

It has been reported that meat obtained from electrically stunned birds was more tender than that obtained from birds which were not stunned (Klose *et al.*, 1972). Within electrical stunning, stunning broilers with either 50 V AC when compared with 200 V AC and filleting breast muscles at either 1, 2 or 4 h post-mortem, resulted in mean texture (Warner-Bratzler shear values) values of 10 vs. 11, 7 vs. 10, and 5 vs. 5, respectively (Dickens and Lyon, 1993). These results show that, irrespective of the stunning voltage, early filleting resulted in tougher meat and that the high voltage stunning produced tougher meat than the low voltage stunning when filleting was performed at 1 and 2 h post-mortem. By contrast, Papinaho and Fletcher (1996) reported that stunning broilers at 125 mA (60 Hz sine wave AC) resulted in significantly tougher breast meat for up to 10 h post-mortem than meat from birds which were stunned with 50 mA (60 Hz sine wave AC) or not stunned at all. Poole and Fletcher (Georgia, 1997, personal communication) also found that stunning broilers with 125 mA (50 Hz sine wave AC) and filleting breasts up to 5 h post-mortem, in comparison with 24 h post-mortem, resulted in tougher meat. However, in the same study, it was reported that stunning broilers with 5–6 mA (500 Hz square wave pulsed DC) and filleting breast at 5 h post-mortem produced tender meat, similar to that filleted at 24 h post-mortem. Craig and Fletcher (1997) found that, when filleting was performed at 24 h post-mortem, the breast meat texture was very similar in broilers stunned with either 125 mA (50 Hz sine wave AC) or 5–6 mA (500 Hz square wave pulsed DC).

Electrical stunning duration (with 100 V 60 Hz sine wave AC) of 0, 5, 10, 20 or 40 s had no effect on Allo-Kramer shear values of cooked broiler breast meat which were filleted at 24 h post-mortem (Papinaho and Fletcher, 1995b). However, when filleting of breast muscles was performed at 1 h post-mortem, stunning duration significantly affected the texture (Young and Buhr, 1997). Young and Buhr (1997) also reported that, under simulated US commercial conditions, increasing the stunning duration from 2 s to 4 or 6 s, and to 8 or 10 s resulted in significant increases in the shear values.

Under commercial conditions, depending on the market demand, poultry processors allow a carcass maturation time of 4–12 h before portioning them. Raj *et al.* (1997) showed that filleting of breasts from electrically stunned broilers (80 mA per bird; 50 Hz clipped sine wave AC) for up to 5 h post-mortem produced tougher meat (based on kg yield force; Table 10.11). Papinaho *et al.* (1995) suggested that, whilst stunning chickens with 120 mA per bird (50 Hz sine wave AC), breast muscles should be aged on the carcass for 10.5 h to produce tender meat (Allo-Kramer shear force of 8 kg g^{-1}) in over 95% of the fillets. Nevertheless, if electrical stunning currents influence the rate of rigor development and thus texture of meat, it will be appropriate to use a constant current stunner (Sparrey *et al.*, 1993) to reduce the variations normally seen under commercial conditions.

When filleting was performed after overnight ageing, broilers stunned with argon-induced anoxia produced slightly more tender breast meat (less kg yield force) than those stunned with either 45% carbon dioxide in air or an electric current (107 mA per bird applied with 50 Hz sine wave AC) (Raj *et al.*, 1990b). This contrasts with other reports which have suggested that accelerated early post-mortem glycolysis usually results in tougher meat (Lee *et al.*, 1979). A subsequent study showed that breast muscles from broilers, which were stunned with anoxia, filleted at 2 and 3 h post-mortem were less tender than those filleted at 5 h post-mortem (Table 10.11). This is probably because rigor tension is greater in chicken breasts held isometrically at 23°C than at 5°C (Wood and Richards, 1974), and a combination of low pH and high temperature at filleting can produce tough meat. It is very likely that in rapidly glycolysing breast muscles the rigor tension continues to exist in the warm

Table 10.11. Effect of stunning method and filleting time on the texture (kg yield force) of cooked broiler breast meat (after Raj *et al.*, 1991, 1997).

Filleting time (h)	Laboratory study		Commercial study	
	90% argon in air	Electrical[a] (107 mA per bird)	30% CO_2 and 60% argon in air	Electrical[a] (80 mA per bird)
2	3.0	NR	1.4	1.7
3	2.6	NR	1.4	1.6
4	NR	NR	1.2	1.5
5	1.9	NR	1.3	1.5
21	1.9	2.0	NR	NR
24	NR	NR	1.2	1.2

[a] Laboratory study: 50 Hz sine wave AC; commercial study: 50 Hz clipped sine wave AC.
NR = not recorded.

carcass. If this tension is reduced by rapid chilling a tender meat could be produced within an hour after slaughter. Indeed, when carcasses of broilers stunned with anoxia were chilled using water and ice and had their breast muscles filleted at 1, 2, 3 or 24 h post-mortem, they all produced tender meat (Raj and Gregory, 1991b). Similarly, tender meat was produced when carcasses from turkeys stunned with anoxia were chilled in water and ice and breast muscles filleted at 2 h post-mortem (Table 10.12).

As mentioned previously, stunning of chickens with a mixture of 30% carbon dioxide and 60% argon retarded the rate of glycolysis early post-mortem, and therefore, filleting of breast muscles from these carcasses at 2 or 3 h post-mortem resulted in relatively tougher meat (Table 10.11). However, these fillets were more tender than those obtained from the

Table 10.12. Effect of stunning method and filleting time on the texture of cooked turkey breast meat (commercial study) (after Raj, 1994a).

Bird type/stunning method	Filleting time (h)			
	2	3	5	18
Hens				
90% argon in air	4.5	4.4	5.5	4.4
CO_2–argon mixture	5.6	4.7	4.5	4.8
Electrical[a]	7.9	8.3	7.2	6.3
16-week-old stags				
Anoxia	5.0	5.5	4.8	4.9
CO_2–argon mixture	5.7	5.8	5.8	5.7
Electrical[a]	9.7	9.1	9.3	5.0
22-week-old stags				
Anoxia	4.0	3.2	4.2	3.5
CO_2–argon mixture	3.9	4.1	3.3	3.9
Electrical[a]	4.6	4.6	5.5	4.5

[a] Applied with a 50 Hz sine wave AC; 150 mA per bird.

electrically stunned broilers filleted at the corresponding times post-mortem. It would appear that, to produce a tender breast meat, filleting of broilers stunned with this gas mixture should be performed at 4 h post-mortem. By contrast, Poole and Fletcher (Georgia, 1997, personal communication) found that breast meat from broilers stunned with this gas mixture and filleted up to 5 h post-mortem produced tougher meat than those filleted at 24 h post-mortem. In the case of turkeys, both argon and carbon dioxide–argon mixture stunning resulted in tender meat when filleting was performed at 2 h post-mortem (Table 10.12). Further research should be carried out under similar stunning, carcass processing, chilling and cooking conditions to clarify the reasons for this difference between chickens and turkeys.

SENSORY PROPERTIES OF MEAT

Eating quality of breast meat evaluated using a trained sensory panel can yield more information than the instrumentally measured texture values. In general, the eating quality of breast meat improves considerably when aged on the carcass. It is known that calcium activated neutral proteinases (calpains) and lysosomal acidic proteinases (cathepsins) degrade myofibrillar and cytoskeletal proteins, and hydrolyse myofibrils, respectively.

Liu *et al.* (1994) showed that structures of chicken semitendinosus muscle endomysium and perimysium disintegrate into thin sheets within 12 h post-mortem, and as a result, gaps appear in the endomysium and perimysium when examined under a light microscope. Under a scanning electron microscope, it was found that, in chicken semitendinosus muscle aged for 12 h at 4°C, the endomysium resolved into individual collagen fibrils and the perimysial sheets separated into collagen fibres (Liu *et al.*, 1995). These structural changes in the connective tissue were minimal until 6 h post-mortem.

As mentioned earlier, stunning methods, particularly anoxia, can result in the development of tenderness early post-mortem. In addition, Fagan *et al.* (1992) found that when isolated chick skeletal muscle was subjected to anoxia the ATP content fell to undetectable concentrations and the muscle suffered a faster rate (35% to 124%) of proteolysis (breakdown of total protein as well as myofibrillar proteins). These scientists have suggested that the calcium-activated proteases (calpains) were involved in the enhanced degradation of total muscle proteins in ATP-depleted tissue. In the same study, it was found that the proteolysis occurring in the ATP-depleted muscles was also mediated through an ATP-independent non-lysosomal process that required calcium. It is likely that, under an argon-stunning situation, anoxia induced at the cellular level results in an efflux of calcium from the sarcoplasmic reticulum and mitochondria and this in association with high carcass temperature during processing enhances proteolysis.

It has been shown that, in comparison with electrical stimulation of broiler carcasses soon after plucking, stunning broilers with anoxia under commercial conditions produced tender breast meat when filleted at 2 h post-mortem (Raj *et al.*, 1992c). Sensory profiling of breast meat from turkeys showed that stunning with argon-induced anoxia resulted in more tender meat with powdery residue, whereas, electrical stunning produced significantly less tender meat with pulpy residue (Raj and Nute, 1995). It is likely that some of these differences in the eating quality are due to the time and extent of activation or inhibition of proteolysis induced by the stunning methods.

REFERENCES

Bigland, C.H. (1964) Blood clotting times of five avian species. *Poultry Science* 43, 1035–1039.

Bilgili, S.F. (1992) Electrical stunning of broilers – basic concepts and carcase quality implications: a review. *Journal of Applied Poultry Research* 1, 135–146.

Cason, J.A., Lyon, C.E. and Papa, C.M. (1997) Effect of muscle opposition during rigor on development of broiler breast meat tenderness. *Poultry Science* 76, 785–787.

Cassens, R.G., Briskey, E.J. and Hoekstra, W.G. (1963) Similarity in the contracture bands occurring in thaw–rigor and in other violent treatments of muscle. *Biomedica* 9, 165–175.

Chiang, W., Solomon, M.B. and Kotula, K.L. (1995) Muscle fibre types of selected muscles from broiler chickens in relation to age and sex. *Journal of Muscle Foods*, 6, 197–210.

Craig, E.W. and Fletcher, D.L. (1997) A comparison of high current and low voltage electrical stunning systems on broiler breast rigor development and meat quality. *Poultry Science* 76, 1178–1181.

Curtin, N.A. (1988) Intracellular pH and relaxation of frog muscle. *Advances in Experimental Medical Biology* 226, 657–669.

Dickens, J.A. and Lyon, C.E. (1993) Effect of two stunning voltages on blood loss and objective texture of meat deboned at various post-mortem times. *Poultry Science* 72, 589–593.

Fagan, J.M., Wajnberg, E.F., Culbert, L. and Waxman, L. (1992) ATP depletion stimulates calcium-dependent protein breakdown in chick skeletal muscles. *American Journal of Physiology* 262, E637–E643.

Froning, G.W. (1995) Colour of poultry meat. *Poultry and Avian Biology Reviews* 6, 83–93.

Ganong, W.F. (1993) In: Ganong, W.F. (ed.) *Review of Medical Physiology*, 6th edn. Lange Medical Publications, Connecticut.

Gregory, N.G. and Wilkins, L.J. (1989a) Effect of stunning current on carcase quality in chickens. *Veterinary Record* 124, 530–532.

Gregory, N.G. and Wilkins, L.J. (1989b) Effect of slaughter method on bleeding efficiency in chickens. *Journal of Science in Food and Agriculture* 47, 13–20.

Gregory, N.G. and Wilkins, L.J. (1990a) Broken bones in chickens: effect of stunning and processing in broilers. *British Poultry Science* 31, 53–58.

Gregory, N.G. and Wilkins, L.J. (1990b) Effect of stunning current on downgrading in turkeys. *British Poultry Science* 30, 761–764.

Gregory, N.G. and Wotton, S.B. (1986) Effect of slaughter on the spontaneous and evoked activity of the brain. *British Poultry Science* 27, 195–205.

Gregory, N.G. and Wotton, S.B. (1990) Effect of stunning on spontaneous physical activity and evoked activity in the brain. *British Poultry Science* 31, 215–220.

Gregory, N.G. and Wotton, S.B. (1991) Effect of electrical stunning on somatosensory evoked potentials in turkey's brain. *British Veterinary Journal* 147, 270–274.

Gregory, N.G., Austin, S.D. and Wilkins, L.J. (1989) Relationship between wing flapping at shackling and red wingtips in chicken carcases. *Veterinary Record* 124, 62.

Gregory, N.G., Wilkins, L.J. and Wotton, S.B. (1991) Effect of electrical stunning frequency on ventricular fibrillation, downgrading and broken bones in broilers, hens and quails. *British Veterinary Journal* 147, 71–77.

Gregory, N.G., Wilkins, L.J., Wotton, S.B. and Middleton, A.V. (1995) Effects of currents and waveforms on the incidence of breast meat haemorrhages in electrically stunned broiler chicken carcases. *Veterinary Record* 137, 263–265.

Griffiths, G.L. (1985) The occurrence of red-skin chicken carcases. *British Veterinary Journal* 141, 312–314.

Griffiths, G.L., MaGrath, M., Softly, A. and Jones, C. (1985) Blood content of broiler chicken carcases prepared by different slaughter methods. *Veterinary Record* 117, 382–385.

Harkema, S.J., Adams, G.R. and Meyer, R.A. (1997) Acidosis has no effect on the ATP cast of contraction in cat fast- and slow-twitch skeletal muscles. *American Journal of Physiology – Cell Physiology* 41, C485–C490.

Heath, G.E., Thaler, A.M. and James, W.O. (1994) A survey of stunning methods currently used during slaughter of poultry in commercial poultry plants. *Journal of Applied Poultry Research* 3, 297–302.

Hillebrand, S.J.W., Lambooy, E. and Veerkamp, C.H. (1996) The effects of alternative electrical and mechanical stunning methods on haemorrhaging and meat quality in broiler breast and thigh muscles. *Poultry Science* 75, 664–671.

HMSO (1995) *The Welfare of Animals (Slaughter or Killing) Regulations*, 1995. Statutory Instrument no. 731, London, HMSO.

Klose, A.A., Sayre, R.N., DeFremery, D. and Pool, M.F. (1972) Effect of hot cutting and related factors in commercial broiler processing on tenderness. *Poultry Science* 51, 634–638.

Kotula, A.W. and Helbacka, N.V. (1966) Blood retained by chicken carcases and cut-up parts as influenced by slaughter method. *Poultry Science* 45, 404–410.

Kotula, A.W., Drewniak, E.E. and Davis, L.L. (1957) Effect of carbon dioxide immobilisation on the bleeding of chickens. *Poultry Science* 36, 585–589.

Kuenzel, W.J., Ingling, A.L., Michael Denbow, D., Wather, J.H. and Schaefer, M.M. (1978) Variable frequency stunning and a comparison of two bleed-out time intervals for maximising blood release in processed poultry. *Poultry Science* 57, 449–454.

Lee, Y.B., Hargus, G.L., Webb, J.E., Rickansurd, D.A. and Hagberg, E.G. (1979) Effect of electrical stunning on post-mortem biochemical changes and tenderness in broiler breast muscles. *Journal of Food Science* 44, 1121–1122.

Leet, N.G., Devine, C.E. and Gavey, A.B. (1977) The histology of blood splashing in lambs. *Meat Science* 1, 229–234.

Liu, A., Nishimura, T. and Takahashi, K. (1994) Structural changes in endomysium and perimysium during post mortem aging of chicken semitendinosus muscle – contribution of structural weakening of intramuscular connective tissue to meat tenderisation. *Meat Science* 38, 315–328.

Liu, A., Nishimura, T. and Takahashi, K. (1995) Structural weakening of intramuscular connective tissue during post-mortem ageing of chicken semitendinosus muscle. *Meat Science* 39, 135–142.

Messina, E.J., Sun, D., Koller, A., Wolin, M.S. and Kaley, G. (1992) Role of endothelium derived prostaglandins in hypoxia-elicited arteriolar dilation in rat skeletal muscle. *Circulation Research* 71, 790–796.

Moran, E.T. and Bilgili, S.F. (1995) Influence of stunning current and convection during slush ice chilling on quality defects with broiler carcases. In: Briz, R.C. (ed.) *Proceedings of the XII European Symposium on the Quality of Poultry Meat*, 25—29 September 1995, Zaragoza, Spain, pp. 315–320.

Papinaho, P.A. and Fletcher, D.L. (1995a) Effect of stunning amperage on broiler breast muscle rigor development and meat quality. *Poultry Science* 74, 1527–1532.

Papinaho, P.A. and Fletcher, D.L. (1995b) Effects of electrical stunning duration on post mortem rigor development and broiler breast meat tenderness. *Journal of Muscle Foods*, 6, 1–8.

Papinaho, P.A. and Fletcher, D.L. (1996) The effects of stunning amperage and deboning time on early rigor development and breast meat quality in broilers. *Poultry Science* 75, 672–676.

Papinaho, P.A., Fletcher, D.L. and Buhr, R.J. (1995) Effect of electrical stunning amperage and peri-mortem struggle on broiler breast rigor development and meat quality. *Poultry Science* 74, 1533–1539.

Papinaho, P.A., Fletcher, D.L. and Rita, H.J. (1996) Relationship of breast fillet deboning time to shear force, pH, cooking loss and colour in broilers stunned by high electric current. *Agricultural and Food Science in Finland* 5, 49–55.

Poole, G.H. and Fletcher, D.L. (1995) A comparison of argon, carbon dioxide and nitrogen in a broiler killing system. *Poultry Science* 74, 1218–1223.

Raj, A.B.M. (1994a) Effect of stunning method, carcase chilling temperature and filleting time on the texture of turkey breast meat. *British Poultry Science* 35, 77–89.

Raj, A.B.M. (1994b) An investigation into the batch killing of turkeys in their transport containers using mixtures of gases. *Research in Veterinary Science* 56, 325–331.

Raj, A.B.M. (1996) Aversive reactions of turkeys to argon, carbon dioxide and a mixture of carbon dioxide and argon. *Veterinary Record* 138, 592–593.

Raj, A.B.M. and Gregory, N.G. (1991a) Efficiency of bleeding of broilers after gaseous or electrical stunning. *Veterinary Record* 128, 127–128.

Raj, A.B.M. and Gregory, N.G. (1991b) Effect of argon stunning, rapid chilling and early filleting on texture of broiler breast meat. *British Poultry Science* 32, 741–746.

Raj, A.B.M. and Gregory, N.G. (1994) An evaluation of humane gas stunning methods for turkeys. *Veterinary Record*, 135, 222–223.

Raj, A.B.M. and Johnson, S.P. (1997) Effect of the method of killing, interval between killing and neck cutting and blood vessels cut on blood loss in broilers. *British Poultry Science* 38, 190–194.

Raj, A.B.M. and Nute, G.R. (1995) Effect of stunning method and filleting time on sensory profile of turkey breast meat. *British Poultry Science* 36, 221–227.

Raj, A.B.M. Gregory, N.G. and Austin, S.D. (1990a) Prevalence of broken bones in broilers killed by different stunning methods. *Veterinary Record* 127, 285–287.

Raj, A.B.M., Grey, T.C., Audsley, A.R.S. and Gregory, N.G. (1990b) Effect of electrical and gaseous stunning on the carcase and meat quality of broilers. *British Poultry Science* 31, 725–733.

Raj, A.B.M., Grey, T.C. and Gregory, N.G. (1991) Effect of early filleting on the texture of breast muscle of broilers stunned with argon-induce anoxia. *British Poultry Science* 32, 319–325.

Raj, A.B.M., Gregory, N.G. and Wotton, S.B. (1992a) Changes in the somatosensory evoked potentials and spontaneous electroencephalogram of hens during stunning with a carbon dioxide–argon mixture. *British Veterinary Journal* 148, 147–156.

Raj, A.B.M., Gregory, N.G. and Wilkins, L.J. (1992b) Survival rate and carcase downgrading after the stunning of broilers with carbon dioxide—argon mixtures. *Veterinary Record* 130, 325–328.

Raj, A.B.M., Nute, G.R., Wotton, S.B. and Baker, A. (1992c) Sensory evaluation of breast fillets from argon-stunned and electrically stimulated broiler carcases processed under commercial conditions. *British Poultry Science* 33, 963–971.

Raj, A.B.M., Gregory, N.G. and Wotton, S.B. (1994) Effect of method of stunning and the interval between stunning and neck cutting on blood loss in turkeys. *Veterinary Record* 135, 256–258.

Raj, A.B.M., Wilkins, L.J., Richardson, R.I., Johnson, S.P. and Wotton, S.B. (1997) Carcase and meat quality in broilers either killed with a gas mixture or stunned with an electric current under commercial processing conditions. *British Poultry Science* 38, 169–174.

Ranatunga, K.W. (1987) Effect of acidosis on tension development in mammalian skeletal muscle. *Muscle and Nerve* 10, 439–445.

Sams, A.R. and Dzuik, C.S. (1995) Gas stunning and post-mortem electrical stimulation of broiler chickens. In: Briz, R.C. (ed.) *Proceedings of the XII European Symposium on the Quality of Poultry Meat*, 25–29 September, Zaragoza, Spain, pp. 307–314.

Schutt-Abraham, I., Wormuth, H.J. and Fessel, J. (1983) Electrical stunning of poultry in view of animal welfare and meat production. In: Eikelenboom, G. (ed.) *Stunning of Animals for Slaughter*, Martinus Nijhoff, Dordrecht, pp. 187–196.

Shorr, E., Zweifach, B.W. and Furchgott, R.F. (1945) On the occurrence, sites and modes of origin and destruction of principles affecting the compensatory vascular mechanisms in experimental shock. *Science* 102, 489–498.

Simmons, N. (1995) The use of high frequency electrical stunning of pigs. PhD Thesis, University of Bristol, UK.

Sparrey, J.M., Paice, M.E.R. and Kettlewell, P.J. (1992) Model of current pathways in electrical waterbath stunners used for poultry. *British Poultry Science* 33, 907–916.

Sparrey, J.M., Kettlewell, P.J., Paice, M.E.R. and Whetlor, W.C. (1993) Development of a constant current waterbath stunner for poultry processing. *Journal of Agricultural and Engineering Research* 56, 267–274.

Veerkamp, C.H. and deVries, A.W. (1983) Influence of electrical stunning on quality aspects of broilers. In: Eikelenboom, G. (ed.) *Stunning of Animals for Slaughter*. Martinus Nijhoff, Dordrecht, pp. 197–207.

Walker, J.M., Buhr, R.J. and Fletcher, D.L. (1993) Investigation of processing factors contributing to haemorrhagic leg syndrome in broilers. *Poultry Science* 72, 1592–1596.

Warren, G.L., Hayes, D.A., Lowe, D.A. and Armstrong, R.B. (1993) Mechanical factors in the initiation of eccentric contraction-induced injury in rat soleus muscle. *Journal of Physiology* 464, 457–475.

Wilson, J.A. (ed.) (1972) *Principles of Animal Physiology*. Macmillan, New York.

Wilson, J.G. and Brunson, C.C. (1968) The effects of handling and slaughter method on the incidence of haemorrhagic thighs in broilers. *Poultry Science* 47, 1315–1318.

Wiskus, K.J., Addis, P.B. and Ma, R. T-I. (1976) Distribution of beta-red, alpha-red and alpha-white fibres in turkey muscles. *Poultry Science* 55, 562–572.

Wood, D.F. and Richards, J.F. (1974) Isometric tension studies on chicken pectoralis major muscle. *Journal of Food Science* 34, 525–529.

Young, L.L. and Buhr, R.J. (1997) Effect of stunning duration on quality characteristics of early deboned chicken fillets. *Poultry Science* 76, 1052–1055.

PART III
Microbiological quality of poultry meat and meat products

CHAPTER 11
Salmonella *infection in poultry: the production environment*

C. Wray, R.H. Davies and S.J. Evans

Central Veterinary Laboratory, New Haw, Addlestone KT15 3NB, UK

INTRODUCTION

More than 2300 different salmonella serovars have been described and although all members of the species are considered to be potentially pathogenic, they differ widely in their host range and pathogenicity. In the veterinary literature a distinction is usually made between infection caused by the two host-adapted serovars, *Salmonella pullorum* (pullorum disease) and *S. gallinarum* (fowl typhoid), the arizona group of salmonellas (arizonosis) and the remainder of the salmonellas (salmonellosis, paratyphoid infection).

Pullorum disease and fowl typhoid were the subject of government-backed control schemes in the United Kingdom and are now infrequent causes of disease. However, in many other countries they are of major importance, resulting in considerable economic losses. They are, however, of little zoonotic importance and will not be considered further.

Paratyphoid infections, generally subclincal, are common in domestic poultry throughout most of the world. Many different serovars have been identified in domestic poultry and one particular serovar may predominate for a number of years before it is replaced by another. Thus, in 1943, *S. thompson* appeared in the UK poultry flock and within two years was the most frequent salmonella isolated from poultry. In the 1970s, *S. agona* was introduced into the country in imported Peruvian fish meal (Turnbull, 1979) and became widespread in poultry and subsequently humans. Likewise, *S. hadar,* first recorded in 1969, affected the turkey industry because it caused disease in table birds which led to food-borne illness in humans (Watson and Kirby, 1984).

During the late 1980s there was a dramatic increase in *S. enteritidis* in poultry and since 1987 this has been the most frequent serovar isolated from poultry in the UK (Fig. 11.1). The increase was associated with the emergence of phage type 4 and a corresponding rise in human illness, with many food poisoning outbreaks having been attributed to poultry products. A similar increase in the prevalence of *S. enteritidis* in both humans and poultry has been observed in many other countries although, in some instances, it has been caused by phage types other than 4, e.g. phage type 13a in the USA. Some countries, such as Australia, have remained free from *S. enteritidis*. Likewise, *S. typhimurium* is another important serovar in poultry (Table 11.1)

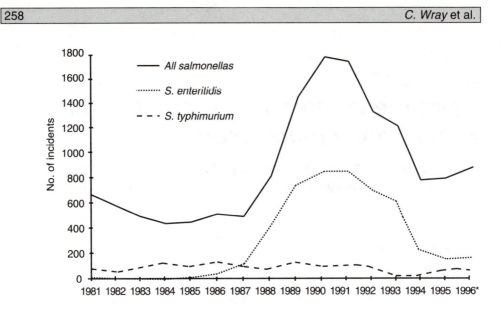

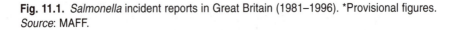

1981 1982 1983 1984 1985 1986 1987 1988 1989 1990 1991 1992 1993 1994 1995 1996*

Fig. 11.1. *Salmonella* incident reports in Great Britain (1981–1996). *Provisional figures.
Source: MAFF.

and currently the presence of DT104, which is often resistant to a number of antimicrobials, is giving cause for concern.

Efforts to control salmonella infections in poultry are, with the exception of those caused by pathogenic serovars, driven by public health considerations rather than expectations that dramatic improvements in production efficiency will be achieved. To this end, the Zoonoses Directive (92/117) aims to control the presence of *S. enteritidis* and *S. typhimurium* in breeder flocks and so prevent vertical transmission to the commercial sector.

Table 11.1. Number of incidents of *S. enteritidis*, *S. typhimurium* and other salmonellas reported under the Zoonoses Order 1989 for the period 1 January–31 December 1996 compared with the same period in 1995.

	S. enteritidis		*S. typhimurium*		Other *Salmonella* spp.	
	1995	1996	1995	1996	1995	1996
Broilers	72	98	48	61	337	431
Broiler breeders	66	45	16	9	208	210
Layers	11	13	5	3	9	11
Layer breeders	6	6	2	1	19	22
Turkeys, ducks and geese	46	16	100	97	232	219
Other birds	27	32	83	70	118	189
Total birds	228	210	254	241	923	1082

ORIGINS OF INFECTION

Once a salmonella with an affinity for poultry has become established in a primary breeding flock, it can infect poultry in other units via hatcheries by both vertical and lateral spread. This can have far ranging and serious effects on the health of both poultry and humans. It is thus of considerable importance to establish how infection can be introduced into a salmonella-free breeding flock given the complex epidemiology (Fig. 11.2).

The poultry industry is separated into egg and meat production enterprises, each of which has its own breeding flock hierarchy. Elite breeder flocks contain the primary genetic stock, whose offspring form the grandparent flocks which, in turn, produce parent breeder flocks. Involvement

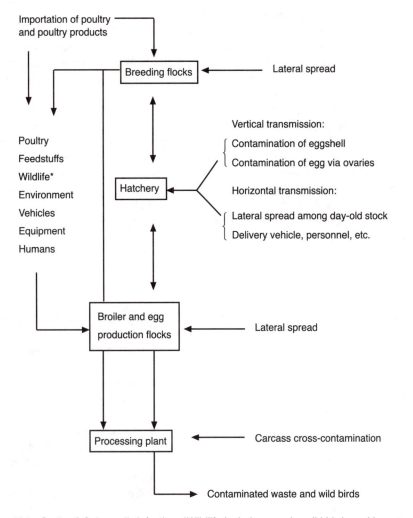

Fig. 11.2. Cycle of *Salmonella* infection. *Wildlife includes vermin, wild birds and insects.

of breeding and production flocks from both sectors of the British Poultry Industry, and the ability of *S. enteritidis* to be transmitted vertically to offspring, may partly explain the widespread nature of the epidemic (O'Brien, 1988; Lister, 1988). However, there have been no confirmed flock infections with *S. enteritidis* in elite or grandparent breeding flocks since the start of compulsory MAFF (Ministry of Agriculture Fisheries and Food) monitoring for salmonella in 1989.

If a breeding flock is infected with salmonellas, a cycle can be established by which the organism passes via the eggs to the progeny and even to chicks hatched from eggs laid subsequently by infected progeny. This cycle can occur by true ovarian transmission, infection within the oviduct or, as is much more likely to happen, through faecal contamination of the egg surface. As the egg passes through the cloaca, salmonella in faeces attach themselves to the warm, wet shell surface and may be drawn inside as it cools. Surface contamination may also occur in the nest boxes.

The possibility of trans-shell invasion of hatching eggs by salmonella is of great concern. Experimentally, substantial trans-shell infection of eggs has been demonstrated, following application of aerosols of salmonella or contact with contaminated litter (Mario-Padron, 1990). Nest box hygiene to reduce contamination and rejection of floor eggs is particularly important to reduce such surface contamination of eggs, which also carries a risk of introducing contamination into the hatchery environment and to personnel and equipment (Bruce and Drysdale, 1990). Damage to the cuticle of the eggshell is important because it allows increased penetration of organisms (Haigh and Betts, 1991). Such damage may occur as a result of commercial handling conditions (Nascimento *et al.*, 1992) or during certain washing procedures (Mayes and Takeballi, 1983). Poor quality shell resulting from adverse nutritional factors or stress may also enhance trans-shell infection (Nascimento and Solomon, 1991).

THE HATCHERY

Modern hatcheries, which are highly automated and have a high throughput of eggs and chicks, are complex operations where many factors interrelate to influence the prevalence of salmonella contamination. Hatcheries can serve as reservoirs of infection and cross-contamination in the hatchery may dramatically increase the prevalence of salmonella-infected chicks leaving the hatchery when compared with the low prevalence of infected eggs entering the hatchery. During the incubation of infected eggs, there is a rise in the number of salmonellas within the egg and in the detectable infection rate (Cason *et al.*, 1991; Hammack *et al.*, 1993). This has no apparent effect on hatchability, so there may be potential for amplification of contamination as salmonellas are released during the hatching process. Bailey *et al.* (1994) demonstrated that a single salmonella-contaminated egg could substantially contaminate other eggs and chicks in the hatching cabinet.

A comparative study of salmonella contamination in 11 commercial hatcheries indicated the main cross-contamination hazard points, but significant reductions in contamination were achievable by good organization, hygiene management and disinfection practices (Davies and Wray, 1994c).

The most important factor in salmonella contamination of a hatchery is the infection status of flocks supplying the eggs. As part of our own studies two hatcheries were sampled before and after elimination of known *S. enteritidis*-infected supply flocks. In both cases, there was no evidence of current *S. enteritidis* contamination within the hatchery at the second visit, although other serotypes were present. In a well-run hatchery there should be little opportunity for long-term persistence of salmonellas at a level that would pose a significant threat to chicks in the absence of an infected egg source. However, if there is potential for high level cross-contamination of eggs and chicks or poor disinfection of incubator ventilation systems, salmonella infection may be perpetuated in future chick crops.

Egg sanitization is the first barrier to the introduction of microbial contamination into the hatchery premises via the egg surface. Egg sanitization on the farm, even where disinfectant fogging was used in the hatchery, was found to be insufficient and further egg treatment by formaldehyde vapour fumigation or further egg sanitization through a well regulated wash machine was required. It was often possible to observe poor removal of litter, feathers and faeces from eggs at certain breeder farms.

Setter incubators are traditionally considered to be low-risk areas for salmonella multiplication and cross-contamination, since eggs are removed before hatching takes place. However, some bursting of eggs and premature hatching does occur. In some hatcheries, there was a high prevalence of salmonella isolation in setters which was associated with poor cleaning due to fixed tray-turning apparatus and failure to remove old shell debris. Fogging with disinfectant was commonly carried out, but was not effective where physical cleaning was poor. More aggressive physical removal of egg debris and disinfection of surfaces were needed in many cases. The system showing least salmonella contamination was single-stage setting which allowed all-in, all-out handling of eggs with effective sanitization between batches. Control of salmonella contamination in setters is important because the warm, humidified air may disseminate salmonella over the surfaces of several batches of eggs within the same incubator.

After 18 days of turning in the setter incubators, the eggs are transferred to hatcher incubators for the final three days of incubation. The transfer from egg trays to hatching baskets is often semiautomatic, using multiple suction cup machines which transfer a whole tray of eggs in one operation. This speeds up the process but the suction heads are sometimes contaminated with salmonellas and so could cause cross-contamination of different batches of eggs. In addition, there appears to be a higher prevalence of broken eggs with some automatic transfer machines so that the surrounding area becomes more contaminated. It is obviously uneconomic to transfer eggs manually in large hatcheries, but tray-turning and emptying devices may be used with advantage in some circumstances. Frequent and effective disinfection of surfaces and suction cups of egg-transfer machines has resulted in improvements in salmonella contamination rate.

Hatching of eggs liberates large quantities of dust and fluff from the chicks which may be highly contaminated with salmonellas (e.g. 10^4 g^{-1}) if eggs from an infected flock are being hatched. The organisms may be circulated within the hatcher by the ventilation system. Chicks from more than one flock may be placed in the same hatcher because of the need to maintain fully stocked incubators and ensure stable incubation conditions. In relation to the high throughput, the hatchers have a larger capacity, but are few in number. This situation may lead to cross-contamination of chicks from different supply flocks.

Effective use of formaldehyde vapour during hatching can be demonstrated, but it is common to find insufficient volumes of formaldehyde solution, irregular replenishment of the solution or formaldehyde containers of insufficient surface area to permit effective vaporization. These errors may allow multiplication of salmonellas in the hatchers.

In many cases, the ventilation system of the hatchers discharges contaminated air into either a common airspace or a poorly sealed dust trap corridor or loft. There are also instances where the air intake fans of pressurized hatchers discharge chick dust to the exterior. This may lead to contaminated air being drawn into the other hatchers in the same airspace, so that chicks from salmonella-free flocks may be at risk from salmonella cross-infection while in the hatcher. As hatching occurs over a 3-day period (days 18–21) there may be ample opportunity for excretion and multiplication of salmonellas before chicks are removed from the hatcher.

Following hatching, chicks are sorted, vaccinated and packed in delivery boxes or crates. When chicks from infected flocks are handled, there is the potential for salmonella contamination of the largely automated handling equipment and its environment via meconium and fluff. If a salmonella-infected flock is handled before a non-infected flock there is a risk of surface cross-contamination of chicks, with subsequent oral infection during preening. It is important to organize all hatchery operations so that eggs and chicks from potentially the least contaminated sources are handled first or eggs from flocks that are known to be infected are hatched on separate days. In some cases present hatchery organization does not allow this degree of prioritization.

The sanitization of chick handling equipment is important to avoid carry-over of salmonella contamination from day to day. In our own investigations, there have been examples of good and poor cleansing and disinfection practices. It is important to remove gross debris before pressure washing, preferably by liquid vacuum suction. The surfaces should then be washed with a detergent sanitizer applied by a power washer set at medium pressure whilst the conveyors are running. Ledges and inaccessible areas should be wiped with disposable cloths soaked in disinfectant and finally all surfaces should be allowed to dry before being sprayed at low pressure with an effective disinfectant applied at the correct concentration for a high-risk salmonella contaminated area (MAFF General Orders rate).

Effective sanitization of egg trays, chick trays and farm trolleys is necessary to avoid carry-over of infection between batches of eggs or chicks. Total elimination of salmonella is particularly important for trays and trolleys that are returned to breeder units, as these may otherwise introduce salmonella from the hatchery to previously uninfected premises.

The efficacy of tray washing appears to vary. Some sanitized trays appear extremely clean whereas others may be contaminated with particles of eggshell, yolk or meconium. It is possible to achieve salmonella-free trolleys and trays using either manual washing or automatic tray washers, but the latter must be set up correctly to clean effectively. The type and concentration of disinfectant used in tray washing also appears to be an important factor, since visibly clean trays can still harbour infection on some occasions.

In some hatcheries, the main ventilation system draws air from areas with a potential source of salmonella contamination, such as the hatcher and chick area, air exhaust ducts or the waste skip, where splashing of macerated egg and dead chick remains can occur. Where such hazards are present, salmonella is always likely to be found in air intake ducts. Because these ducts are high-speed intakes there can be very little dust to sample, so the presence of salmonellas may reflect a larger number of organisms drawn back into the building to be distributed to a variety of areas. In many cases, coarse filtration of air is used, but this is unlikely to restrict the access of small, contaminated dust particles.

In most cases, it would be possible to upgrade the filtration of air. Effective screening of the air intake plant is also beneficial and spread of contamination from exhaust ducts can be reduced by the use of sanitary traps. Ideally, all hatcheries should be designed so that air is drawn in from the opposite side of the building to that on which stale air and waste are discharged. Similarly, recirculation of air to conserve heat should be discouraged unless effective bacteriological filters are used.

There are many other areas such as transport vehicles, personnel, chick-holding accommodation, waste management, segregation of 'dirty' and 'clean' areas, avoidance of backtracking and personal hygiene measures and facilities which are also important in controlling salmonella contamination in hatcheries.

ENVIRONMENTAL CONTAMINATION

Persistent environmental contamination of houses is an important factor in the maintenance of *S. enteritidis* and other salmonellas in poultry flocks (Kradel and Miller, 1991; Baggesen *et al.*, 1992). The effective decontamination of salmonella-infected houses before repopulation is a highly important consideration in a Hazard Analysis Critical Control Point approach for poultry units. A high standard of disinfection is necessary to avoid infection of poultry placed in previously infected houses, because it has been shown experimentally that an infective dose of salmonella for chickens can be less than five cells (Milner and Shaffer, 1952) or 100 cells for adult birds following conjunctival inoculation (Humphrey *et al.*, 1992). Intercurrent disease may make the birds even more susceptible (Arakawa *et al.*, 1992; Holt, 1993; Nakamura *et al.*, 1995). A number of analytical studies have associated salmonella infection with poor hygiene standards at poultry sites (Opitz, 1992; Henzler and Opitz, 1992; Fris and van den Bos, 1995). The tendency for persistent infection on the farm is widely recognized and in a case control study of British poultry breeding flocks, *S. enteritidis* PT4 infection was associated with a history of salmonella at the poultry site, highlighting the importance of the farm environment in the epidemiology of infection (Evans and Sayers, unpublished observations). Similar findings were reported following a study of broiler flocks in Denmark (Angen *et al.*, 1996).

Salmonellas may persist in dry livestock buildings for many months (Bailey, 1993; Bale *et al.*, 1993) and our own studies (Davies and Wray, 1996a) have confirmed the ability of these organisms to survive for long periods (Table 11.2). Samples were obtained for a 12-month period from a poultry house, which had contained birds naturally infected with *S. enteritidis*. There was a high isolation rate of salmonella from samples taken two weeks before depletion of the flock, particularly at ground level and in nest boxes. One week after removal of all the birds, no salmonellas were found in litter or droppings picked from the litter surface, although feed troughs, nest boxes and other areas were still contaminated. The rapid decline in prevalence of salmonella isolations from litter and faeces suggests that continued deposition of salmonellas from infected birds may be necessary to maintain contamination of litter. The prevalence of salmonellas remained low until the removal of the litter at 30 weeks, when 41% of the 36 swabs taken from the floor were contaminated with salmonellas (Table 11.2), even though salmonellas were not isolated from bulk litter removed from the house. However, the organism was present in small pockets of spilt litter, which remained outside the house after depletion. Similar results were obtained from two broiler breeder sites, where salmonellas were detected in fan dust outside the house, whereas swabs taken within the house were negative. Further studies in occupied poultry houses (Davies and Wray, 1996b) found a threefold higher salmonella isolation rate from nest box floors and dust on in-house slave feed hoppers than from drinkers, chain feeders, slats, perches or dust on beams and ventilation ducts. In broiler breeder houses, salmonellas were isolated from egg sorting tables and 75% of the egg collecting trolleys that were sampled.

Table 11.2. Persistence of *S. enteritidis* in an empty poultry unit.

Sample site	Two weeks before depletion	After litter removal at 30 weeks after depopulation
Drinkers	3/4[a]	0/3
Ground swabs	4/4	15/36
Litter	4/4	0/20
Walls	3/4	4/12
Dust on beams	2/4	2/12
Total	16/20 (80%)	21/83 (25.3%)

[a]No. of *Salmonella*-positive samples/total no. of samples.

DISINFECTION STUDIES

A high standard of disinfection is necessary to avoid infection of poultry placed in a previously infected house and studies carried out at the Central Veterinary Laboratory and in the field have identified many potential problems during disinfection of poultry units that were naturally contaminated with *S. enteritidis* (Davies and Wray, 1995a). Sampling carried out on cleaned and disinfected poultry houses after infected flocks had been slaughtered, showed persistence of *S. enteritidis* in the environment of 16 of 20 houses. Cleansing and disinfection regimens using formaldehyde, either as part of a terminal disinfectant spray strategy or as a fogging agent after the use of other products, were associated with the lowest level of persistent salmonella contamination. Thus, *S. enteritidis* was not found to have persisted in five of the nine houses in which a formaldehyde disinfectant spray or fogging treatment had been used. In another six of the houses, *S. enteritidis* was only found on equipment that had not been treated with formaldehyde, and in another house only 1 of 90 samples was positive. The other two houses in which formaldehyde had been used were heavily reinfested by *S. enteritidis*-infected mice. There appeared to be a relationship between the standard of cleansing and the level of persistent salmonella when a tar–oil mixture spray and a peroxygen compound fog was used. However, when a synthetic phenolic compound was used as a spray, salmonellas were not isolated from treated surfaces, even in the presence of large quantities of organic matter and the organism was only detected on equipment that had not been disinfected.

The prevalence of salmonella contamination was significantly increased in a contaminated house following ineffective cleansing and disinfection (Table 11.3). Kradel and Miller (1991) also observed increased contamination leading to persistent poultry flock infection following environmental carry over of salmonella.

The poor results of some cleansing and disinfection regimens lend support to those that believe in leaving poultry litter *in situ*, which is claimed to increase colonization resistance of chicks to salmonella (Corrier *et al.*, 1993), but which may lead to a build up of a wide range of harmful organisms and degrade the principle of all-in, all-out stocking as a means of breaking disease cycles.

Table 11.3. Persistence of *S. enteritidis* in a broiler house after cleansing and disinfection.

Sample site	Before sanitization (%)	After sanitization (%)
Floor	4/7[a] (57.0)	6/8 (75.0)
Walls	0/5 (–)	4/7 (57.1)
Post bases	0/5 (–)	5/8 (62.5)
Chain feeders	1/8 (12.5)	3/6 (50.0)
High beams and pipes	1/6 (16.7)	0/8 (–)
Total	6/31 (19.3)	18/37 (48.6)

[a]No. of *Salmonella*-positive samples/total no. of samples.

It was generally observed that the standard of cleaning of poultry houses by farm staff was inferior to that of contractors (Table 11.4). The level of supervision by site and field management was low, resulting in missed areas and in errors that could compromise the disinfection of the site.

Further work is necessary, however, to confirm that these regimes are effective over a wide range of situations. Use of disinfectants, especially formaldehyde, necessitates that all safety requirements are met, especially the use of a respirator to protect the operator. Although effective cleansing and disinfection carries a cost, improvements in broiler growth rates have been reported in formaldehyde-treated houses (Allen, 1993).

THE ROLE OF WILDLIFE

Elimination of the persistent contamination of some poultry breeder units has been one of the most difficult problems in controlling *S. enteritidis* and other salmonella serotypes in poultry flocks in Great Britain and other countries (Baggesen *et al.*, 1992; Brown *et al.*, 1992). Such persistent contamination may be caused by failure of disinfection routines or the presence of wildlife carriers or vectors.

Role of Rodents

Although *S. enteritidis* infection in mice on poultry units was reported more than 15 years ago (Krabisch and Dorn, 1980), the significance of mice as vectors of *S. enteritidis* on poultry units has only received widespread attention relatively recently (Henzler and Opitz, 1992). Naturally infected mice, captured at depletion on poultry units where *S. enteritidis* infection had been confirmed in the birds, excreted the organism for up to 18 weeks (Davies and Wray, 1995b). Excretion was intermittent and reactivation of infection occurred during periods of stress. The prevalence of *S. enteritidis* in individual faecal pellets was usually low (< 10 colony-forming units (cfu)) but one pellet contained 10^2–10^3 organisms. More recent work has identified levels of 10^5–10^6 cfu in some faecal pellets. Salmonella contamination in the environment may be amplified by mice defecating into feed troughs and on egg-collection belts and may be spread further throughout the house by automated feeding systems, egg conveyors and manure removal equipment.

Table 11.4. Persistence of *Salmonella* after cleansing and disinfection.

No of units	Application by	No. of samples positive/ total no. of samples (%)
7	Farm staff	185/1238 (14.9)
13	Contractor	143/1921 (7.4)

S. enteritidis-infected mice were detected in a single poultry house for more than two years after depopulation and they constituted a reservoir of infection for the next flock. Infected, dead mice or droppings were found on 50% of broiler breeder or layer breeder units that were investigated after cleaning and disinfection. Many areas on poultry units may become infected with rodents and an intensive and sustained rodent control programme is necessary for the control of salmonella. The programme needs to be well planned, flexible, continuous and its effectiveness monitored (WHO, 1994). Trapping of rodents may also be used to monitor salmonella contamination, because mice remain infected even after environmental contamination becomes difficult to detect by standard sampling techniques.

Role of Birds

Salmonella infection has been detected in many species of wild bird. At hatcheries and poultry-processing plants salmonellas were detected in a number of different species of wild birds, which may contaminate clean equipment left outside the buildings (Davies and Wray, 1994a).

Role of Insects

Flies have frequently been shown to be contaminated with salmonella and Edel *et al.* (1973) found that 1.5% of 202 fly traps examined were contaminated with the organism. Blowfly larvae (*Lucilia serricata*) were also found to be contaminated with salmonellas and our studies have shown that maggots are a potent vehicle of salmonella infection for chickens (Davies and Wray, 1994b). Maggots, which may contain up to 10^6 cfu of salmonella depending on the substrate, are attractive to chickens and, when ingested, the cuticle has a protective effect so that the bactericidal activity of gastric acidity etc. is by-passed.

It has been suggested that mealworm beetles (*Alphitobius diaperinus*) may also be important in the persistence and transmission of salmonella infections on poultry units (Baggesen *et al.*, 1992; Brown *et al.*, 1992). In our studies 500 live *Alphitobius* beetles were collected before cleansing and disinfection on two poultry units, and although the environmental contamination with salmonella was high the organism was not isolated from any of the beetles. Likewise we failed to infect the beetles by artificial contamination with 10^3 cfu of salmonella, although Geissler and Kösters (1972) found that beetles artificially infected with 10^9 cfu excreted salmonellas for 15 days.

BIOSECURITY

Staff on farms and visitors can carry salmonellas mechanically from one unit to another on contaminated equipment, footwear, clothing and hands. As a consequence, visitors to livestock units should be restricted to those on essential business and adequate protective clothing should be provided and hygienic procedures adhered to.

The farm should be located away from other poultry holdings, where circumstances permit, and visitors should park away from the buildings, preferably outside the holding. No visitor should enter a poultry building unless wearing disposable overall clothing, or overall clothing which is capable of being laundered and boots which are capable of being cleansed and disinfected. On leaving a poultry building, the person should immediately cleanse and disinfect boots and wash hands. Further details of biosecurity may be found in the Codes of Practice for the prevention and control of salmonella in poultry flocks (MAFF).

STATUTORY ASPECTS OF THE CONTROL OF SALMONELLA IN GREAT BRITAIN

In 1989, a new Zoonoses Order replaced and broadened the scope of the previous order which was first enacted in 1975. The main provisions of the Zoonoses Order (HMSO, 1989a) are the requirement to report the results of tests which identify the presence of salmonella, the provision of a culture of the salmonella for MAFF, the taking of live birds and other samples for diagnostic purposes, imposition of movement restrictions and isolation requirements, as well as a requirement for the cleaning and disinfection of premises and vehicles. The Order also applies the provision of the Animal Health Act (HMSO, 1981a) with regard to the compulsory slaughter of salmonella-infected poultry flocks and payment of compensation.

To combat *S. enteritidis* infection in poultry, the Poultry Breeding Flocks and Hatcheries (Testing and Registration) Order was enacted in 1989 (HMSO, 1989b). Both orders required the testing of poultry for salmonella on a regular basis. The purpose was to prevent transmission of salmonella through eggs and to reduce vertical transmission of salmonellas so that chickens for commercial rearing did not take infection on to customers' premises. The two orders were revoked in 1993 with the implementation of the Poultry Breeding Flocks and Hatcheries Order (HMSO, 1993) which brought salmonella control measures in poultry into line with the European Union Directive 92/117/EEC. This requires the regular monitoring of breeding flocks and hatcheries for *S. enteritidis* and *S. typhimurium* by a prescribed programme using methods laid down in the Order.

Since 1993, there has been no statutory requirement to monitor turkeys, ducks or geese, or the commercial generations of domestic fowl. Flock owners have, however, been encouraged to adopt good management practices for the control of salmonellas by following voluntary codes of practice that have been produced by the Ministry in collaboration with the poultry industry and the veterinary profession.

SALMONELLA IN ANIMAL FEEDS

Feedstuffs have always been a potential source of salmonella for poultry and the Processed Animal Protein Order (HMSO, 1989c) requires those processing animal protein to be registered with the Ministry and to test each day's consignment for salmonella in an authorized laboratory. If salmonella is isolated the processor is required to ensure that no contaminated material is incorporated into animal feedstuffs. As part of its package of control measures, the Ministry, with the cooperation of the feeding stuffs industry, introduced a number of voluntary codes of practice for the production, storage, handling and transport of animal feeding stuffs.

The Importation of Processed Animal Protein Order (HMSO, 1981b) prohibits the landing in Great Britain of any processed animal protein or any product containing processed animal protein except under the authority of a licence. The conditions imposed in the import licence reflect the likely contamination status of imported materials. In some countries, these conditions may require detention of every imported consignment at the port of landing until negative salmonella test results have been obtained.

DETECTION

Salmonella can be isolated from bacteraemic birds by direct culture but the caecum is the most likely site for isolation in adult birds for which selective enrichment is usually needed. However, the standard culture methods may lack sensitivity and more sensitive, rapid techniques have been developed to allow a greater throughput of samples (Davies and Wray, 1994c). Population screening methods must be capable of detecting low-incidence infections of poultry, which are common, and methods have been developed to sample the environment as an indirect indicator of flock infection.

Various isolation methods are in current use and most involve selective enrichment in selenite, tetrathionate or Rapport–Vassiliadis medium with incubation at 37–42°C and the use of selective plating media, such as MacConkey, deoxycholate citrate or brilliant green agar. Pre-enrichment in buffered peptone water, before selective enrichment in semisolid media such as Diassalm and plating on Rambach agar has been shown to be the most sensitive method.

Various serological tests are available for the detection of salmonella in poultry. The enzyme-linked immunosorbent assay (ELISA) is used in many countries for the identification of flocks infected with *S. enteritidis,* although bacteriological confirmation is recommended due to the lack of specificity. Two systems are in current use, the indirect ELISA and the competitive double antibody blocking ELISA, the former being favoured for monitoring purposes in Britain (WHO, 1994). One disadvantage of using a serological test is that positive results do not necessarily mean that the bird is still infected and negative results can be obtained in the early stages of infection prior to the development of an immune response. Interpretation of serological tests is further complicated by vaccination of flocks.

MONITORING FOR SALMONELLAS

Monitoring should be carried out at all stages of the production cycle. In breeding flocks and hatcheries it is mandatory, as indicated in the Breeding Flocks and Hatcheries Order (HMSO, 1993) if the breeding flock has more than 250 birds and the hatchery an incubator capacity of 1000 eggs or more. More intensive sampling can be carried out by checking fluff from the interior surfaces of the hatchers and broken eggshells from the trays. Surface swabs from different parts of the hatchery and sampling of macerated waste should assist in checking for the presence of salmonellas as well as the effectiveness of cleansing and disinfection.

At the rearing site, the presence of salmonellas in replacement birds can be checked by culturing of chick box-liners or swabs from the bottom of the boxes, chicks dead on arrival and those culled or dying within a few days of arrival. During the rearing period, bulked litter samples and dust from various sites, e.g. exhaust fans, provide the most convenient samples for monitoring. When breeders are in lay, the most reliable samples are nest-box floor swabs, nest-box litter, dust from internal feed hoppers and swabs from egg sorting tables and corridors; for elite birds more frequent sampling is desirable. Laying flocks may be sampled by using drag swabs in the manure pit, dust samples, swabs of the manure scraper and spilled debris from the egg collection belt. In the case of barn layers, litter, dust samples and nest boxes should be sampled.

After depopulation, and when cleansing and disinfection have been carried out, buildings should be checked for persistence of salmonellas. Samples should include large fabric swabs of earth floor surfaces or floor sweepings from concrete floors, nest-box floors, slave feed hoppers, beams, pipes and electrical fittings.

There is now evidence that the measures taken to eradicate *S. enteritidis* infection in the British poultry industry have had some success. Primary breeder flocks are free of infection and there is a declining trend in reports from parent breeding flocks (Fig. 11.3). However, eradication is still likely to be remote. Therefore, attention has also been directed at interventions to reduce the chance of infection or to eliminate infections that do occur. The most feasible are competitive exclusion with antibiotic treatment and vaccination. Competitive exclusion refers to colonization control in the live bird by the establishment of protective populations of intestinal bacteria (Nurmi and Rantala, 1973). Despite success under experimental conditions, this approach has shown mixed results in the field in its ability to protect against salmonella infection (Goren *et al.*, 1988; Mead, 1991; Mulder and Bolder, 1991). In general, protection is superior with undefined cultures that contain a broad range of bacteria (Stavric *et al.*, 1991), although there may be a risk of spreading pathogens to recipient birds. The use of antibiotic treatment is generally considered unwise due to the risk of selecting resistant strains of bacteria (particularly if quinolone drugs are used). Recent trials in British breeder flocks infected with *S. enteritidis* have shown that a combination of antibiotic treatment and competitive exclusion reduced the prevalence of infection but did not eliminate the organism (Reynolds *et al.*, 1997). Control by vaccination is

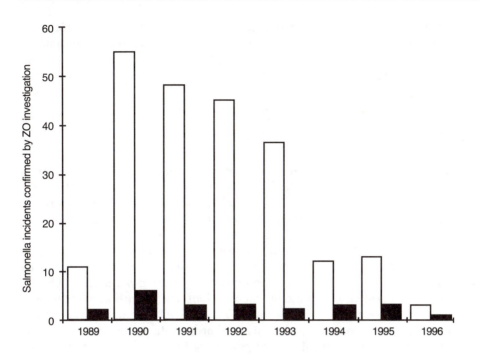

Fig. 11.3. Confirmed *Salmonella* incidents in broiler breeding flocks in Great Britain (1989–1996). ZO, Zoonoses Order 1989; □, *Salmonella enteritidis*; ■, *S. typhimurium*. Source: MAFF.

still in the developmental stages, although an inactivated vaccine is available in the UK and has been used successfully in breeding flocks. One disadvantage of vaccination is its interference with the results of serological monitoring. All three methods of intervention are likely to be most successful when used as part of a comprehensive salmonella control programme, with the main emphasis on a high level of disease security and hygiene.

CONCLUSIONS

Salmonella control presents a major challenge to all involved in animal production. During the *S. enteritidis* PT 4 epidemic, it became apparent that control must be based on a detailed knowledge of the epidemiology of infection and a specific control programme for each individual unit. An integrated programme is necessary covering all aspects of the supply chain from primary breeding flocks to the final product and it should include all those involved in poultry production. Many strategies were tried and tested e.g. slaughter, immunization, use of antibacterials. None was successful on its own, but improved hygiene and disease security, combined with vaccination has had the most impact on the *S. enteritidis* status of the UK poultry parent breeder sector and biosecurity measures alone have been effective in maintaining freedom from the organism in primary breeding flocks. There is a danger, however, that vaccination for one particular serotype will create a niche for other serovars to emerge. Thus, future control measures must concentrate on eliminating or reducing all salmonella serotypes by comprehensive disease security precautions assisted, perhaps, by the use of multivalent salmonella vaccines in specific cases.

THE FUTURE

As the prevalence of human salmonellosis continues to increase, there is recognition that a 'farm to fork' approach is necessary to reduce pathogens, and Good Manufacturing Practices (GMPs) using Hazard Analysis Critical Control Point (HACCP) principles are being increasingly used to effect a reduction. Using the HACCP system applied to the critical control points on farms and supplies of feed and services will be beneficial in future. As we have shown earlier, the prevalence of salmonella in the hatchery can be reduced by a comprehensive planning and sanitization programme. On the farm, it is necessary to combine effective biosecurity with monitoring and our studies have shown (Davies and Wray, 1996b) that monitoring of the litter and environment is more reliable than sampling individual birds. It is important that the critical control points are identified for each individual farm and that the application of HACCP is maintained by key-point process monitoring. There are, however, still many unanswered questions on the most effective and economic means of controlling *Salmonella* in the poultry industry. This is an area where more investigative bacteriology, using the principles of Best Practice Analysis, is required to identify existing effective measures (and errors) and to disseminate information on effective techniques.

REFERENCES

Allen, P.C. (1993) Effects of formaldehyde fumigation of housing on carotenoid pigmentation in three breeds of chickens. *Poultry Science* 72, 1040–1045.

Angen, O., Skov, M.N., Chriel, M., Agger, J.F. and Bisgaard, M. (1996) A retrospective study of *Salmonella* infections in Danish broiler flocks. *Preventive Veterinary Medicine* 26, 223–237.

Arakawa, A., Fukaton, T., Baba, E., McDougald, L.R, Bailey, J.S. and Blankenship, L.C. (1992) Influence of coccidosis on colonisation in broiler chickens under floor pen conditions. *Poultry Science* 71, 59–63.

Baggesen, D.C., Olsen, J.E. and Bisgaard, M. (1992) Plasmid profiles and phage types of *Salmonella typhimurium* isolated from successive flocks of chickens on three parent farms. *Avian Pathology* 21, 569–579.

Bailey, J.S. (1993) Control of *Salmonella* and *Campylobacter* in poultry production, a summary of work at Russell Research Centre. *Poultry Science* 72, 1169–1173.

Bailey, J.S., Cox, N.A. and Berreang, M.E. (1994) Hatchery acquired *Salmonellae* in broiler chicks. *Poultry Science* 73, 1153–1157.

Bale, J., Bennett, P.M., Beringer, J.E. and Hinton, M.H. (1993) The survival of bacteria exposed to desiccation on surfaces associated with farm buildings. *Journal of Applied Bacteriology* 75, 519–528.

Brown, D.J., Olsen, J.E. and Bisgaard, M. (1992) *Salmonella enteritidis* infection, cross-infection and persistence within the environment of a broiler parent stock unit in Denmark. *Zentralblatt für Bakteriologie* 277, 129–138.

Bruce, J. and Drysdale, E.M. (1990) Egg hygiene: routes of infection In: Tullett, S.G. (ed.) *Avian Incubation*. Butterworth, London, pp. 257–267.

Cason, J.A., Cox, N.A. and Bailey, J.S. (1991) Survival of *Salmonella typhimurium* during incubation and hatching of inoculated eggs. *Poultry Science* 70 (Suppl. 1), 152.

Corrier, D.E., Hargis, B.M., Hinton, A. and Deloach, J.R. (1993) Protective effect of used poultry litter and lactose in the feed ration on *Salmonella enteritidis* colonisation of Leghorn chicks and hens. *Avian Diseases* 37, 47–52.

Davies, R.H. and Wray, C. (1994a) *Salmonella* pollution in poultry units and associated enterprises. In: Dewi, I.A.P., Axford, R.F.F., Marai, I.F.M. and Umed, H. (eds) *Pollution in Livestock Systems*. CAB International, Wallingford, pp. 137–166.

Davies, R.H. and Wray, C. (1994b) Use of larvae of *Lucilia serricata* in colonisation and invasion studies of *Salmonella enteritidis* infection in poultry Flair No 610. In: Pusztai, A., Hinton, M.H. and Mulder, R.W.A.W. (eds) *The Attachment of Bacteria to the Gut*. COVP-DLO, Het Spelderholt, pp. 117–123.

Davies, R.H. and Wray, C. (1994c) An approach to reduction of *Salmonella* infection in broiler chicken flocks through intensive sampling and identification of cross-contamination hazards in commercial hatcheries. *International Journal of Food Microbiology* 24, 147–160.

Davies, R.H. and Wray, C. (1994d) Evaluation of a rapid cultural method for identification of *Salmonellas* in naturally contaminated veterinary samples. *Journal of Applied Bacteriology* 77, 237–241.

Davies, R.H. and Wray, C. (1995a) Observations on disinfection regimens used on *Salmonella enteritidis* infected poultry units. *Poultry Science* 74, 638–647.

Davies, R.H. and Wray, C. (1995b) Mice as carriers of *Salmonella enteritidis* on persistently infected poultry units. *Veterinary Record* 137, 337–342.

Davies, R.H. and Wray, C. (1996a) Persistence of *Salmonella enteritidis* in poultry units and poultry food. *British Poultry Science* 37, 589–596.

Davies, R.H. and Wray, C. (1996b) Determination of an effective sampling regime to detect *Salmonella enteritidis* in the environment of poultry units. *Veterinary Microbiology* 50, 117–127.

Edel, W., van Schothorst, M., Guinee P.A.M. and Kampelmacher, E.H. (1973) Mechanisms and prevention of *Salmonella* infection in animals In: Hobbs, B.C. and Christian, J.H.B. (eds) *The Microbiological Safety of Food*. Academic Press, London, pp. 247–256.

Fris, C. and van den Bos, J. (1995) A retrospective case control study of risk factors associated with *Salmonella enteritidis* infection on Dutch broiler farms. *Avian Pathology* 24, 255–272.

Geissler von, H and Kösters, J. (1972) Die hygienische Bedeutung des Getreidesehim melkäfers (*Alphitobius diaperinus* Panz) in der Geflügelmast. *Deutsche Tierartzliche Wochenschrift* 79, 177–181.

Goren, E., de Jong, W.A., Doornenbal, P., Bolder, N.M, Mulder, R.W.A.W. and Jansen, A. (1988) Reduction of *Salmonella* infection of broilers by spray application of intestinal microflora: a longitudinal study. *Veterinary Quarterly* 10, 249–255.

Haigh, T. and Betts, W.B. (1991) Microbial barrier properties of hen egg shells. *Microbios* 68, 137–146.

Hammack, T.S., Sherrod, P.S., Bruce, V.R., June, G.A., Satchell, F.B. and Andrews, W.H. (1993) Growth of *Salmonella enteritidis* in grade A eggs during prolonged storage. *Poultry Science* 72, 373–377.

Henzler, D.J. and Opitz, H.M. (1992) The role of mice in the epizootiology of *Samonella enteritidis* infection on chicken layer farms. *Avian Diseases* 36, 625–631.

HMSO (1981a) The Animal Health Act 1981. *Statutory Instrument 1975* No. 1030.

HMSO (1981b) Importation of Processed Animal Protein Order. *Statutory Instrument* No. 677.

HMSO (1989a) The Zoonoses Order 1989. *Statutory Instrument 1989* No. 285.

HMSO (1989b) The Poultry Breeding Flocks and Hatcheries (Registration and Testing) Order 1989. *Statutory Instrument 1989* No. 1963.

HMSO (1989c) The Processed Animal Protein Order 1989. *Statutory Instrument 1989* No. 661.

HMSO (1993) The Poultry Breeding Flocks and Hatcheries Order 1993. *Statutory Instrument 1993* No. 1898.

Holt, P.S. (1993) Effect of induced molting on the susceptibility of white leghorn hens to a *Salmonella enteritidis* infection. *Avian Diseases* 37, 412–417.

Humphrey, T.J., Baskerville, A., Chart, H., Rowe, B. and Whitehead, A. (1992) Infection of laying hens with *Salmonella enteritidis* PT4 by conjunctival challenge. *Veterinary Record* 131, 386–388.

Krabisch, P. and Dorn, P. (1980) Zur epidemiologischen Bedeuntung von Lebendvektoren bei der Verbreitung von Salmonellen in der Geflügelmast. *Berliner and Munchener Tierartzliche Wochenschrift* 92, 232–235.

Kradel, D.C. and Miller, W.L. (1991) *Salmonella enteritidis* observations on field related problems. In: *Proceedings of the Fortieth Western Poultry Disease Conference,* Acapulco, pp. 146–150.

Lister, S.A. (1988) *Salmonella enteritidis* infection in broilers and broiler breeders. *Veterinary Record* 123, 350.

Mario-Padron, N. (1990) *Salmonella typhimurium* penetration through the egg-shell of hatching eggs. *Avian Diseases* 34, 463–465.

Mayes, F.J. and Takeballi, M.A. (1983) Microbial contamination of the hen's egg: a review. *Journal of Food Protection* 46, 1092–1098.

Mead, G.C. (1991) Developments in competitive exclusion to control *Salmonella* carriage in poultry. In: Blankenship, L.C. (ed.) *Colonization of Human Bacterial Enteropathogens in Poultry.* Academic Press, New York, pp. 91–104.

Milner, K.C. and Shaffer, M.F. (1952) Bacteriologic studies of experimental *Salmonella* infections in chicks. *Journal of Infectious Diseases* 90, 81–85.

Mulder, R.W.A.W. and Bolder, N.M. (1991) Experience with competitive exclusion in the Netherlands. In: Blankenship, L.C. (ed.) *Colonization of Human Bacterial Enteropathogens in Poultry.* Academic Press, New York, pp. 77–90.

Nakamura, M., Nagamine, N., Takahashi, T., Norimatsu, M., Suzuki, S. and Sato, S. (1995) Intratracheal infection of chickens with *Salmonella enteritidis* and the effect of feed and water deprivation. *Avian Diseases* 39, 853–858.

Nascimento, V.P. and Solomon, S.E. (1991) The transfer of bacteria (*Salmonella enteritidis*) across the eggshell wall of eggs classified as 'poor quality'. *Animal Technology* 42, 157–165.

Nascimento, V.P., Cranstown, S. and Solomon, S.E. (1992) Relationship between shell structure and movement of *Salmonella enteritidis* across the egg shell wall. *British Poultry Science* 33, 37–48.

Nurmi, E. and Rantala, M. (1973) New aspects of *Salmonella* infection in broiler production. *Nature* 241, 210–211.

O'Brien, J.D.P. (1988) *Salmonella enteritidis* infection in broiler chickens. *Veterinary Record* 122, 214.

Opitz, H.M. (1992) Progress being made in *Salmonella enteritidis* reduction on the farm. *Poultry Digest* March, 16–22.

Reynolds, D.J., Davies, R.H., Richards, M. and Wray, C. (1997) Evaluation of combined antibiotic and competitive exclusion in broiler breeder flocks infected with *Salmonella enterica* serovar enteritidis. *Avian Pathology* 26, 83–95.

Stavric, S., Gleeson, T.M. and Blanchfield, B. (1991) Efficacy of undefined bacterial treatments in competitive exclusion of *Salmonella* from chicks. In: Blankenship, L.C. (ed.) *Colonization of Human Bacterial Enteropathogens in Poultry.* Academic Press, New York, pp. 323–330.

Turnbull, P.C.B. (1979) Food poisoning with special reference to *Salmonella* – its epidemiology, pathogenesis and control. *Clinical Gastroenterology* 8, 663–714.

Watson, W.A. and Kirby, F.D. (1984) The *Salmonella* problem and its control in Great Britain. In: *Proceedings of the International Symposium on Salmonella.* American Association of Avian Pathologists, Kennett Square, USA, pp. 35–47.

WHO (1994) Wray, C. and Davies, R.H. (eds) *Guidelines on Detection and Monitoring of Salmonella Infected Poultry Flocks with Particular Reference to Salmonella enteritidis.* WHOZoon/94/173.

CHAPTER 12
Hygiene during transport, slaughter and processing

R.W.A.W. Mulder
DLO Institute for Animal Science and Health, PO Box 15, 8200 AB Lelystad, The Netherlands

INTRODUCTION

Poultry meat is by far the most popular food product worldwide. Several factors contribute to the popularity of this product, of which sensory, dietary and economic factors are the most important. This is mainly due to the extensive development of the poultry industry in the last 30–40 years, which brought the food poultry meat from being a rather exclusive product, only available to a limited class of consumer, to the popular, cheap and wholesome meat within everyone's budget. There are no primary religious restrictions associated with the consumption of poultry meat, but it has to be realized that, due to religious considerations, hygiene during the slaughter process sometimes can be negatively influenced.

Hygiene aspects of poultry production and processing relate to the presence (or absence) of potentially pathogenic as well as of spoilage microorganisms. In both cases their presence may result in cases of human food-borne disease or in spoilage of the product, which, as a consequence, results in considerable economic losses to society and industry.

Foods of animal origin, and poultry products in particular, are often found contaminated with potentially pathogenic microorganisms such as *Salmonella* spp., *Campylobacter* spp., *Escherichia coli*, *Listeria monocytogenes* and *Staphylococcus aureus*. On some occasions *Yersinia enterocolitica*, *Aeromonas* spp. and *Clostridium perfringens* also seem to be important pathogens. However, *Salmonella* spp. and *Campylobacter* spp. and, to a lesser extent, *Listeria monocytogenes* are considered the major food-borne disease-causing pathogens in poultry.

Epidemiological reports all over the world incriminate poultry meat as a source for outbreaks of human food poisoning. As poultry meat is usually not eaten raw, these outbreaks are caused by secondary contamination, from poultry, introduced during the preparation of food. The aim of the poultry industry is to find ways to avoid contamination of live poultry and poultry products with these potentially pathogenic microorganisms, as their presence makes the industry very vulnerable. Figure 12.1 provides a scheme for routes of contamination in the poultry industry from animal–human–environment to consumers and vice versa.

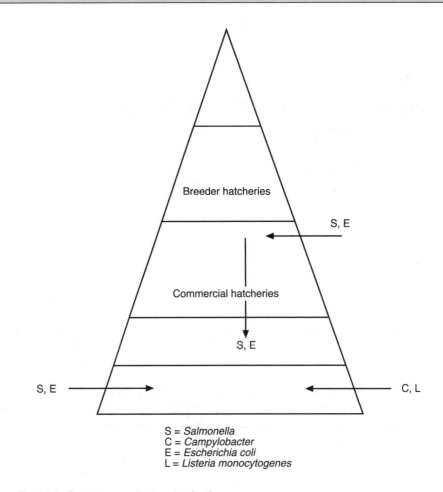

Breeder hatcheries

S, E

Commercial hatcheries

S, E

S, E

C, L

S = *Salmonella*
C = *Campylobacter*
E = *Escherichia coli*
L = *Listeria monocytogenes*

Fig. 12.1. Routes on product contamination.

Contamination of consumer-ready products with microorganisms of public health significance the initial contamination of live birds and the care taken during slaughter. However, intervention measures, which can be taken by industry to avoid contamination of the consumer-ready product, exert more effect when they start with the live bird. It has to be mentioned that research activities in this field have mainly concentrated on pathogenic microorganisms and, in this respect, the ecology of spoilage microorganisms has been neglected.

Preventative measures to reduce the level of contamination with potentially pathogenic microorganisms during the grow-out period should focus on the control of husbandry practices as well as on the use of technologies and products known to be effective against the colonization of these microorganisms (Mulder, 1997). The aim should be to deliver live poultry free of pathogens. However, at present, the processing industry has to cope with contaminated flocks coming to the processing plant, and their main task then is not to spread the contamination further.

The poultry product chain can be described in terms of the Hazard Analysis Critical Control Point (HACCP) concept, identifying critical points along the production chain. Although the application of HACCP in the live-bird phase is questionable, several examples in the processing phase, from transport to scalding, evisceration, chilling and cutting can be found. Again critical control points are defined with regard to the presence or absence of potentially pathogenic microorganisms and do not mention spoilage organisms.

The influence of transport of the live birds to the slaughterhouse on contamination of the consumer-ready product has not been studied intensively. Some researchers have concluded that there is an increased excretion of potentially pathogenic microorganisms, as a result of stress during catching and transport, which could result in additional contamination of the final product (Mulder, 1995).

The application of feed withdrawal practices can be of help in lowering the microbial input to the slaughterhouse, as these empty the intestinal tract and so gut breakage during slaughter will not cause extra cross-contamination (Bilgili, 1988). However, these stress effects (increased shedding of *Salmonella* and/or *Campylobacter*) were not always measurable in the final product.

In relation to the slaughter process, special emphasis has been placed on developments in scalding, plucking and evisceration of the carcass. With multistage cleaning and scalding, followed by plucking, and combined scalding and plucking, cross-contamination between carcasses is reduced. Further, new evisceration equipment, which separates carcasses from the viscera and giblets, has improved the microbiological quality of carcasses with respect to pathogens. The effects on spoilage organisms are not as clear. Earlier studies, in which the effect on microbial counts of varying scalding temperatures in conjunction with the use of different chilling methods (water, air etc.) was assessed, resulted in a longer shelf-life of the product.

The development of automatic cut-up lines increases productivity. However, there is the difficulty of cleaning the equipment during and after production hours.

STRESS FACTORS

Stress is observed during fattening, catching and loading, transport and holding at the slaughter plant. Stress can also be accompanied by symptoms such as damage to the intestinal tract and a lower level of immunity. Factors influencing the intestinal microflora are summarized in Table 12.1, although the effects on the microflora are not well understood. A disturbance of the microflora can occur which changes the incidence of microorganisms present and lowers resistance to infection. This change can be readily detected in the upper part of the small intestine where the composition of the microflora is more aerobic. Another consequence of stress is the increase in shedding of caecal material and therefore an increased spreading of bacteria, contributing to external contamination of the birds. *Salmonella* spp. and *Campylobacter* spp.

Table 12.1. Factors causing an imbalance in the intestinal microflora.

Deprivation/fasting	Antibiotics
Consumption of spoiled feed	Malabsorption
Change of feed	No secretion of acids
Stress	Insufficient peristaltic activity

can be present in healthy birds and in the intestinal tract the number of colony-forming units can range from 10^2 to 10^3 g^{-1} for *Salmonella* and from 10^6 to 10^7 g^{-1} for *Campylobacter*. Increased shedding due to whatever circumstance therefore has to be avoided.

FEED WITHDRAWAL

Feed withdrawal before catching and crating has been used to avoid carcasses becoming contaminated with microorganisms originating from the upper and lower digestive tract, crop and intestines. Normally chickens empty their caeca every 24 h, but, because of changes in environmental conditions, excretion patterns change, e.g. stress associated with fasting (Duke *et al.*, 1969) and transportation (Mitchell and Kettlewell, 1994). Withdrawal of feed and water prior to transport influences gut contents and the emptying of the digestive tract of birds. Withdrawal of feed 8–12 h before slaughter minimizes the faecal contamination of carcasses (Papa and Dickens, 1989) and causing chickens stress, under conditions simulating the practice of feed withdrawal and live haulage, results in a delayed caecal retention of another 24 h (Moran and Bilgili, 1990).

Withdrawal of feed and water may result in gut breakage during processing causing contamination of carcasses and the slaughter environment. Bilgili and Hess (1997) reported a higher incidence of faecal contamination due to increased intestinal fragility after feed withdrawal times of 14 h and longer.

This aspect is becoming more important as the USDA/Food Safety Inspection Service Pathogen Reduction Programme includes both a mandatory testing for salmonellas and *E. coli*, a so-called 'zero-tolerance' with respect to visual contamination. Visual faecal contamination does not predict the presence of salmonellas and *E. coli*, but makes their presence likely. This 'zero-tolerance' rule will change evisceration technology and carcass washing procedures from that currently used. Contamination due to intestinal breakage will be controlled more and more, so from this point of view, visual faecal contamination will be decreased. Contamination caused by microorganisms present in the crop and the way the cropping equipment performs during the slaughter process will probably become more important (Mulder, 1998).

TRANSPORT

The increase in salmonella-contaminated broilers after transport has been described by several authors. Some authors used artificially infected birds (Moran and Bilgili, 1990), others used birds contaminated under normal circumstances (Bolder and Mulder, 1983). In the latter case, *Salmonella* serotypes on slaughtered products were similar to those isolated from the live birds, indicating intestinal origin.

The literature suggests that the following aspects are important:

1. the time between crating and holding before slaughter;
2. the number of chickens per square metre in the crate;
3. the opportunity for movement;
4. the temperature during transport.

Some studies, with excessively prolonged transportation times, even showed no effect on the intestinal carrier rate of pathogenic microorganisms, e.g. salmonellas, although the organisms were more often isolated from the liver and body cavity, suggesting an increased systemic infection from the gut. Most data relate to the spreading or shedding of salmonellas. Therefore a study to demonstrate the influence of feed withdrawal, holding time, transport and slaughter on *Campylobacter* contamination of birds and consumer-ready products is worthy of mention (Jacobs-Reitsma *et al.*, 1998). Tables 12.2 and 12.3 summarize some of these results. There are no effects of feed withdrawal or any other stress factor applied to the birds on *Campylobacter*. Probably the high colony-forming units of campylobacters in the intestinal tract make the effects difficult to measure.

Table 12.2. Campylobacters (log cfu g^{-1} (standard deviation)) in caecal contents of broilers with or without feed withdrawal before and after transport (Jacobs-Reitsma *et al.*, 1998).

Flock	Before transport		After transport	
	Ad lib feed	No feed	Ad lib feed	No feed
A	NE	NE	7.5 (0.75)	7.8 (1.04)
B	NE	NE	6.6 (1.27)	7.7 (1.09)
C	7.6 (0.30)	7.9 (0.78)	8.1 (0.63)	7.1 (0.90)
D	7.5 (0.48)	8.0 (0.72)	7.8 (0.65)	8.3 (0.50)

cfu, Colony-forming units; NE, not estimated.

Table 12.3. Campylobacters (log cfu g^{-1} (standard deviation)) in faecal material in transport crates from broilers with or without feed withdrawal (Jacobs-Reitsma *et al.*, 1998).

Flock	Ad lib feed	No feed
A	6.2 (0.35)	6.9 (0.07)
B	5.1 (0.21)	8.0 (0.07)
C	6.7 (0.21)	5.9 (0.21)
D	6.2	6.4 (0.42)

cfu, Colony-forming units.

SLAUGHTER AND PROCESSING TECHNOLOGY

Many factors influence the contamination of live and processed birds. The microorganisms transferred to carcasses are a reflection of the types and numbers of organisms acquired by the birds at rearing, during the period of catching and transport to the processing plant and the care taken during slaughter. Preventive measures to reduce the numbers of salmonellas, other potentially pathogenic microorganisms and spoilage microflora in the live bird should be encouraged. Implementation of existing and new processing technology will help to reduce the further spread of microorganisms over carcasses and equipment (Mead, 1983; Mulder et al., 1993).

The degree of mechanization of the individual processing steps will determine the extent of involvement of human labour. Modern poultry processing implies a high rate of throughput. Slaughter capacities of more than 6000 birds per hour can only be realized with completely mechanized and automated processing lines. From a microbiological point of view, several steps are critical in controlling the microbiological contamination of products and equipment (Hupkes, 1996). The condition of the birds before slaughter has an enormous influence on the faecal contamination of feathers and skin during processing. Cleaning and disinfecting of transport crates or containers after each journey is therefore necessary and should be optimized in terms of energy, water and chemicals.

The HACCP steps in processing following transport, holding, hanging, scalding, plucking and evisceration are considered critical. There are developments in poultry processing which influence the hygienic quality of the process and consequently the products. Multistage cleaning and scalding and combined scalding and plucking have reduced microbial counts for both carcasses and scald water. The use of this equipment also reduces the possibilities for cross-contamination (Mulder et al., 1977). Aspects of energy and water conservation are included in these developments.

Developments in new evisceration technology and the automatic cleaning and disinfecting of evisceration equipment are also expected to have a considerable impact on the microbiological quality of products. The new evisceration technology automatically removes the intestinal pack and transfers it to a synchronously running organ line. No contact between carcass and product is possible. After this hearts, lungs and livers are removed automatically. From a hygiene point of view this new technology offers the possibility to produce products without cross-contamination, although published data are not yet available. For all machines used during opening and evisceration, cleaning in-place systems have been developed. These developments also mean that cross-contamination from equipment to product is less likely. In this respect the amount of water, detergents and chemicals should be optimized. Re-use of water is still forbidden by present European Union directives, but the development of recirculation processes could be effective in reducing total water consumption in poultry slaughterhouses.

REFERENCES

Bilgili, S.F. (1988) Research note: Effect of feed and water withdrawal on shear strength of broiler gastro-intestinal tract. *Poultry Science* 67, 845–847.

Bilgili, S.F. and Hess, J.B. (1997) Tensile strength of broiler intestines as influenced by age and feed withdrawal. *Journal of Applied Poultry Research* 6, 279–283.

Bolder, N.M. and Mulder, R.W.A.W. (1983) Contamination des carcasses de poulets pas des Salmonelles: la role des caises de transport. *Courier Avicole* 39, 23–25.

Duke, G.E., Oziuk, H.E. and Hawkins, L. (1969) Gastrointestinal transit-times in normal and bluecomb diseases turkeys. *Poultry Science* 49, 835–842.

Hupkes, H. (1996) Automation and hygiene in relation to poultry processing. In: Hinton, M.H. and Rowlings, C. (eds) *Proceedings of a Meeting in Concerted Action CT94-14565: Microbial Control in the Meat Industry*. University of Bristol Press, Bristol, pp. 95–98.

Jacobs-Reitsma, W.F., Bolder, N.M. and Mulder, R.W.A.W. (1998) The influence of pre-slaughter stresses on the incidence and extent of *Campylobacter* in poultry and poultry products. In: Franchini, A. and Mulder, R.W.A.W. (eds) *Proceedings COST Action 97 'Pathogenic Micro-organisms in Poultry and Eggs' Meeting*. Rome, Italy, pp. 3–6.

Mead, G.C. (1983) Significance of the intestinal micro-flora in relation to meat quality in poultry. In: *Proceedings of the 6th European Symposium on Quality of Poultry Meat, Ploufragan, France*, pp. 107–122.

Mitchell, M.A. and Kettlewell, P.J. (1994) Road transportation of broiler chickens: induction of physiological stress *World's Poultry Science Journal* 50, 57–59.

Moran, E. and Bilgili, S.F. (1990) Influence of feeding and fasting market age broilers on caecal access to an oral dose of *Salmonella*. *Journal of Food Protection* 53, 205–207.

Mulder, R.W.A.W. (1995) Impact of transport and related stresses on the incidence and extent of human pathogens in pig-meat and poultry. *International Journal of Food Safety* 15, 239–246.

Mulder, R.W.A.W. (1997) Safe poultry meat production in the next century. *Acta Veterinaria Hungarica* 45, 307–315.

Mulder, R.W.A.W. (1998) Technology for zero tolerance regulations. *World Poultry* 14, 30–31.

Mulder, R.W.A.W., Dorresteijn, L.W.J. and van der Broek, J. (1977) Kruisbesmetting tijdens het broeien en plukken van slachtkuikens. *Tijdschrift voor Diergeneeskunde* 102, 619–629.

Mulder, R.W.A.W., Kan, C.A. and Bolder, N.M. (1993) Microbiology of poultry meat: challenges and perspectives. In: *Proceedings 11th European Symposium of the Quality of Poultry Meat*, Tours, France, pp. 473–477.

Papa, C.M. and Dickens, J.A. (1989) Lower gut contents and defecatory responses of broiler chickens as affected by feed withdrawal and electrical treatment at slaughter. *Poultry Science* 68, 1478–1484.

CHAPTER 13
The decontamination of carcass meat

M.H. Hinton and J.E.L. Corry
Division of Food Animal Science, School of Veterinary Science,
University of Bristol, Langford, Bristol BS40 5DU, UK

INTRODUCTION

Animals carry many microorganisms on their outer surfaces and in the alimentary tract. Some of the organisms are potentially hazardous to human health although they are usually carried asymptomatically by the animals. Others, derived mainly from the environment, are cold tolerant and cause spoilage of meat during chill storage. Fresh meat is an ideal medium for the growth of spoilage organisms, whereas pathogens survive, but usually do not multiply, provided that temperature abuse is avoided.

Raw meat, particularly poultry meat, remains an important source of human infection with campylobacters and salmonellas and one approach to controlling the spread of these pathogens to the human population is to decontaminate the final raw product. Various decontamination techniques are summarized below and some are listed in Table 13.1. The ideal method will have the following attributes:

- it will not change appearance, smell, taste or nutritional properties of the meat;
- it will leave no residues; it will pose no threat to the environment;
- it will encounter no objections from consumers or legislators;
- it will be cheap and convenient to apply;
- it will improve the shelf-life by inactivating spoilage organisms as well as pathogens;
- it will be compatible with the use of modified atmosphere packaging.

GAMMA IRRADIATION AND ELECTRON ACCELERATORS

Gamma Irradiation

A dose of 2–3 kGy will decontaminate meat from salmonellas, campylobacters and *Escherichia coli* 0157 : H7 (Ingram and Farkas, 1977; Monk *et al.*, 1995). Its safety to the consumer is not seriously questioned (WHO, 1981) although its

Table 13.1. Older, newer and novel methods for decontaminating raw meat: some of their advantages and disadvantages.

	Effect on smell and taste	Changes in appearance	Effect on nutritional quality	Residues	Effect on the environment	Consumer resistance	Cost	Ability to penetrate
γ-irradiation	No	Slight	No	No	Requires radioactive isotopes	Considerable	High	Yes
Electrons	No	Slight	No	No	No	So far no	Low	A little
Steam or hot water dips or sprays	No	Transitory changes	No	No	No	Unlikely	Low	No
Acid dips or sprays	Not at low conc.	Transitory changes	No	Very little	A little	Unlikely	Medium	No
Trisodium phosphate	No	No	No	Very little	A little	Unlikely	Medium	No
Ultraviolet light	No	No	No	No	No	Unlikely	Low	No
Microwaves	No	Transitory changes	No	No	No	Low	No	A little
Air ions	No	No	No	No	?	Unlikely	Low	No
High pressure	No	Yes	No	No	No	Unlikely	High	Yes
Ultrasonic energy	No	No	No	No	No	Unlikely	?	Probably not into solids – effective on solids in liquid

use, for example, for meat preparations is specifically forbidden in the EU by Directive 94/65/EC (1994). Gamma irradiation has the advantage of being able to penetrate large pieces of meat or whole poultry and being applicable to packaged or unpackaged chilled, frozen or dried foods, causing very little visible change, with only minimal, or no, organoleptic effect (Lagunas-Solar, 1995). The reasons why this technique is not used appear to be:

1. the distrust by the public of any process that depends on the nuclear industry;
2. a lack of knowledge by the public in general concerning food-borne infections and the effectiveness of irradiation.

There are genuine logistical problems in using cobalt-60 as a radiation source because (1) there are limited supplies available at present and (2) it would not be practicable for each slaughterhouse or food processing factory to have its own irradiation unit.

Electron Accelerators

A preferred option might be to use electron accelerators which require no isotope. These are used, particularly in France, to decontaminate raw chicken portions. Their main disadvantage is that electrons with the required energy level (up to 10 MeV) do not penetrate more than 1–2 cm, so large pieces of meat or whole poultry carcasses cannot be treated in this way.

COLD WATER WASHING

The washing of carcasses or portions should be done as soon as possible after the exposure of a 'fresh' surface so that bacterial cells do not have time to become firmly adherent. This concept is equally applicable when steam, hot water or antibacterial solutions are used for decontamination.

In poultry processing, the washing of carcasses at intermediate points during the various stages of production is to be recommended, thus removing contaminants before attachment can occur. The process is not particularly effective, however, typically reducing bacterial numbers by less than 50-fold. When washing is delayed until after evisceration, an even smaller proportion of the organisms present can be removed.

STEAM OR HOT WATER DIPS OR SPRAYS

Dips

Smith and Graham (1978) found that immersion in hot water at 80°C for 10 s gave a 10- to 1000-fold reduction in counts from beef and sheep carcasses. This treatment gave a cooked appearance that disappeared almost completely after a few hours of chill-storage.

Sprays

Graham (1979) and Graham *et al.* (1978) developed a commercial-scale hot water spray cabinet for sheep carcasses which was adapted for beef by Powell and Cain (1987). These delivered water at 20–300 kN m^{-2} at about 90°C, which gave a meat surface temperature of about 80°C (sheep at 300 carcasses h^{-1}) or 83°C (beef at 135 carcasses h^{-1}). Reductions in coliforms from 10- to 1000-fold were achieved.

'Deluge' or Waterfall

This approach involving low-pressure water at 80°C was found to be more effective than the spray cabinet (Davey and Smith, 1989; Davey 1989, 1990).

Steam

Morgan *et al.* (1996) have studied the pasteurization effect of steam for microorganisms on the surfaces of poultry. Steam has a higher heat capacity than the same amount of water and can inactivate bacteria in a much shorter time than that required for 'cooking' the flesh. In order to prevent cooking steam must condense and then re-evaporate rapidly from the surface. The application of steam under vacuum has been investigated and its use is associated with an increase in the shelf-life of poultry meat (Klose and Bayne, 1970). More recently the technique has been found to be effective in killing pathogenic *E. coli* present on beef (Dorsa *et al.*, 1996).

ACID DIPS OR SPRAYS

Certain organic acids have antibacterial properties and several acids have been recommended for decontamination purposes including acetic, adipic, formic, lactic, propionic and succinic acids. Of these agents acetic and lactic acids have been most thoroughly investigated for the decontamination of meat and poultry.

Organic acids are more effective as undissociated molecules and this means that the operational pH value has to be ≤ 5.5. The antimicrobial effect of these acids is more marked on fat surfaces than on lean since the latter has a greater buffering capacity. Organic material such as blood and intestinal contents will also tend to reduce the antimicrobial effects. For this reason, treatment systems involving recirculation of the acid solution are unlikely to be effective.

Laboratory-scale trials have indicated that lactic and acetic acids (at 1.2–3.0% w/v) are effective as sprays or dips, at low (15°C or 25°C) or high (52–55°C) temperatures (Smulders, 1987, 1995; Anderson and Marshall, 1989; Dickson, 1992; Cutter and Siragusa, 1994). 'Buffered' lactic acid, obtained by adding sodium hydroxide until a pH value of 3.0 is achieved, has been reported to be effective at 10% lactic acid concentration (e.g. Zeitoun and Debevere, 1990). In practice, spray treatment of hot meat appears most effective (Smulders, 1995), since use of dips can cause accumulation of dirt and debris that inactivate the acids (Cherrington *et al.*, 1991). In general, Gram-negative bacteria are more susceptible to acids than Gram-positive species (Cherrington *et al.*, 1991). Salmonellas and campylobacters should be reduced to very low numbers, but this treatment might be less effective against *E. coli* O157 : H7 which has been reported to be unusually resistant to acids (Brachett *et al.*, 1994; Hardin *et al.*, 1995). The advantage of acid washes is that there is a residual antimicrobial effect which extends shelf-life, whereas shelf-life in water-washed carcasses is sometimes actually reduced due to the increased wetting of the meat.

The combination of acid treatment and modified atmosphere packaging has been shown to have an additive effect when used for the packaging of poultry portions (e.g. Zeitoun and Debevere, 1991, 1992).

TRISODIUM PHOSPHATE

Trisodium phosphate (TSP) at 8% has a pH value of > 12. Of the various phosphates available TSP is the most effective antimicrobial agent (Gudmunsdottir *et al.*, 1993; Hwang and Beuchat, 1995). The mode of action appears to depend mostly on the high pH which lyses Gram-negative bacteria including coliforms, salmonellas, campylobacters and pseudomonads on the skin of chickens (M.H. Hinton and J.E.L. Corry, 1997, unpublished observations). It is the subject of a US patent (Bender and Brotsky, 1992) and is marketed as 'Avguard' with the specific aim of reducing numbers of salmonella on poultry. It is used as a dip immediately post-water-chilling or pre-air-chill. Several minutes should elapse before TSP is rinsed off in order to allow the product to act. The product can be recycled but care must be taken in handling the resultant effluent since the high levels of phosphate may pose a pollution problem.

A small-scale study indicated that immersion of poultry carcasses for 15 s in 10% TSP reduced the numbers of thermotolerant campylobacters present by 20-fold (Federighi *et al.*, 1995) whereas other studies have reported a 10- to 30-fold reduction in the numbers of salmonellas and *E. coli* on lean meat with a 10-fold higher lethality on fat. Combined hot water treatment and TSP increases their effectiveness in an additive manner (de Ledesma *et al.*, 1996) whereas the addition of Tween 80 to the TSP solution appears to enhance the removal of psychrotrophs and salmonellas, but not *Listeria monocytogenes* (Hwang and Beuchat, 1995).

CHLORINE AND CHLORINE DIOXIDE

Chlorine, an oxidizing agent which is more active in slightly acidic conditions, is effective as an environmental decontaminant for controlling cross-contamination during the water chilling of poultry carcasses and reducing contamination on equipment but shows little activity when applied directly to carcasses, since chlorine is inactivated rapidly by contact with organic matter. Chlorine dioxide is more effective than chlorine, but it can only be used at relatively low concentrations because of possible unpleasant effects on personnel.

Staphylococcus aureus may persistently colonize poultry defeathering equipment and some strains, particularly those that are endemic in particular processing plants, have been shown to be relatively resistant to the action of chlorine (Mead and Adams, 1986; Bolton *et al.*, 1988).

The toxicity of chlorine, and its possible mutagenicity, have contributed to its use being banned in some countries, including many of those in Europe.

ELECTROMAGNETIC WAVES

Ultraviolet Light

Ultraviolet (UV) light is used to disinfect surfaces in packaging lines or food processing environments but does not appear to have been used routinely on meat or other foods. Its effectiveness is a function of the intensity of the light and the time of exposure. A major disadvantage is its low penetration, such that shadows or crevices are likely to protect microbes. Continuous exposure to low levels of UV during chill-storage of carcass meat, using reflecting surfaces on the walls of the cold store, has been reported to double shelf-life (Anon, 1970; Kaess and Weidemann, 1973), possibly due to an extended lag phase (Reagan *et al.*, 1973). Salmonellas, *E. coli* and campylobacters are all relatively sensitive to UV. The treatment can lead to oxidative rancidity of fat and this is a further constraint to its use as a decontaminant of meat.

Microwaves

The effect seems to be mostly one of heating and hence treatment sufficient to inactivate salmonellas on meat is likely to result in a semi-cooked appearance (Teotia and Miller, 1975; Fung and Cunningham, 1980). However, the greater penetrating power of microwaves indicates that they would be more effective than UV light against bacteria in crevices and also on prepackaged meat.

VISIBLE LIGHT

The use of short pulses of broad-spectrum light at very high intensity has been proposed as a means of inactivating microorganisms. The effect is likely to be thermal and, despite a lack of specific information, the process appears to suffer from the same limitations as UV light, when applied to meat.

AIR IONS

This technique, which will have no effect as a means of decontaminating meat, could be applied to the air during chill storage of unwrapped carcasses where it significntly reduces the multiplication of the surface flora (Croegaert *et al.*, 1986). Manufacturers have also claimed that the method is effective against microbes in food processing areas (Gysin, 1986).

HIGH PRESSURE

There is potential to use this technique for products such as minced meat, although the cost will be high and the process may cause changes in appearance. Pressure is generally effective against vegetative cells, with spores being more resistant. Combinations of high pressure with mild heat treatment and/or preservatives are more promising alternatives (Carlez *et al.*, 1993, 1994; Knorr, 1995).

ULTRASONIC ENERGY

This seems to be effective only when used in combination with other agents such as mild heat, or with heat plus high pressure (Sala *et al.*, 1995). Although of limited application to carcasses, ultrasound, which is more effective in liquid systems, may facilitate the loosening of bacteria from the surfaces of poultry carcasses during chilling in chlorinated water (Lillard, 1994). Ultrasonic energy may also prove suitable for cleaning implements such as knives, shackles and steel mesh gloves that are difficult to clean by other means.

OSCILLATING MAGNETIC FIELD PULSES

Oscillating magnetic field pulses have been little studied in the present context, but their use is reported to result in reductions of 100- to 1000-fold in vegetative cells and spores of various microorganisms. Advantages include minimal heating of the meat and the possibility of treating packaged products.

COMBINATION TREATMENTS

Although some of the treatments listed above have been investigated in combination with others (e.g. ultrasonic energy and high pressure with raised temperature) there is plenty of scope for investigating other synergistic effects. Of particular interest for the raw meat industry would be to investigate combinations of acid or TSP dips or sprays with electromagnetic waves, (or ultrasonic energy for poultry) and possibly the effect of air ions during chill-storage of red meat.

CONCLUSIONS

The principal method for increasing the shelf-life of raw meat and poultry is by chilled storage. The method is frequently combined with one or more other procedures to provide a series of 'hurdles'. Decontamination presents one such 'hurdle' and there is likely to be growing interest in this approach to increasing shelf-life and product safety in the years to come.

Decontamination must not be seen as an alternative to high standards of good manufacturing practice which are clearly an essential feature of hygienic meat production. Certainly none of the available methods will sterilize meat that is to be sold fresh or render it free of microbial pathogens. Some procedures, such as organic acid and TSP treatment, will merely reduce microbial numbers slightly, typically 100-fold or less, although this may be sufficient to increase product shelf-life when combined with satisfactory chill storage.

The most effective methods of decontamination involve heat. There is, however, a fine line between killing the microorganisms and cooking the surface layers of the product. Systems which are capable of applying high temperatures for a short time, for example steam under vacuum, are worthy candidates for further investigation and may prove of considerable benefit to the meat industry in the future.

It was suggested by Szczawinska *et al.* (1991), with reference to irradiation, that a reduction in or elimination of the 'natural' microflora of the meat might increase the risk of food poisoning since any recontamination of the product after treatment could allow food poisoning pathogens to multiply more rapidly should there be any temperature abuse during distribution and display of the product. Irradiation is not in general use for decontaminating fresh meat and time will tell if this 'pessimistic' view is justified in the context of other methods of decontamination, particularly those which do not have any residual action after treatment is completed.

REFERENCES

Anderson, M.E. and Marshall, R.T. (1989) Interaction of concentration and temperature of acetic acid solution on reduction of various species of micro-organisms on beef surfaces. *Journal of Food Protection* 52, 321–315.

Anon. (1970) Storage of meat under ultraviolet light (UV). *CSIRO Meat Research Newsletter* 70, no. 2.

Bender, F.G. and Brotsky E. (1992) Process for treating poultry carcasses to control salmonella growth. US Patent 5,143,739 September 1, 1992, Int. Cl A23L 3/34 A22C 21/00.

Bolton, K.J., Dodd, C.E.R., Mead, G.C. and Waites, W.M. (1988) Chlorine resistant strains of *Staphylococcus aureus* isolated from poultry processing plants. *Letters in Applied Microbiology* 6, 31–34.

Brachett, R.E., Hao, Y.Y. and Doyle, M.R. (1994) Ineffectiveness of hot acid sprays to decontaminate *Escherichia. Journal of Food Protection* 57, 198–203.

Carlez, A., Rosec, J., Richard, N. and Cheftel, J. (1993) High pressure inactivation of *Citrobacter freundii, Pseudomonas fluorescens* and *Listeria innocua* in inoculated minced beef muscle. *Lebensmittel-Wissenshaft und Technologie* 26, 357–363.

Carlez, A., Rosec, J., Richard, N. and Cheftel, J. (1994) Bacterial growth during chilled storage of pressure treated minced meat. *Lebensmittel-Wissenshaft und Technologie* 27, 48–54.

Cherrington, C.A., Hinton, M., Mead, G.C. and Chopra, I. (1991) Organic acids: chemistry, antibacterial activity and practical applications. *Advances in Microbial Physiology* 32, 87–108.

Croegaert, T., de Zutter, L. and Van Hoof, J. (1986) Influence of air ionisation on the microbial contamination of carcasses during refrigeration. *Proceedings of the 32nd European Meeting of Meat Research Workers*, Gent, Belgium, pp. 193–195.

Cutter, C.N. and Siragusa, G.R. (1994) Efficacy of organic acids against *Escherichia coli* 0157:H7 attached to beef carcass tissue using a pilot scale model carcass washer. *Journal of Food Protection* 57, 97–103.

Davey, K.R. (1989) Theoretical analysis of two hot water cabinet systems for decontamination of sides of beef. *International Journal of Food Science and Technology* 24, 291–304.

Davey, K.R. (1990) A model for the hot water decontamination of sides of beef in a novel cabinet based on laboratory data. *International Journal of Food Science and Technology* 25, 88–97.

Davey, K.R. and Smith, M.G. (1989) A laboratory evaluation of a novel hot water cabinet for the decontamination of sides of beef. *International Journal of Food Science and Technology* 24, 305–316.

de Ledesma, A.M.R., Reimann, H.P. and Farver, T.B. (1996) Short-time treatment with alkali and/or hot water to remove common pathogenic and spoilage bacteria from chicken wing skin. *Journal of Food Protection* 59, 746–750.

Dickson, J.S. (1992) Acetic acid action on beef tissue surfaces contaminated with *Salmonella typhimurium. Journal of Food Science* 57, 297–301.

Directive 94/65/EC (1994) Laying down the requirements for the production and placing on the market of minced meat and meat preparations. *Official Journal of the European Communities* L368, 10–31.

Dorsa, W.J., Cutter, C.N. and Siragusa, G.R. (1996) Effectiveness of a steam–vacuum sanitiser for reducing *Escherichia coli* O157 : H7 inoculated on beef carcass tissue. *Letters in Applied Microbiology* 23, 61–63.

Federighi, M., Cappelier, J.M., Rossero, A., Coppen, P. and Denis, J.C. (1995) Assessment of the effect of a decontamination process of broiler carcasses on thermotolerant campylobacters. *Sciences des Aliments* 15, 393–401.

Fung, D.Y.C, and Cunningham, F.E. (1980) Effect of microwaves on micro-organisms in foods. *Journal of Food Protection* 43, 641–650.

Graham, A. (1979) A hot shower for clean carcasses. *Australian Refrigeration Air Conditioning and Heating* 33, 33–35.

Graham, A., Cain, B.P. and Eustace, I.J. (1978) An enclosed hot water spray cabinet for improved hygiene of carcass meat. *CSIRO Meat Research Report* no. 11/78.

Gudmunsdottir, K.B., Marin, M.L., Allen, V.M., Corry, J.E.L. and Hinton, M. (1993) The antibacterial activity of inorganic phosphates. In: Löpfe, J., Kan, C.A. and Mulder, R.W.A.W. (eds) *Prevention and Control of Pathogenic Micro-organisms in Poultry and Poultry Meat Processing. 11.* Contamination with Pathogens in Relation to Processing and Marketing. Agricultural Research Service (DLO-NL), Beekbergen, pp. 95–100.

Gysin, C. (1986) How ionisation benefits the food industry. *Meat Industry* 59, 29.

Hardin, M.D., Acuff, G.R., Lucia, L.M., Oman, J.S. and Savell, J.W. (1995) Comparison of methods for decontamination of beef carcass surfaces. *Journal of Food Protection* 58, 368–374.

Hwang, C.A. and Beuchat, L.R. (1995) Efficiency of selected chemicals for killing pathogenic and spoilage microorganisms on chicken skin. *Journal of Food Protection* 58, 19–23.

Ingram, M. and Farkas, J. (1977) Microbiology of food pasteurised by ionising radiation. *Acta Alimentaria* 6, 123–185.

Kaess, G. and Weidemann, J.F. (1973) Effect of ultra-violet irradiation on the growth of micro-organisms on chilled beef slices. *Journal of Food Technology* 8, 59–69.

Klose, A.A. and Bayne, H.G. (1970) Experimental approaches to poultry meat surface pasteurisation by condensing vapours. *Poultry Science* 49, 504–511.

Knorr, D. (1995) Hydrostatic pressure treatment of food: microbiology. In: Gould, G.W. (ed.) *New Methods of Food Preservation.* Chapman & Hall, London, pp. 159–175.

Lagunas-Solar, M.C. (1995) Radiation processing of foods: an overview of scientific principles and current status. *Journal of Food Protection* 58, 186–192.

Lillard, H.S. (1994) Decontamination of poultry skin by sonification. *Food Technology* 48, 72–73.

Mead, G.C. and Adams, B.W. (1986) Chlorine resistance of *Staphylococcus aureus* isolated from turkeys and turkey products. *Letters in Applied Microbiology* 3, 131–133.

Monk, J.D., Beuchat, L.R. and Doyle, M.P. (1995) Irradiation inactivation of food-borne micro-organisms. *Journal of Food Protection* 58, 197–208.

Morgan, A.I., Goldberg, N., Radewonuk, E.R. and Scullen, O.J. (1996) Surface pasteurization of raw poultry meat by steam. *Food Science and Technology* 29, 447–451.

Powell, V.H. and Cain, B.P. (1987) A hot water decontamination system for beef sides. *CSIRO Food Research Quarterly* 47, 79–84.

Reagan, J.O., Smith, G.C. and Carpenter, Z.L. (1973) Use of ultraviolet light for extending the retail caselife of beef. *Journal of Food Science* 38, 929–931.

Sala, F.J., Burgos, J., Condon, S., Lopez, P. and Raso, J. (1995) Effect of heat and ultrasound on micro-organisms and enzymes. In: Gould, G.W. (ed.) *New Methods of Food Preservation.* Chapman & Hall, London, pp. 176–204.

Smith, M.G. and Graham, A. (1978) Destruction of *Escherichia coli* and salmonellae on mutton carcasses by treatment with hot water. *Meat Science* 2, 119–128.

Smulders, F.J.M. (1987) Prospectives for the microbial decontamination of meat and poultry by organic acids with special reference to lactic acid. In: Smulders, F.J.M. (ed.) *Elimination of Pathogenic Organisms from Meat and Poultry.* Elsevier, Amsterdam, pp. 319–344.

Smulders, F.J.M. (1995) Preservation by microbial decontamination; the surface treatment of meats by organic acids. In: Gould, G.W. (ed.) *New Methods of Food Preservation.* Chapman & Hall, London, pp. 253–282.

Szczawinska, M.E., Thayer, D.W. and Phillips, J.G. (1991) Fate of unirradiated salmonella in irradiated mechanically deboned chicken meat. *International Journal of Food Microbiology* 14, 313–324.

Teotia, J.S. and Miller, B.F. (1975) Destruction of salmonellae on poultry meat with lysozyme, EDTA, X-ray, microwave and chlorine. *Poultry Science* 54, 1388–1394.

WHO (1981) Wholesomeness of Irradiated Food. Report of a Joint FAO/IAEA/WHO Expert Committee. *Technical Report 651.* WHO, Geneva.

Zeitoun, A.A.M. and Debevere, J.M. (1990) The effect of treatment with buffered lactic acid on microbial decontamination and on shelf life of poultry. *International Journal of Food Microbiology* 11, 305–312.

Zeitoun, A.A.M. and Debevere, J.M. (1991) Inhibition, survival and growth of *Listeria monocytogenes* on poultry as influenced by buffered lactic acid treatment and modified atmosphere packaging. *International Journal of Food Microbiology* 14, 161–170.

Zeitoun, A.A.M. and Debevere, J.M. (1992) Decontamination with lactic acid/sodium lactate buffer in combination with modified atmosphere packaging effects on the shelf-life of fresh poultry. *International Journal of Food Microbiology* 16, 89–98.

CHAPTER 14
Strategies for extending the shelf-life of poultry meat and products

L.F.J. Woods and P.N. Church

Food Technology Section, Leatherhead Food Research Association, Randalls Road, Leatherhead, Surrey KT22 7RY, UK

INTRODUCTION

The concept of shelf-life is intimately linked with that of quality. The latter is a subjective term used to describe certain attributes of a product and how these compare with the expectations of the consumer. If a food product meets the needs of the consumer we can say that it is of acceptable quality. However, foods are perishable by nature and numerous changes occur during their processing and storage. These changes can adversely affect the quality attributes of the food and, after storage for a certain period, one or more attributes may reach a level that is undesirable. At that point, the food is considered unsuitable for consumption and is said to have reached the end of its shelf-life. If the quality expectations of the consumer are not met, re-purchase of the product is unlikely – some consumers will switch to competitors' products and others may complain.

The changes that occur in meat are generally enzymic or chemical and are influenced by a number of environmental factors such as temperature, humidity, oxygen and light, which result in physical, chemical or microbiological changes leading to deterioration. If the shelf-life of a food is to be extended, it is important to understand the changes that occur in the food, so that ways of slowing down these changes can be found.

Physical changes in the food can result in negative effects on shelf-life. While the bird is whole, the individual muscles are essentially sterile inside, but physical changes associated with boning and mincing, for example, will contaminate the meat and favour bacterial growth. Release of enzymes during these physical processes can also have an effect on product quality, particularly during long-term, frozen storage. In the case of frozen foods, temperature fluctuations can lead to a build-up of ice crystals; sublimation of water from exposed parts can cause localized dehydration (freezer burn). This condition is not only unsightly but may accelerate other quality problems such as oxidative rancidity.

Chemical changes that occur in meat are generally associated with enzymic action, although the chemical oxidation of fat, resulting in flavour changes, can lead to a reduction in shelf-life. The presence of unsaturated fatty acids in a food is a major reason for rancidity, if the food is exposed to oxygen, and free radicals formed during the ensuing reactions can lead not only to rancidity but also loss of vitamins, alteration of colour and degradation of proteins (see Chapter 8). As well as requiring the presence of oxygen, lipid oxidation is affected by water activity and occurs faster at lower water activity. Oxygen also affects the colour of meat by formation of oxymyoglobin, and changes in the oxygen content of the meat will influence its colour and acceptability. The presence of nitrite can result in the formation of nitrosomyoglobin, which has a pink colour; this may be desirable (as in some cured turkey products) or undesirable, as a result of chemical contamination during processing or more commonly microbial reduction of nitrate to nitrite, due to excessive holding times prior to cooking. Whatever the cause of unwanted pinking, the consumer perceives that the product is undercooked and hence is unlikely to purchase it.

Maillard reactions, which generally occur during cooking at high temperatures (particularly roasting and grilling), cause colour and flavour changes in meat. These changes may confer attributes on the food which are required in cooked products, although the extent to which they occur must be controlled. Some Maillard products have antioxidant activity and may help to reduce the production of warmed-over flavour (WOF) which is caused by fat oxidation (Bailey *et al.*, 1987). One useful strategy in minimizing oxidative rancidity is to supplement the diet of the birds with α-tocopheryl acetate (see Chapters 5 and 8).

A major factor in determining product shelf-life is the growth of microorganisms and the changes that result. The types of microbiological change that occur in poultry meat fall into two categories. First, the growth of non-pathogenic microorganisms can lead to off-flavours and odours, and release of enzymes by the bacteria can also change the structure of the meat. Secondly, any growth of pathogenic microorganisms is a major concern and can lead to illness and even death. Various measures are commonly used to reduce or prevent microbial growth in foods. These include altering the environmental temperature – either lowering it to slow down growth, or increasing it to destroy microorganisms. Other measures include controlling the water content, altering the environmental gases or changing the pH of the food by the direct addition of acid or by fermentation. Microbial growth rate is dependent on temperature and models have been established that allow the prediction of growth over a range of temperatures for foods of different composition. Such models are useful in helping to predict the shelf-life of foods in terms both of food spoilage and food-poisoning risks.

Shelf-life remains an important factor for meat and meat products and as improvements are made in the chill chain, increasing shelf-life, fewer deliveries and lower wastage can have a significant impact on the success or failure of a food product. This chapter considers those factors that affect shelf-life and strategies that may be used to increase the life of a product without increasing the risk to the consumer.

RAW POULTRY MEAT

The microbiological status of the raw material is crucial in determining shelf-life; any technique that can reduce the initial microbial load will have a beneficial effect. For example, alternative methods of evisceration (e.g. Russell and Walker, 1997), when evaluated in different processing plants, have shown potential for reducing bacterial contamination of chicken carcasses.

Preventing the contamination of carcasses with *Aeromonas* spp., an enterotoxigenic organism, is particularly important with regard to poultry; the species *A. hydrophila*, *A. sobria* and *A. caviae* are the most common. The organism is psychrotrophic and grows well in stored chicken at 5°C. Carcasses can become infected via water, poultry faeces and food handlers, but the organism is destroyed by cooking (Izatnagar, 1996).

The literature on the decontamination of poultry carcasses is extensive and many different treatment compounds have been considered. The spraying of chicken carcasses with trisodium phosphate before chilling has been shown to bring about a >3 log reduction in *Salmonella typhimurium* (Li *et al.*, 1997); however, the binding of bacterial cells to skin appears to increase their resistance. Tamblyn and Conner (1997), in experiments with organic acids, found that concentrations of >4% acids were required to reduce numbers by at least 2 log, and that cells bound to chicken skin were more resistant than free cells in suspension.

Work by Li and Slavik (cited by Bjerklie, 1997) has shown that the application of an electric current to poultry carcasses while passing through a treatment bath containing an organic acid can further reduce the number of bacteria on the skin. The electric current has the additional effect of killing bacteria that accumulate in the treatment bath, which is a further aid to maintaining the cleanliness of the carcasses. Alternative strategies to reduce the risk of cross-contamination during chilling include prepackaging in vacuum packs, and, more recently, spray chilling. Spray-chilling systems use a combination of water sprays and air for the initial stages of chilling (e.g. spraying for *c.* 90 s at 15-min intervals during the first 8 h of chilling) and then air only for the rest of the chilling cycle. Besides appearing to reduce the risk of cross-contamination, spray chilling is claimed to offer other advantages such as preventing excessive moisture pick-up (see Veerkamp, 1989).

The addition of biopreservative cultures to the spray water has been recommended as a means of further improving product shelf-life and safety. Although cultures have been used successfully in reduced-nitrite bacon (Tanaka *et al.* 1980), problems of excessive acid production, greening and slime formation have been encountered (Church, 1993). Also, even though suitable cocktails of cultures may be found for particular applications, unfavourable publicity from the news media may lead to the strategy becoming unacceptable, just as media handling of food irradiation caused its commercial failure.

Airborne transfer of microorganisms in poultry-slaughtering plants has been studied recently (Lutgring *et al.*, 1997) and a number of factors, including air-flow, factory design, temperature and humidity, were found to be important in developing bio-aerosols that could contaminate carcasses. Such contamination would have an effect on the spoilage and safety of the product. This work underlines the importance of factory design and separation of different operations within the factory. The layout and control of air-flow between departments can have a significant impact on the microbiological status of the product. The flow of materials, equipment and personnel also needs to be considered.

The importance of temperature in determining the shelf-life of a perishable product has already been mentioned, and the industry has worked hard to establish a robust chill chain that allows the product to be transported under controlled temperature conditions.

Generally, these systems operate in the range 0–5°C. However, by reduction of the temperature to as near the freezing point as possible, the shelf-life of fresh poultry can be significantly extended. Sawaya *et al.* (1997) have shown that storing poultry carcasses at –2°C, extends the shelf-life for up to 11 days in comparison with a temperature of +2°C. However, the cost of establishing a chill chain capable of maintaining such low temperatures would be significant. Monitoring and maintenance of temperature would become critical if shelf-life relied on a single factor such as temperature; the consequences of a refrigeration breakdown could be costly both in a commercial sense and from the point of view of food safety.

PRESERVATIVES

Preservatives have been used extensively over the years to increase the shelf-life of meat products. In the past, the use of these compounds at high concentrations has resulted in adverse effects on flavour and texture. Combinations of preservatives and other chemicals at concentrations that alone would not extend shelf-life offer the possibility of minimizing organoleptic changes, while still giving useful product durability.

Antimicrobial food preservatives are those that inhibit or retard the growth of spoilage and pathogenic microorganisms and can therefore be used to enhance the shelf-life and safety of foods. However, current consumer trends are towards foods that contain minimal numbers and amounts of additives, including preservatives, and which, therefore, are preserved by the use of refrigeration. The perceived benefits of these types of food are that they are healthier and more nutritious because they are natural, as opposed to more highly processed foods.

The effectiveness of chemical preservatives is dependent on a wide variety of factors, including their chemical structure, the concentration used, the microorganisms present, the type and form of the microorganism (whether vegetative cell or spore), phase of growth (whether lag or log), the composition (e.g. water activity) and pH of the food, and the temperature and period of storage. In general, the use of chemical preservatives is controlled and, in the case of poultry products, only certain preservatives and additives are permitted for use in the EU.

Given certain concerns about the use of chemical food preservatives, the use of so-called 'biopreservatives' has been suggested as an alternative approach (Ray and Daeschel, 1992). These preservatives are made by micro-organisms that are already widely used in the manufacture of foods, such as fermented meats and yoghurt, and have proven records in relation to food safety. Biopreservatives can be used either as isolated chemicals in pure form or, by growing the organism in the food, they can be produced *in situ*. Direct addition of producing cells to meat has been used to inhibit the growth of Gram-negative spoilage bacteria in ground beef and in cooked, mechanically deboned poultry meat. The addition of *Pediococcus cerevisiae* or *Lactobacillus plantarum* inhibited *Pseudomonas* spp., *Salmonella typhimurium* and *Staphylococcus aureus* (Raccach and Baker, 1978).

As previously mentioned, high levels of the bacteria are required, and possible taint problems have limited the use of this technique. The bio-preservatives from lactic acid bacteria have been studied widely and this group of protein complexes, collectively called bacteriocins, has been characterized and their antimicrobial spectrum described (see, for example, Green *et al.*, 1997). The use of bacteriocins may offer more consistent results in comparison with live cultures and also may prove more acceptable to consumers.

A recent examination of some commercially available preparations for extending the shelf-life of cooked chicken breast (Rozum and Maurer, 1997) gave disappointing results in that, after addition in injected brine, only one preparation, a pediocin-containing material produced from fermented corn syrup, showed an increase in shelf-life; the other materials, which were sodium lactate, liquid smoke and another pediocin, showed no effect.

Part of the action of lactic acid bacteria is the production of organic acids, particularly acetic, propionic and lactic acids. The preservation of foods by fermentation or direct addition of acids has been widely used for many traditional foods. One of the benefits of marinading is that the acids involved can result in an extension of shelf-life.

However, as with all strategies, problems can arise; for example, organic acids are generally ineffective with meat with high microbial counts since the lag phase, when inhibitory effects are greatest, is very short. Meat is also an excellent buffer and will resist attempts to alter its pH to that required for optimum inhibition. Since meat is a nutrient source, it can encourage the growth of bacteria and, since these vary widely in their sensitivity to acids, a resistant flora can be selected. Flavour changes caused by the simultaneous addition of herbs and spices can produce a variety of other beneficial effects, including inhibition of microbial growth and oxidative rancidity.

MARINADING

Marinading is a traditional technique used to tenderize and improve the flavour of meat. A wide range of marinaded products as well as liquid and dry marinades is available. Marinades can be either oil-based or water-based, with the latter being either acidic and containing organic acids or neutral and containing salts and polyphosphates. Marinades are intended to give a distinctive flavour to meat products and to enhance tenderness by increasing water binding and hence yield.

The essential feature of marinading is the increase in water binding of the meat, brought about by decreasing its pH below the isoelectric point. In studies of beef muscles, minimum hydration occurred at pH 5.0, which corresponds to the mean isoelectric point of the major myofibrillar proteins, with maximum hydration occurring at values of pH 3.5 and 10.5. It is thought that this water binding is related to the swelling of the muscle fibres, which also occurs maximally at these two pH values. A likely explanation is that the addition of acid below the isoelectric point protonates negatively charged carboxyl groups in the protein to break hydrogen bonding to amino groups; the overall increase in positive charges also leads to electrostatic repulsion and opening up of the protein structure. This creates extra space for more water to be bound. This effect is greatest at pH 3.5, below which no more carboxyl groups are available; however, at this pH, the product would be considered too acidic by most consumers (Gault, 1991).

Another potential disadvantage of marinading is that the colour of marinaded meat is different from that of fresh meat. The lower pH results in formation of metmyoglobin which is brown and has a lower colour intensity; sarcoplasmic proteins are leached from the surface of acid-marinaded meat, resulting in a pale appearance. In extreme cases, precipitation of the proteins by acid can cause a white appearance on the surface of the meat similar to that of cooked meat.

The addition of organic acids and the changes in pH associated with marinading can help to extend the shelf-life of the product. The acid used to alter the pH will also be a factor. Acetic acid is effective at inhibiting bacteria since, having a pK of 4.75, it is in the undissociated form at marinade pH. The undissociated form of the acid is the active inhibitor. Although some bacteria are resistant to acid, others, particularly food-poisoning organisms, are inhibited, and so marinading can increase the safety of a food as well as extending shelf-life.

An examination of some commercial marinades (Gault, 1991) showed that they had little effect on meat pH and hence tenderness and that the greatest effect was on the flavour of the meat. This indicates that, at the time, the potential of marinading to improve texture of meat and to extend shelf-life had not been fully realized. More recently, spices as well as the organic acids in marinades have been shown to have antimicrobial activities and to extend the shelf-life of beef, mutton and chicken carcasses (Ziauddin *et al.*, 1996).

PHYSICAL APPROACHES

Heating

There are at least two reasons why heat processing is carried out. The first is to cook the product. This process involves aspects of the palatability and acceptability of the food. Denaturation of the proteins and softening of the collagen make meat more pleasant to eat and more easily digestible. The colour of the product is important to the consumer and this is influenced by cooking, as is the flavour.

The second reason for heat processing is to preserve the product and extend its shelf-life. Heat destroys certain microorganisms and can therefore be used to prevent or delay spoilage and to reduce the risk of food poisoning. Recent approaches have involved mild heat processes in order to minimize thermally induced quality losses. Better process control can result in optimization, with minimum use of heat. Techniques such as electrical resistance (ohmic) heating, high-frequency heating and microwave heating have been used to bring about rapid temperature rises in treated products which helps to shorten processing time and maintain product quality.

Microwaves have found a number of food-processing applications, including tempering, drying, pasteurization and sterilization of products. A shelf-life of 6 weeks at 4°C has been claimed for hot-filled products that have been treated with microwaves prior to cooling. Advances in equipment design, which have largely overcome problems of runaway and inadequate heating, offer savings in time, energy, space and labour costs. Depending on the product, microwaves also offer the potential for greater automation and increased production rates during processing.

As with microwaves, ohmic heating relies on the physical properties of the food. In this case, the electrical resistance is used to generate heat as a current is passed through the food by means of electrodes. This system is particularly suited to the continuous heating of liquids since, in foods that have an homogeneous electrical conductivity, heating is predictable and uniform. If particles are present, however, differences in conductivity between the solid and liquid will give rise to non-uniform heating.

Sous Vide

This type of processing was originally designed for the catering market and involves the pasteurization of a prepared meal in its pack followed by rapid chilling and refrigerated storage for distribution. The meal is usually reheated before serving. Because sous vide products are packed under vacuum and are not given a botulinum cook, there is some concern about the possible growth of *Clostridium botulinum*; for this reason, guidelines have been published concerning the heat processing that such products should receive.

A major selling point for sous vide products is the improved flavour and texture compared with those of foods made by the more usual technologies; this comes about as a result of the in-pack cooking and minimal heat process.

High-intensity Light

The use of intense pulses of light to kill microorganisms on the surfaces of foods and on packaging has been investigated (Dunn *et al.*, 1995) and has been patented as the 'PureBright' process. This system uses short pulses of high-intensity white light to bring about a microbial kill of 1–3 logs on meat surfaces. All types of microorganisms are affected by the treatment, which has been shown to be beneficial for meats, seafood and baked goods. Microbial reductions of 9 logs for vegetative cells and 7 logs for spores have been reported when the treatment was used on packaging. A drawback of this system is that uneven surfaces and indentations can be shielded from the light and have reduced exposure. It is also possible that the increase in free radicals caused by the light could promote rancidity in some foods, such as poultry, although such effects have not been reported. A patent exists for a machine designed to sterilize meat on all surfaces using UV light (Newman, 1994), in which the meat is mechanically turned while exposed to the light.

High Pressure

Large and rapid pressure changes are known to cause disruption of bacterial cell walls, leading to destruction of viability. Systems for applying pressure changes to foods have therefore been suggested as ways in which shelf-life can be extended. Some foods undergo very small physical changes during the process, and so undesirable side-effects can be minimized with the right choice of raw materials.

Other Techniques

Other techniques that have been investigated as a means of reducing the microbial load on meat surfaces include rapid freeze–thaw cycling, air ionization, oscillating magnetic field pulses, electrostimulation, steam under vacuum and sonication. By use of these techniques, microbial reductions have ranged from 0.3 to 6 logs. James *et al.* (1997), in their extensive review of decontamination methods, concluded that the most cost-effective methods for improving the microbial quality of meat were:

1. development of an automatic hot water decontamination cabinet for red meat carcasses;
2. development of the optimum organic acid treatment;
3. development of a steam condensation decontamination unit for small carcasses.

PACKAGING

Packaging is often overlooked as a means of extending product shelf-life. The most commonly used techniques rely on the removal of oxygen and elevation of carbon dioxide within the pack, linked to good temperature control. Both vacuum packing and modified-atmosphere packing are widely used. In vacuum packing, an oxygen-deficient environment is created around the product, which reduces the rate of microbial growth. Other factors, such as the storage temperature, the properties of the packaging film and the efficiency of oxygen removal, will influence the degree of shelf-life extension. Modified- and controlled-atmosphere packaging systems employ an elevated level of carbon dioxide to inhibit microbial growth either in the presence or absence of oxygen.

In the case of red meats, high-oxygen modified-atmosphere packaging (60–80% O_2, 40–20% CO_2) can be used to enhance colour and extend the chilled retail display life. However, such systems are not suitable for prolonged chilled storage since a low-oxygen atmosphere is required to slow the development of spoilage organisms (Hotchkiss et al., 1985).

Saturated carbon dioxide systems, with residual oxygen levels below 0.1%, have been successful in extending the life of red meats over that achieved in vacuum under similar storage conditions. Gill et al. (1990) demonstrated that, in carbon dioxide, chicken carcasses did not spoil until 7 weeks at 3°C and 14 weeks at –1.5°C, compared with 2 and 3 weeks, respectively, under vacuum. However, Bohnsack et al. (1988), although showing an extension of shelf-life, were reluctant to suggest this method for retail packs since colour changes brought about by discoloration of the oxymyoglobin resulted in a product that was considered unacceptable to the consumer. It may be that combination systems, a strategy used for red meats, in which retail packs in oxygen-permeable film are packed in a 'mother' bag of carbon dioxide for long-term storage, could be used. Removal of the packs from the 'mother' bag prior to retail display would allow colour to be developed as oxygen from the air diffused into the pack.

Types of Gas

The precise choice of gas mixture used in modified-atmosphere packaging is influenced by the types of microorganism that are capable of growing on the product, the sensitivity of the product to O_2 and CO_2, and colour-stabilizing requirements (e.g. the preservation of oxymyoglobin in fresh meat and of nitrosomyoglobin in cured meat products). The gases normally used are those found in the atmosphere – oxygen, carbon dioxide and nitrogen. A wide variety of other gases has been investigated experimentally for their potential to extend shelf-life. The gases that have been considered include argon, carbon monoxide, chlorine, helium, hydrogen, nitric oxide, ozone and sulphur dioxide. Of these other gases, carbon monoxide has been used to pack lettuce in America to inhibit browning reactions, and for packing meat in Norway and fish in the tropics. Nitrous oxide, which is used as a gas propellant in aerosol creams, may also find further commercial applications, since it is claimed to inhibit fat oxidation. It may prove useful in combination with argon to inhibit the development of rancidity during processing operations. However, the use of gases other than O_2, CO_2 and N_2 has been limited by safety concerns, legislation, adverse consumer response, cost and negative effects on the organoleptic properties of packed products.

For meats that require high levels of oxygen to maintain colour and therefore an appearance acceptable to the consumer, packing in an atmosphere with high oxygen is common. Application of high-pressure oxygen, to obtain meat supersaturated with oxygen, has been claimed to improve colour stability and reduce drip for red meats. With paler meats such as chicken, the effect on colour would probably not be so great, although reducing drip could help presentation.

In an aerobic atmosphere with up to 25% CO_2, poultry has an increased shelf-life, and concentrations over 25% are also beneficial, although unpleasant flavours can develop in the cooked meat. Fresh poultry packed in 50% N_2 and 50% CO_2 can be kept for 7 days (Paine and Paine, 1992).

Developments in modified-atmosphere packaging were reviewed by Church (1994) and several areas with potential to improve the safety and shelf-life of foods were identified. Control of oxygen levels in the packs by use of scavengers or improved, high-barrier films remains an area of interest. When very low oxygen levels are required and the packaging film is permeable to oxygen, then oxygen absorbers or scavengers can be used to mop up the gas as it enters the pack. If, for example, oxygen scavengers are present in a carbon dioxide-atmosphere pack, they will compete with the meat for oxygen. Chemical oxidation of the meat, leading to formation of metmyoglobin can result in product deterioration as surface browning occurs. Although, in theory, the scavenger will prevent discoloration, it should be remembered that the oxygen absorption capacity of the meat and the scavenger is related to their surface area and, unless the scavenger is particularly effective or has a large surface, discoloration can still occur since oxygen absorption may be too slow to prevent irreversible colour changes.

There has been resistance to the use of in-pack scavengers, particularly in the USA, due to fears of litigation should accidental ingestion of the scavenger occur, and, for this reason, incorporation of the scavenger in the packaging film is an attractive idea. One recent example of this (Anon., 1997) is a film in which a light-activated scavenger has been incorporated. This system is activated by exposure to light of particular wavelengths and is claimed to remove oxygen in the headspace of the pack, as the gas penetrates during storage.

In controlling the level of oxygen or other gases in the pack, the gas permeability of the packaging film is important. This in turn is affected by the type of film, the thickness and any coatings (e.g. anti-fog) that have been applied to it. At present, only aluminium foil provides an absolute, flexible barrier to oxygen, but it does not allow the consumer to see the product. Some foil packs have windows of different material, but this allows some oxygen ingress. Other clear, high-barrier films are being developed, particularly glass- and silica-coated types, and aluminium oxide coatings have also been investigated. It has been suggested that environmental legislation will encourage the use of oxide-coated films rather than foils and metallized films.

The incorporation of a scavenger in the packaging film has already been mentioned. Impregnation of the film with stabilizer additives such as α-tocopherol has also been suggested and shown to reduce film yellowing and 'aroma-scalping' in cereal products. Other possibilities, such as the incorporation of organic acids into the film to reduce surface microbial growth and therefore extend shelf-life, could be developed.

Although they do not extend shelf-life *per se*, in-pack indicators can be used to inform customers about the state of the pack contents before opening. Changes in the gas composition during storage can provide an indirect indication of the condition of the product. Carbon dioxide- and oxygen-sensitive labels, which change colour at set gas concentrations, could have potential as non-destructive prespoilage indicators, and could be used to detect faulty packs and product tampering. Time–temperature indicators, which show storage abuse of product, also fall into this category of in-pack indicators.

Edible Packaging

Edible coatings have been suggested as a means of extending shelf-life by preventing migration of moisture and other components from one part of the food to another. They can be used, for example, in the separation of sauces from meat, for separating enzymic activity or acid dressing from meat and for keeping cured meat away from uncured meat to prevent colour problems. Films made from corn zein have been used in experiments with sliced, cooked turkey breast (Herald *et al.*, 1996), and reduced the amount of lipid oxidation, as measured by hexenal content and stale/warmed-over aroma, compared with similar product packed in polyvinyl chloride film. Unfortunately, the zein imparted an off-flavour and aroma to the product. Edible coatings could also be impregnated with antimicrobial and antioxidant agents to extend shelf-life further.

SAFETY IMPLICATIONS OF EXTENDED SHELF-LIFE

In any consideration of extending the shelf-life of foods, the potential health hazard posed by the growth of the cold-tolerant pathogens *Aeromonas hydrophila*, *Clostridium botulinum*, *Listeria monocytogenes* and *Yersinia enterocolitica* should be considered.

The growth rate of *L. monocytogenes* is similar under aerobic and anaerobic conditions, although growth is inhibited by carbon dioxide, particularly in oxygen-free atmospheres containing >75% carbon dioxide. *A. hydrophila* responds in a similar way to *L. monocytogenes* and so hazards from these microorganisms can be reduced by use of high-concentration carbon dioxide atmospheres.

Y. enterocolitica shows reduced growth in vacuum packs compared with aerobic packs, and is inhibited by carbon dioxide.

The most serious cause for concern in any anaerobically packed meat product is the non-proteolytic and psychotrophic strains of *C. botulinum* and, of these, type B is the most important since the others in this group (type E) are associated with fish. These non-proteolytic forms of *C. botulinum* are able to grow and form toxin at temperatures as low as 3.3°C. In a report on vacuum packaging and associated processes, the Advisory Committee on the Microbiological Safety of Food (ACMSF, 1992) considered that growth of psychrotrophic *C. botulinum* in vacuum-packed, prepared, chilled foods with a shelf-life of greater that 10 days was a definite possibility and that, in order to prevent this, such foods should be subject to one or more controlling factors at levels to prevent growth and toxin production. Examples of such factors are heating, reduction of pH or water activity, or addition of salt or preservatives.

STRATEGIES

A number of different ways to extend product shelf-life can be considered, where the potential exists for this to be achieved on a laboratory scale and sometimes in factory situations. In establishing suitable strategies, there are two broad approaches, although there is some overlap between them.

The first approach is in the use of 'old' and established technologies. In this case, it is largely a matter of making improvements in existing practices, including the control of temperature for example. Even without the use of 'superchilling', there is potential for better control of meat temperature from the point of slaughter. This can be achieved by simple measures, such as better education of workers and training to increase awareness of the importance of temperature, establishing and enforcing correct material flow within production areas and the use of intermediate chill rooms between stages in a process.

Together with better education to improve temperature control, hygiene training is also very important, and awareness of its impact on product quality and shelf-life should again be emphasized. The introduction of the Hazard Analysis Critical Control Point (HACCP) system and the discipline that this encourages in examining the food production process will have a positive effect on shelf-life and quality. Factory cleaning, which is generally done outside office hours when senior management are absent, can be perceived as mundane and unimportant when, in reality, it is a key part of factory operations. A hygienic production environment will have a direct impact on microbial levels and hence on shelf-life. Equipment design is important and makes a contribution to the overall standard of factory hygiene. Now that more operations are being carried out by machines, e.g. cutting and portioning, it is particularly important that machines are easily cleanable and do not contaminate product with stale débris.

Marinading is another old technology which could be further exploited; most marinades are applied to the product to alter flavour and have little impact on, for example, the pH of the meat. This means that any improvement in texture and extension of shelf-life is small. Further investigation of marinades and their application could have marked benefits in shelf-life and quality attributes of the food.

In summary, the established techniques that could provide benefit in the area of shelf-life extension are:

- low-temperature storage;
- gas packing;
- marinading;
- hygienic production;
- HACCP programmes.

Having considered the application of old technologies to extending shelf-life we can now consider some of the newer and less widely known approaches that might benefit the product. Strategies to improve shelf-life inevitably aim to prevent/reduce microbial contamination or to decontaminate exposed surfaces where bacteria build up during processing.

Microbial contamination of poultry meat should be minimized during processing and this may be achieved, as suggested above, when factory operations are suitably improved. Again, HACCP is a vital tool in achieving this. Ultimately, the establishment of a 'clean' working environment and the application of some high-care principles to standard production situations could give benefits. However, poultry carcasses are contaminated with micro-organisms on the outside and this cannot be avoided. It is a reflection of the need to retain the skin following slaughter.

Greater use of filtered air and stricter control of hygiene disciplines would contribute to a decrease in the microbial load on the product during processing.

Decontamination and use of irradiation are dealt with elsewhere and will not be considered in detail here; however, high-intensity light is one new approach that does show potential and may be worth considering as part of a strategy to extend shelf-life.

Modified-atmosphere packing has been used in various forms for some time and has shown benefits in relation to shelf-life and presentation to the consumer. Further advances are still possible, not only with developments in packaging films but also in the incorporation of scavengers and other compounds in the films. This use of functional packaging films will be an important aspect in the future and is likely to show substantial growth.

The newer approaches may be summarized as follows:

- supplementation of animal diets with functional ingredients, e.g. vitamin E;
- combination treatments – use of microbiological and chemical 'hurdles';
- improved slaughter and cutting – introduction of more controlled processing lines;
- high-intensity light and other decontamination treatments for surfaces;
- scavengers in packaging and sparging/blanketing in inert gases during storage;
- edible films impregnated with functional ingredients.

If the relationship between cost and goal/benefit is correct, any particular strategy should succeed. Ultimately, the success or failure of the strategy will be reliant on greater cooperation and communication between the various sectors of the poultry industry throughout the production chain. One weak link due to either lack of understanding of each sector's requirements or, more commonly, human error will result in failure. Therefore, future strategies are likely to become increasingly dependent on automation, which minimizes the possibilities of human error. Price, flexibility and speed are no longer stumbling blocks for this particular strategy. Machines capable of deboning poultry carcasses, which cost £60,000 a few years ago, are now available for £15,000 with improved hygiene and greater flexibility.

REFERENCES

ACMSF (1992) *Report on Vacuum Packaging and Associated Processes*. Advisory Committee on the Microbiological Safety of Food, HMSO, London.

Anon. (1997) Major packaging technology breakthrough. *Food Australia* 49, 177.

Bailey, M.E., Shin-Lee, S.Y., Dupuy, H.P., St Angelo, A.J. and Vercellotti, J.R. (1987) Inhibition of warmed-over flavour by Maillard reaction products. In: St Angelo, A.J. and Bailey, M.E. (eds) *Warmed-over Flavor of Meat*. Academic Press, New York, pp. 237–267.

Bjerklie, S. (1997) Zapping down bacterial counts. *Meat Processing* 36, 46–47.

Bohnsack, U., Knippel, G. and Höpke, H.-U. (1988) The influence of a CO_2 atmosphere on the shelf-life of fresh poultry. *Fleischwirtschaft* 68, 1553–1557.

Church, P.N (1993) Meat products. In: Parry, R.T. (ed.) *Principles and Applications of Modified Atmosphere Packaging of Food*. Blackie Academic and Professional, London, pp. 229–268.

Church, P.N. (1994) Developments in modified-atmosphere packaging and related technologies. *Trends in Food Science and Technology* 5, 345–352.

Dunn, J., Ott, T. and Clark, W. (1995) Pulsed-light treatment of food and packaging. *Food Technology* September, 95–98.

Gault, N.F.S. (1991) Marinaded meat. In: Lawrie, R. (ed.) *Developments in Meat Science*, Vol. 5. Elsevier, London, pp. 191–246

Gill, C.O., Harrison, J.C.L. and Penney, N. (1990) The storage life of chicken carcasses packaged under carbon dioxide. *International Journal of Food Microbiology* 11, 151–158.

Green, G., Dicks, L.M.T., Bruggeman, G., Vandamme, E.J. and Chikindas, M.L. (1997) Pediocin PD-1, a bactericidal antimicrobial peptide from *Pediococcus damnosus* NCFB 1832. *Journal of Applied Microbiology* 83, 127–132.

Herald, T.J., Hachmeister, K.A., Huang, S. and Bowers, J.A. (1996) Corn zein packaging materials for cooked turkey. *Journal of Food Science* 61, 415–417, 421.

Hotchkiss, J.H., Baker, R.C. and Qureshi, R.A. (1985) Elevated carbon dioxide atmospheres for packaging poultry. II. Effects of chicken quarters and bulk packages. *Poultry Science* 64, 333–340.

Izatnagar, C.A.R.I. (1996) *Aeromonas* in poultry products. *Poultry International* 35, 121–122.

James, C., Goksoy, E.O. and James, S.J. (1997) *Past, Present and Future Methods of Meat Decontamination*. MAFF Fellowship, University of Bristol, Langford, UK.

Li, Y., Slavik, M.F., Walker, J.T. and Xiong, H. (1997) Pre-chill spray of chicken carcasses to reduce *Salmonella typhimurium*. *Journal of Food Science* 62, 605–607.

Lutgring, K.R., Linton, R.H., Zimmerman, N.J., Peugh, M. and Heber, A.J. (1997) Distribution and quantification of bioaerosols in poultry-slaughtering plants. *Journal of Food Protection* 60, 804–810.

Newman, P.B.D. (1994) Method and apparatus for reducing microbial loads. *International Patent Application PCT/GB94/00898.*

Paine, F.A. and Paine, H.Y. (1992). *A Handbook of Food Packaging*, Blackie Academic and Professional, London.

Raccach, M. and Baker, R.C. (1978) Lactic acid bacteria as an antispoilage and safety factor in cooked, mechanically deboned poultry meat. *Journal of Food Science* 41, 703.

Ray, B. and Daeschel, M. (1992) In: *Food Preservatives of Microbial Origin,* CRC Press, Boca Raton, Florida, USA.

Rozum, J.J. and Maurer, A.J. (1997) Microbiological quality of cooked chicken breasts containing commercially available shelf-life extenders. *Poultry Science* 76, 908–913.

Russell, S.M. and Walker, J.M. (1997) The effect of evisceration on visible contamination and the microbiological profile of fresh broiler chicken carcasses using the Nu-Tech evisceration system or the conventional streamlined inspection system. *Poultry Science* 76, 780–784.

Sawaya, W.N., Abu-Ruwaida, A.S., Dashti, B.H., Hussain, A.J. and Al-Othman, H.A. (1997) Marketing of eviscerated broiler carcasses under supercooled conditions. *Fleischwirtschaft* 77, 365–371.

Tamblyn, K.C. and Conner, D.E. (1997) Bactericidal activity of organic acids against *Salmonella typhimurium* attached to broiler chicken skin. *Journal of Food Protection* 60, 629–633.

Tanaka, N., Meske, L.M., Doyle, M.P. and Traisman, E. (1980) Plant trials of bacon prepared with lactic acid bacteria, sucrose and reduced amounts of sodium nitrite. *Journal of Food Protection* 43, 450–457.

Veerkamp, C.H. (1989) Chilling, freezing and thawing. In: Mead, G.C. (ed.) *Processing of Poultry.* Elsevier Applied Science, London, pp. 103–125.

Ziauddin, K.S., Rao, H.S. and Fairoze, N. (1996) Effect of organic acids and spices on quality and shelf-life of meats at ambient temperatures. *Journal of Food Science and Technology (Mysore)* 33, 255–258.

PART IV
Poultry meat products

CHAPTER 15
On-line assessment of poultry meat quality

H.J. Swatland

Department of Animal and Poultry Science, University of Guelph, Ontario N1G 2W1, Canada

INTRODUCTION

The outstanding success of the modern poultry industry has been built on efficient production, highly mechanized processing and customer appreciation of white meat. Having built the industry up, however, it is less obvious what to do next for an encore. In the building phase, decisions based on quantitative data have been very important: breeding and feeding have been evaluated from growth rates, animal health from pathology statistics and secondary processing from product yield. Thus, overall efficiency has been measured extensively within the industry, not just in academic research. But although there has been a lot of talk about meat quality, it is seldom checked and rarely measured because it is much more difficult to measure product quality than product weight. Thus, so far, little attempt has been made to measure and manipulate meat quality in the poultry industry. The poultry industry has looked after the birds, but it has been left to the birds to look after the meat quality.

If decisions are dictated by meat yield but are blind to meat quality, the risk is obvious. Efficiency of production may go up while product quality may come down. For example, rapid muscle growth in many different types of meat animals is achieved by the radial growth of fast-contracting muscle fibres, containing few mitochondria and lipid droplets, whereas slow-contracting fibres with numerous mitochondria and lipid droplets make a major contribution to tenderness, succulence and taste (Swatland, 1994). Thus, situations may occur, such as that detected by Grey *et al.* (1986), in which turkeys with slow growth may develop more tender meat than those with faster growth. Fast-contracting fibres loaded with glycogen may also be poised for a precipitous glycolytic decline in pH after slaughter (Vanderstoep and Richards, 1974; van Hoof, 1979), causing processing problems with paleness and high fluid losses (Barbut, 1996; McCurdy *et al.*, 1996; Santé *et al.*, 1996).

An ideal solution would be to develop high-speed, non-destructive sensors for commercially important traits of poultry meat quality. Computer and tracking technology is already adequate to allow that information to be used

© CAB *International* 1999.
Poultry Meat Science (eds R.I. Richardson and G.C. Mead)

for making management decisions to improve future product quality (information feed-back to producers), as well as for making maximum use of the current product (information feed-forward for niche marketing and manufacturing process control). Thus, if we wish to compete on the basis of meat quality, first we must develop ways to measure meat quality on-line. Methods must be rapid and non-destructive: there is no time on-line for conventional laboratory methods. Thus, the biophysical attributes of meat quality offer more than the biochemical attributes, because they are more readily measurable optically and electronically.

This chapter surveys some quality traits amenable to on-line assessment in poultry meat, then delves into the concepts and technology of specific case studies. It is only possible for a brief glimpse of the technology involved, but further information is readily available (Swatland, 1995a). Development of on-line sensors for meat quality is closely integrated with development of meat yield sensors and robotics, but these topics are too extensive to incorporate into this short chapter.

REVIEW OF ON-LINE QUALITY TRAITS

Toughness and Sarcomere Length

Much is known about the optical properties of muscle at the ultrastructural level from biophysical studies on the molecular basis of contraction (Martin Jones et al., 1991; Jacquemond et al., 1996). However, on-line measurements can only be made realistically if the muscle is in a bulk state, that is, with a probe pushed into or against a whole muscle to interface with thousands of muscle fibres simultaneously. At the ultrastructural level, the transverse striations of myofibrils are caused by the regular longitudinal arrangement of sets of thick myofilaments (10–12 nm in diameter) and thin myofilaments (5–7 nm in diameter), with each thick myofilament surrounded by six thin myofilaments where thick and thin myofilaments overlap.

When a living muscle fibre contracts, the thick filaments slide between the thin filaments so that the I band gets shorter. The length of the A band remains constant. If a muscle is at its resting length, the gap between opposing thin filaments at the mid-length of the sarcomere causes a pale H zone in the A band. Thus, at the ultrastructural level, there are many ways to assess sarcomere length and to deduce from this, the degree of meat toughness attributable to rigor bonding between overlapping thick and thin myofilaments (Arafa and Chen, 1978; Dunn et al., 1993, 1995). Although it is well known that cold-shortening can occur in poultry muscle (De Fremery, 1966), the impact on customer perception of toughness in commercial poultry meat is uncertain. However, since the whole meat industry is moving strongly towards more rapid refrigeration in order to reduce microbial risks, even if cold-shortening is not already a concern, one day it might be.

Conditioning and Z-line Integrity

Other features of the myofibril are detectable by light microscopy under optimum conditions and, more easily, by electron microscopy. A thin Z line or Z disc occurs at the middle of the I band. The sarcomere length is generally taken as the distance from one Z line to the next. The Z line is a complex structure formed from woven protein filaments and it extends as a partition across the myofibril, anchoring the thin filaments. Z-line degradation by calpains contributes to ageing or conditioning of meat and produces highly desirable increases in taste and tenderness. In red meat, other components of the cytoskeleton (such as vinculin, desmin and nebulin) are also involved, because Z-line degradation is quite late (3 or 4 days in beef; Taylor *et al.*, 1995). In poultry, post-mortem autolysis is far more rapid than in red meat, with not just Z-lines, but whole I bands degenerating by 4 h (MacNaughtan, 1978). Z-line integrity can be assessed by polarized light under laboratory conditions (Swatland, 1989), but the motive to exploit this as a bulk optical method to assess Z-line integrity is far less pressing for poultry meat than it is for beef.

Connective Tissue

Although myofibrillar autolysis is rapid in poultry meat (12–24 h; De Fremery, 1966), relative to red meat it is, of course, not rapid enough for those who pay for the refrigerated storage. Thus, it is the later optical changes of conditioning that are of interest in the poultry industry. A reliable sensor could be used to minimize holding time while attaining specified levels of tenderization. According to Liu *et al.* (1994a, b) the later aspects of tenderization in poultry muscle (> 4 h, after early myofibrillar tenderization) are a result of endomysial and perimysial disruption, with previously strong layers of connective tissue separating into individual fibres. Connective tissue collagen is also responsible for chicken meat from older birds being tough, although the relationship is quite complex (Nakamura *et al.*, 1975). For connective tissue collagen, we can draw on the now fairly well developed on-line technology for detecting connective tissue in beef, where fluorometry via fibreoptics enables us to monitor both the intramuscular distribution of collagen as well as its heat-stable pyridinoline cross-links (Swatland, 1995a).

Paradoxically, however, strong connective tissue is not always the problem and, in products such as processed turkey rolls, the opposite seems to be the case. As turkeys grow heavier, their muscle fibres outgrow their surrounding connective tissues (Swatland, 1990). Perhaps this is an advantage if the bird is to be roasted whole (although a flaky texture may be associated with dryness in the mind of the customer), but it definitely causes problems in making cooked turkey rolls. The end product then may become a heap of crumbled meat flakes rather than a supple slice of meat for a sandwich.

Adipose Distribution

Although the chicken has responded to genetic selection and optimum nutrition by efficiently producing muscle it has, nevertheless, increased its deposition of abdominal fat (Cartwright, 1991). Redistribution of this fat to an intramuscular location for the development of a self-basting product would be welcome, particularly for those in customer-service departments who have to deal with the 'rubber-chicken' complaints. Or, as we might say more politely, principal component analysis shows that the 'fattiness factor' is one of the three main determinants of cooked chicken meat texture (Fritjers, 1976). Assessment of fat content by near-infrared (NIR) spectroscopy is well known (Norris, 1984) and much of the technology is easily adaptable for the bulk state using fibreoptics (Conway *et al.*, 1984). With the wide commercial base already developed in infrared spectroscopy, it is not the sensor technology that needs development for an immediate application in the poultry industry, but the means of applying it.

Muscle Pathology

Muscle pathology is another uncertainty in the quantity–quality balance of poultry meat production, with a variety of ominous consequences of rapid muscle growth, including deep pectoral myopathy (Siller, 1985), focal myopathy (Wilson *et al.*, 1990) and ascites (Julian, 1993). Interestingly, this is an area in which on-line testing received an early application (Jones, 1977). The spectra of affected muscle are easily recognized using a fibreoptic probe (Swatland and Lutte, 1984). Carcasses with septicaemia can also be detected by fibreoptic spectrophotometry (Chen, 1992; Chen and Massie, 1993).

Muscle Colour

The first stage in developing a successful quality assurance programme is to visit the complaints department to identify the problems with the greatest impact on the final customer. Residual redness in cooked poultry would rank highly on any list. The problem has been investigated from many perspectives, including old suspects such as nitrite, as well as newer ones such as *Fusarium* (Mugler *et al.*, 1970; Ahn and Maurer, 1990; Trout, 1990; Claus *et al.*, 1994; Young and Lyon, 1994; Wu *et al.*, 1994; Millar *et al.*, 1994). In fresh poultry meat, oxidation of myoglobin may be faster than in red meat (Froning, 1972), with a corresponding effect on the appearance of the product to the customer. Appropriate detection technology is well known, using fibreoptic spectrophotometry or video analysis (Swatland, 1995a) so, again, it is the commercial motive and delivery system rather than the sensors that await development for routine on-line use.

Fat Colour

Accumulation of carotenoid pigments in chicken skin and adipose tissue (Stone *et al.*, 1971) is an important attribute in the appearance of poultry when presented to the customer (Yacowitz *et al.*, 1978). Yellowness also is affected secondarily by scalding temperature (Heath and Thomas, 1973). Appropriate on-line methods are available for carotene content in beef fat, either a fibreoptic probe or video image analysis (Swatland, 1995a) and could be available for use on poultry with little modification. Opportunities for niche marketing by sorting could exist. Mainstream supermarket customers want their poultry to be white, whereas those with an interest in nutrition and health now view yellow carotenoid pigments in a more favourable light. Sorting the product could keep both groups happy at little extra cost. Oiliness is a quality defect in poultry skin (Fletcher and Thomason, 1980), as it is in pork fat and possibly could be monitored on-line by a combination of translucency and temperature measurements as it is in pork fat (Swatland, 1995a).

Pale, Soft, Exudative (PSE)

The PSE condition is a major problem in pork, where much effort has been directed towards its detection on-line (Swatland, 1995a). Almost any factor that leads to an acceleration or prolongation of postmortem glycolysis is likely to create PSE, with a variety of known causes ranging from mutations in the calcium release channels of the sarcoplasmic reticulum, to stress before slaughter and reflex activity during slaughter, all of which may lead to a similar end result – PSE. Poultry meat is no exception (Vanderstoep and Richards, 1974; Wood and Richards, 1975; Froning *et al.*, 1978; van Hoof, 1979; Barbut, 1996; McCurdy *et al.*, 1996; Santé *et al.*, 1996). Rapid glycolysis in turkey breast meat can be detected by a loss of electrical impedance (Aberle *et al.*, 1971). Loss of impedance results from a loss of membrane capacitance combined with the high conductivity of fluid exudate. Under some conditions, the tenderness of turkey meat can be detected electrically (Ranken and Shrimpton, 1968).

Taste and Odour

Although little or nothing has been done yet to monitor poultry meat taste objectively on-line, technology for the detection of volatiles is evolving very rapidly (Dickinson *et al.*, 1996; White *et al.*, 1996) and could eventually make this a practical possibility. Chemiluminescence methods have been developed for conditioning of beef (Yano *et al.*, 1996a) and for meat spoilage (Yano *et al.*, 1996b) and probably would be equally applicable to the characteristic spoilage odours of chicken meat (Cox *et al.*, 1975). Semiconductor gas sensors also are suitable for use on meat (Berdagué and Talou, 1993).

Emulsifying Capacity

A key feature of the suitability of poultry meat for further processing is its emulsifying capacity, essentially, the availability of its salt-soluble proteins to bind together meat fragments and trap fat globules when coagulated by heat (Cunningham and Froning, 1972). Predictions can be made directly by electrical impedance, or indirectly from the fact that rapid or extensive glycolysis (PSE-like conditions) and high intrinsic lipid levels both tend to reduce emulsifying capacity. Skin content reduces emulsifying capacity and can be monitored by UV fluorescence (Swatland and Barbut, 1991).

NEEDLE FLUOROMETRY AND COMPRESSION RHEOLOGY FOR CONNECTIVE TISSUE

Concepts

This first case study (Swatland, 1995d) looks at the possibility of needle fluorometry for connective tissue in poultry meat. The key point here is that poultry are the smallest of the meat animals and every thing must be scaled down in size to the dimensions of a hypodermic needle, otherwise there is too much damage to the commercial carcass. Much of the recent increase in turkey meat consumption may be attributed to increased consumption of processed products such as cooked turkey rolls. Can needle fluorometry tell us anything useful about the suitability of turkey breasts for further processing?

The principle of needle fluorometry is that UV light is directed into the meat through an optical fibre mounted in the needle. As the needle moves through the meat, the layers of connective tissue fluoresce, with endomysium creating a background ripple and perimysium distinct peaks. The fluorescence is captured by the same optical fibre that excited it. As the fluorescence passes back into the apparatus, it is separated from the UV excitation at a dichroic mirror, then measured. In this case study, the fluorescence patterns obtained from the moving needle are compared with non-destructive rheological testing of breast muscles – a technique which itself could also be adapted as an on-line method of product evaluation. In essence, therefore, one on-line method for connective tissue is being compared with another. If they are both working, the results should be correlated in a logical manner.

Technical Details

Twelve turkey breast muscles (pectoralis plus supracoracoideus, initial weight 1622 ± 158 g, pH 6.05 ± 0.08) were measured optically at the point of maximum thickness, perpendicular to the long axes of muscle fibres. The needle fluorometer is shown in Fig. 15.1. A plastic optical fibre (type HFBR-EUS, Hewlett-Packard, Palo Alto, California) with 1 mm outside

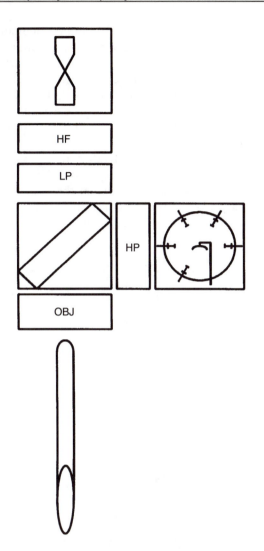

Fig. 15.1. Needle fluorometer for measuring connective tissue fluorescence in poultry meat. UV light from a xenon arc passes through a heat filter (HF), a low-pass filter (LP), through a dichroic mirror, and is launched into the optical fibre to the needle by a microscope objective (OBJ) lens. Fluorescence captured by the optical fibre is reflected off the dichroic mirror, through a high-pass filter, and on to a photomultiplier.

diameter was glued into a hypodermic needle (16 gauge, 1.6 mm outer diameter, 38 mm length) with epoxy resin and the protruding end was trimmed to the cutting angle of the needle (15°) under a dissecting microscope. Light from a 100 W mercury arc was passed through a heat-absorbing filter, through a short pass filter (< 400 nm), reflected off a dichroic mirror (cut-off 395 nm) and was launched into the optical fibre. Fluorescence collected from the sample by the optical fibre was transmitted through the dichroic mirror, through a long-pass filter (> 420 nm) and on to a photomultiplier. The depth of the needle tip in the sample was found from a potentiometer geared to a plate pressed against the sample surface by a weak spring.

The rheological properties of the muscles were measured by compression applied perpendicularly to the muscle fibres (Fig. 15.2). A series of weak compression cycles (30 cycles at 5 s intervals at 24°C) was used with a maximum force cut-off at 4.3 ± 0.5 N to avoid excessive damage on the first test cycle. Weak, repetitive testing was chosen to maximize the sensitivity of the test to the connective tissues holding muscle fibres together laterally (mainly epimysium and perimysium). The descent of the compression plate is shown in Figs 15.3 and 15.5 as distance moved downwards relative to the platform supporting the sample. Thus, when the plate had compressed the sample and the platform was pushed down, there was no further increase in distance, because both compression plate and platform moved down together.

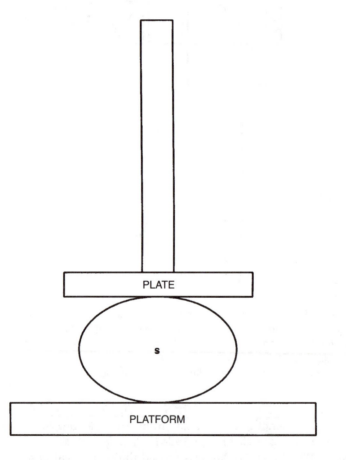

Fig. 15.2. Non-destructive compression testing of turkey meat. A plate pushes down on a sample (S) of turkey breast meat supported on a platform. To avoid damage to the sample, the platform drops when a certain force is reached. As in the next figure, the force applied to the sample is plotted against the distance between the plate and the platform.

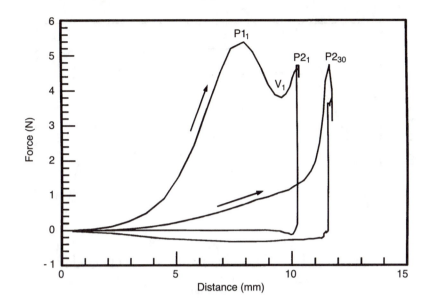

Fig. 15.3. First and last of 30 compression cycles of a sample of turkey pectoralis muscle. The arrows show the direction around the hysteresis loop. The features noted are the first peak (P1$_1$), valley (V$_1$), and second peak (P2$_1$) on the first cycle, and the second peak (P2$_{30}$) on the last cycle.

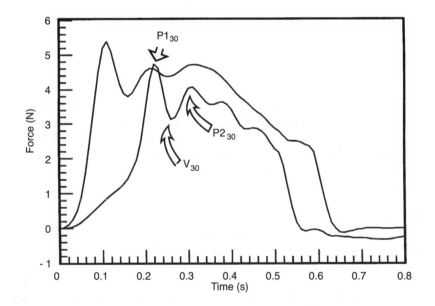

Fig. 15.4. Time sequence analysis of the force data from Fig. 15.3, showing the first and last cycles, noting the first peak (P1$_{30}$), valley (V$_{30}$), and second peak (P2$_{30}$) of the last cycle.

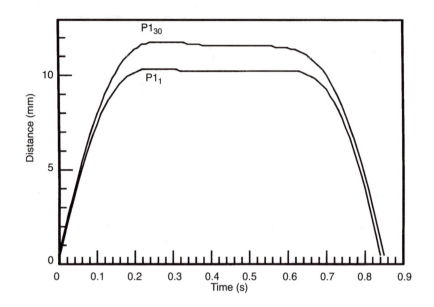

Fig. 15.5. Time sequence analysis of the distance data from Fig. 15.3, showing the first (lower line) and last cycles (upper line), reaching a distance plateau at the first peak ($P1_1$ and $P1_{30}$) where the force cut-off mechanism was activated.

The force acting on the platform supporting the sample is shown on the y-axis in Figs 15.3 and 15.4. The release mechanism responded to the rheology of the sample, giving an early release for relatively hard samples and a late release for relatively soft samples.

Results

A typical compression test is shown in Fig. 15.3, where the arrows show the direction around the hysteresis loop (caused by compression followed by elastic recoil of the sample). In the first compression cycle (subscript 1), there was a steep slope (412 ± 313 N mm^{-1}) to reach the first peak ($P1_1$ at 6.4 ± 6.9 mm, 4.3 ± 0.5 N). Then the force cut-off was activated, to give an initial drop in force to a valley (V_1 at 7.3 ± 6.9 mm, 3.6 ± 0.2 N). A second peak occurred ($P2_1$ at 7.8 ± 7.0 mm, 4.2 ± 0.4 N) as the descending compression plate caught up with the released platform, just before the compression plate started to rise to finish the cycle. After 30 compression cycles (only one or two would be used on-line), the sample had been flattened and much of its elasticity destroyed and P1 and V were lost, leaving only the second peak ($P2_{30}$ at 8.5 ± 7.1 mm, 3.9 ± 0.5 N). There was a decrease in the work area under the curve from 13.7 ± 4.7 mJ in cycle 1, to 5.6 ± 2.9 mJ in cycle 30. After 30 cycles, $P1_{30}$ and V_{30} were still present, only hidden by the method of presentation in Fig. 15.3. In Fig. 15.4, the same data as those of Fig. 15.3 are shown with respect to time and $P1_{30}$, V_{30} and $P2_{30}$ are visible in cycle 30.

Another temporal analysis of the data in Fig. 15.3, is given by Fig. 15.5 which shows the distance–time relationship. For cycle 1 (the lower in Fig. 15.3), the sample was compressed until the force cut-off mechanism was activated, giving a plateau of almost constant distance as the platform supporting the sample was pushed down by the vertically descending compression plate. At mid-cycle (between 0.4 and 0.5 s in Fig. 15.5), the plate started to rise and was followed by the sample platform. In cycle 1, there was relatively little compression of the sample, so that the compression plate descended approximately 10 mm until the force-cut-off mechanism was activated. After 30 cycles, the sample depth had been compressed by approximately 1.8 mm, so that the compression plate was able to descend further before activating the force-cut-off mechanism at approximately 11.8 mm at $P1_{30}$. In other words, very little damage had been done to the sample with as many as 30 compression cycles. With a couple of compression cycles, the method might be compared to squeezing a muscle sample tightly between thumb and forefinger, simulating the 'magic thumb' of the expert master butcher.

An example of a fluorescence signal is shown in Fig. 15.6, where the way-in signal made as the probe penetrated the sample is shown as a solid line and the way-out signal as the probe was withdrawn is shown by solid squares imposed on a line. Because surface epimysial connective tissues have an important effect, the probe was programmed to take readings above the muscle surface, prior to penetration. These data formed a plateau from 0 to 10 mm,

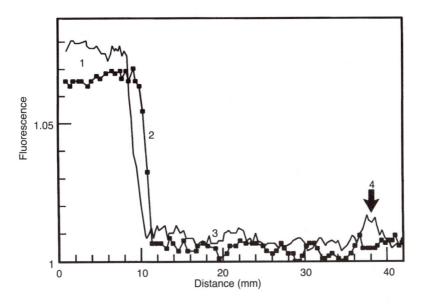

Fig. 15.6. Connective tissue fluorescence signals on the way-in (line) and way-out (line with squares for each data point) of a sample of turkey pectoralis muscle, showing the needle above the muscle (1), penetrating or leaving the muscle (2), within the muscle (3) and hitting a seam of perimysium within the muscle (4).

Table 15.1. Simple correlations of compression with fluorescence in turkey breast muscle.

Compression	Area cm^{-1}	Fluorescence	
		Mean peak height	Maximum peak height
Slope to P1$_1$	0.82[b]	0.77[b]	0.77[b]
P1$_1$ distance	−0.87[c]	−0.83[c]	−0.97[c]
P1$_{30}$ distance	−0.86[c]	−0.80[b]	−0.96[c]
V$_1$ distance	−0.87[c]	−0.83[c]	−0.97[c]
V$_{30}$ distance	−0.86[c]	−0.81[b]	−0.96[c]
P2$_1$ distance	−0.86[c]	−0.83[c]	−0.96[c]
P2$_{30}$ distance	−0.86[c]	−0.81[b]	−0.96[c]
P2$_1$ force	0.73[b]	0.64[a]	0.71[b]

[a]$P \leq 0.025$, [b]$P \leq 0.005$, [c]$P \leq 0.0005$.

approximately (Fig. 15.6, 1), with a major effect on the area under the signal (0.21 ± 0.07 fluorescence units cm^{-1}).

With initial penetration into the sample there was a sharp decrease in fluorescence (Fig. 15.6, 2; 0.09 ± 0.03 fluorescence units). For the signal processing algorithm, this edge was counted as a peak and appears as the maximum peak height in Table 15.1. Within the sample, there were numerous (5.8 ± 1.5 peaks cm^{-1}) small peaks (0.024 ± 0.010 fluorescence, 0.49 ± 0.14 mm half-width) generated by minor connective tissues, mostly endomysium and perimysium (Fig. 15.6, 3), punctuated by occasional, irregular, large peaks of perimysium (Fig. 15.6, 4).

There was a logical pattern in the correlations of compression parameters with UV probe parameters (Table 15.1). Variation in distance was the most important feature (because the apparatus had a force cut-off mechanism). Thus, all the correlations of compression distance with UV probe signals were negative, indicating that samples with a high connective tissue content (large signal area cm^{-1}, large mean peak height and peak 1 height) reached P1, V and P2 sooner, at a lesser distance, than did samples with a low connective tissue content. When the distance of P1$_1$ was small (because of a high connective tissue content), this increased the slope to P1$_1$ so that slope to P1$_1$ was correlated positively with connective tissue content.

On the first compression cycle, samples with a high connective tissue content (large signal area cm^{-1}, large mean peak height and peak 1 height) reached a greater force before the force cut-off mechanism was activated, so that UV probe signals were correlated positively with P2$_1$ force. Thus, samples with a high connective tissue content (as indicated by UV fluorescence) were more firm and less readily deformed.

When the breasts were secondarily processed to make cooked turkey rolls, the frequency of fluorescence peaks in raw samples was correlated with the maximum force required for penetration of the cooked product ($r = 0.74$, $P < 0.005$) and with Young's modulus ($r = -0.71$, $P < 0.005$). The mean height of strong fluorescence peaks was correlated with the tensile strength of the cooked product ($r = 0.72$, $P < 0.005$).

Conclusions

Within the normal range of turkey breast muscle quality for Ontario, both potential methods of on-line testing were capable of detecting the connective tissue integrity of samples. With compression testing alone, it would not have been possible to prove that rheological properties originated from connective tissue rather than myofibrils. With needle fluorometry alone, it would not have been possible to prove that differences in connective tissue distribution had a measurable effect on product rheology.

These techniques would be ideal for a plant where only part of the total production was being used for secondary processing as cooked turkey rolls. Thus, the soft weak ones would be ideal for sale as fresh breasts (because they would be very tender when cooked by the customer), whereas the hard, strong ones would be ideal for making cooked turkey rolls for thin slicing (because the slices would not fall apart).

If the main conclusion one can make from such studies is that both rheological testing and needle fluorometry contain useful information about meat quality, is it possible to obtain both types of information simultaneously? A technique that has proved useful in the on-line measurement of connective tissue in beef is to use the needle itself as a mechanical probe. As it cuts through the meat it often pauses and bounces when it encounters connective tissue, as shown by a dynamic analysis of the needle velocity. In Fig. 15.7, the way to read the results of dynamic analysis is as follows.

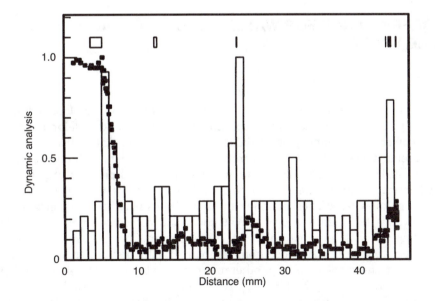

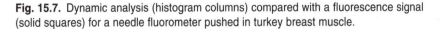

Fig. 15.7. Dynamic analysis (histogram columns) compared with a fluorescence signal (solid squares) for a needle fluorometer pushed in turkey breast muscle.

1. The normalized optical signal for the UV fluorescence of connective tissue is shown by solid squares. Each square shows one measurement, but often they are superimposed.

2. The histogram columns across the bottom of the graphics frame show the normalized frequency of data collection in each millimetre of meat depth. The higher the histogram column, the longer the probe pauses at the depth indicated for that column.

3. At the top of the graphics frame, above the normalized data, are rectangular blocks whose x-axis coordinates show the depth at which the probe paused. Most blocks are narrow (where the probe stops at one depth), but a wide block indicates a long sequence of disordered data in the reverse direction to the overall direction of the probe.

Thus, a tall histogram column without a matching block at the top of the frame shows where the probe is moving slowly, but always follows the overall direction of movement. A tall column topped by a narrow block shows where the probe stops momentarily. A column topped by a wide block shows where the probe bounces as it encounters a strong elastic structure. A more detailed explanation of the technique is available (Swatland, 1995a), but the pattern in Fig. 15.7 is fairly obvious: when the needle hits connective tissue and the fluorescence signal rises, the probe slows down and may pause or bounce. Thus, it can be useful to glean the maximum amount of information possible from any on-line measuring technique. If one has paid to install a sensor, why not maximize the information it can produce? The more information the better.

NIR BIREFRINGENCE FOR WATER-HOLDING CAPACITY AND COOKING LOSSES

Concepts

NIR reflectance spectroscopy (Norris, 1984) is widely used in the food industry and the apparatus is readily available commercially. It works well for a variety of commercially important predictions but is not very attractive from an academic perspective because correlations of spectral data with quality traits are usually empirical. Multivariate analysis or a neural network may tell us what wavelengths to use and how to weight them to make a prediction, but we seldom know why. Thus, although the statisticians may have a chance to be innovative, the science involved may wither away to become empirical, merely testing a hypothesis that engineers from company A have produced more reliable apparatus than those from company B. At worst, simply moving the apparatus from one room to another may require a total recalibration resulting in different wavelengths for the predictions. The method described for our second case study attempts to improve on this situation by taking into account the plane of polarization of the NIR. The commercial objective in this case is to predict water-holding capacity and cooking losses in turkey breast meat.

Well known to all those who have rotated two pairs of Polaroid sunglasses, if there are two plane polarizers (fixed polarizer and rotatable analyser), maximum transmittance occurs when the analyser is rotated parallel to the polarizer and the minimum is when the analyser is perpendicular to the polarizer. But if the polarizer is at 0°, when the analyser is at 90°, then a birefringent muscle fibre at 45° between the polarizer and analyser rotates light so that it can now pass through the analyser. The brightest bands are in the A bands, where thick (myosin) and thin (actin) filaments overlap. But maximum transmittance is now at an analyser angle >90°, because of the optical path difference of the muscle fibre. When the pH of the muscle fibre is decreased towards its isoelectric point, the optical path difference increases and the analyser angle of maximum transmittance increases. In other words, with polarized NIR the signal from sarcomere length is superimposed (depending on analyser azimuth) on the signal determined by protein pH and lipid content.

Technical Details

Light from a 12 V, 100 W halogen source was passed through an 800-nm interference filter (Fig. 15.8, λ) and into a fibreoptic light guide acting as a depolarizer. Light then passed through a polarizing filter (Fig. 15.8, P), through an aperture (diameter 9 mm), through the sample (Fig. 15.8, S), through an analyser (Fig. 15.8, A) and on to a photodiode (Fig. 15.8, PD). The photodiode was a flat-response silicon detector (90% output at 800 nm). Analyser rotation (0 to 180° in steps of 5°) and photometer reading were automated via an IEEE488 microcomputer bus.

The apparatus was checked by calculating extinction coefficients at different wavelengths,

$$k = \log_{10} (T_0 / T_{90})$$

where T_0 is with the analyser parallel to polarizer and T_{90} is with the analyser perpendicular to the polarizer. Values for k at increasing wavelengths were 1.21 at 500 nm, 1.52 at 600 nm, 1.69 at 700 nm, 1.65 at 750 nm, 1.56 at 800 nm, 0.43 at 850 nm and 0.05 at 900 nm. Thus, at 800 nm, the polarizer–analyser combination was as effective as with visible light, but could not have been used above 800 nm.

Portions (200 g) of 12 turkey breasts were chopped for 1.5 min in a food processor to evaluate water-holding capacity. Samples (5 g) were mixed with 8 ml 0.6 M NaCl, incubated for 30 min at 0°C and centrifuged at 7000 g to find the portion of fluid retained by the sample. Other samples (20 g) were cooked (0.75°C min⁻¹) in sealed test tubes (25 × 120 mm) to a temperature of 72°C in a water bath. The amount of liquid separating during cooking was measured and reported as percentage cooking loss.

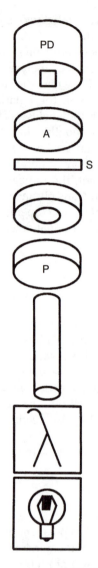

Fig. 15.8. Apparatus for the measurement of the transmittance of polarized NIR through a sample of turkey meat showing the polarizer (P), sample (S), analyser (A) and photodetector (PD).

Results

The range in sarcomere length (determined by laser diffraction) in the samples was relatively low (1.69 ± 0.21 mm) and no significant effect of sarcomere length on NIR birefringence was detected (although such an effect would have been expected if some of the samples had been cold-shortened). It is well known that non-polarized NIR contains useful information about lipid and pigment concentration in meat: can polarization be used to improve on this? If sarcomere length and myofibrillar birefringence make no meaningful contribution to NIR transmittance, then correlations of NIR transmittance with properties such as water-holding capacity and cooking loss should be unaffected by analyser angle (provided that, when crossed with the polarizer, there is sufficient intensity NIR to make reasonable use of the dynamic range of the photodetector – as was the case).

Mean cooking loss was 0.40 ± 0.25 ml per 20 g sample. As Fig. 15.9 shows, when analyser angle was changed, the correlation coefficient of transmittance with cooking loss followed the expected sine function. This shows that the polarized NIR was interacting in a meaningful way with the sample, improving on the base-line correlation of $r = 0.61$ to attain $r = 0.81$ by adding information on myofibrillar birefringence which, in turn, was strongly affected by sarcomere length.

At optimum analyser angles, NIR birefringence was correlated with pH ($r = 0.82$, $P < 0.0005$). Because water-holding capacity is determined by pH, the strongest correlations of NIR birefringence with water-holding capacity were for samples mounted at 315°, close to the pH response angles, $r = 0.85$, $P < 0.0005$, at 30°. Prediction of water-holding capacity from NIR birefringence at one angle of measurement would not be as precise as with pH ($r^2 = 0.85$ for pH vs 0.72 for NIR birefringence), but several birefringence angles were available for stepwise regression, giving $R = 0.92$ for the correlation of birefringence with water-holding capacity and elevating the adjusted R^2 to 0.82. Mean water-holding capacity ($57.0 \pm 10.3\%$) was correlated with pH ($r = 0.92$, $P < 0.0005$), although none of the samples was PSE.

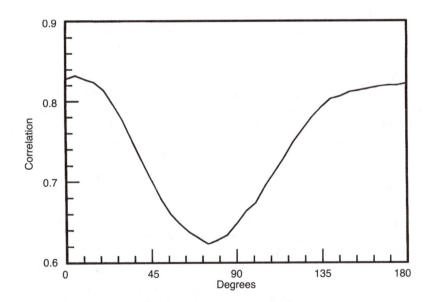

Fig. 15.9. The azimuthal distribution of the simple correlation of polarized NIR transmittance with turkey breast cooking losses.

Conclusion

Cooking losses are very important factors for meat processors because they are directly related to profitability. Thus, even at the levels of performance found in these trials, NIR birefringence could be used to sort turkey breasts, diverting raw materials to different products. A serious criticism of the methodology described here is that it required a thin slice of muscle to be taken for measurement, thus taking time and causing damage. However, since making these measurements (Swatland and Barbut, 1995) it has been shown that the method can be made to work as a probe, by mounting the crossed polarizers on the end of optical fibres (Swatland, 1996). Thus, the method is now non-destructive and fast enough for serious consideration for industrial use.

LIGHT SCATTERING FOR PALENESS AND COLOUR

Concepts

For most situations relating to muscle, paleness is a function of microstructural light scattering, whereas colour is a function of the concentration and chemical state of myoglobin and its derivatives in solution between the scattering elements of the microstructure. Being amenable to biochemical spectroscopy of dissolved chromophores, the myoglobin contribution to meat colour is better known than paleness. The principles of colorimetry are well known (Billmeyer and Saltzman, 1981) and commercial instrumentation is readily available for remote video measurement of food product colour, which is the ultimate on-line method for speed and non-destructiveness. Thus, the major focus of this case study is the on-line measurement of light scattering in meat, with colour as a secondary consideration.

To explain the paleness of meat with a rapid or extensive pH decline post-mortem, such as PSE pork, Bendall and Wismer-Pedersen (1962) proposed that light scattering at a low pH is caused by protein denaturation, comparable to the denaturation of egg albumen by heat. Thus, with cooking, albumen changes from a transparent liquid to a soft, white solid. By analogy, as the acidity of meat develops after slaughter, some of the transparent, soluble meat proteins may be denatured and the resulting increase in light scattering may increase the paleness of the meat. Evidence in support of this hypothesis is now quite convincing (Fischer et al., 1979; Stabursvik et al., 1984), but only when the pH decline is rapid or extended. Protein precipitation, therefore, may be regarded as a major cause of scattering, but a mechanism that is only really important at a low pH or when the pH acts on meat proteins that are still near body temperature. How can we account for pH-dependent differences in scattering at pH values above those at which protein precipitation is expected? In another early hypothesis, suggested by Hamm (1960) and supported by Offer et al. (1989), it was proposed that shrinkage of myofibrils at a low pH should increase the refractive index difference between the myofibrils and their surrounding sarcoplasm. This would act to increase the scattering of light from the myofibrillar surface. This second hypothesis (pH-related changes in reflection at the myofibrillar surface) is attractive because it may explain the differences in light scattering between normal and DFD (dark, firm and dry) meat but, so far, little experimental evidence has been published in support.

Myofibrils account for much of the volume in meat, starting at about 80% and declining to 50% as the pH declines post-mortem. Thus, even small optical changes within the myofibrils are likely to have a measurable effect on the bulk optical properties of meat. Myofibrils are strongly birefringent, as indicated by the naming of A (anisotropic) and I (isotropic) bands and this enables them to be investigated with polarized light to study the changes in refractive index in response to pH. Measurements on individual muscle fibres show that the optical path difference (between rays following different refractive pathways allowed by birefringence) tends to increase when pH is decreased (Swatland, 1989). Thus, light scattering in meat may involve at least three different processes (protein denaturation, reflective scattering at the myofibrillar surface and refractive scattering as light passes through myofibrils). Protein denaturation caused by a low pH in meat is irreversible, whereas the other mechanisms can be experimentally reversed by manipulating pH (Swatland, 1995b).

Described below are two possible on-line methods for measuring scattering in poultry meat. It should be borne in mind that the degree of muscle paleness itself may be relatively unimportant, but it may be a secondary predictor of water-holding capacity, which is always important because it translates directly into profitability.

Laser Scattering

Many different food commodities are sorted rapidly, using various types of optical sensors involving lasers and video, so why not poultry meat? Birth *et al.* (1978) proposed that meat could be sorted with a laser beam directed from above while below the meat a photodiode would scan from 0° (in line with the laser beam) to 45° to one side of the axis. Thus, the length of the light path through the meat is not constant (Fig. 15.10). A more convenient approach might be to have the laser beam passing upward through the sample to a video camera above, using a mask to protect the camera from the direct beam and allowing detection of the light scattered in the sample around the main beam (like looking at the solar corona during an eclipse of the sun).

Birth *et al.* (1978) adapted the Kubelka–Munk analysis of light scattering so that, with the upper surface of a muscle sample illuminated by a helium–neon laser,

$$\log M_T = A - Br$$

where M_T is the radiant exitance on the lower surface, A is the intercept and B

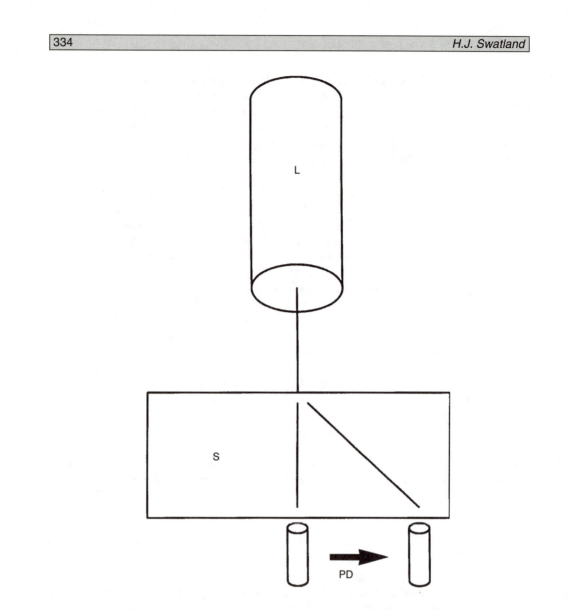

Fig. 15.10. The original laser scattering layout proposed by Birth *et al.* (1978) with the laser (L) beam impinging downwards through the sample (S) and the photodetector (PD) scanning across below the sample.

is the slope of a regression (light intensity versus distance) and r is the path length through the meat. Birth *et al.* (1978) showed that

$$B = \log 2 \, (S + K)$$

where S is a scatter coefficient (cm^{-1}) and K is the absorption coefficient (cm^{-1}). B was given no special name but might be called a spatial measurement of scattering. It was shown that spatial measurements of scattering at 632 nm (the wavelength of a red helium–neon laser) was a useful measure of light scattering in meat. Meat is far more complex than the relatively simple situations for which the Kubelka–Munk analysis was intended and one would expect an additive effect on spatial measurements of scattering by both myofibrillar scattering and chromophore absorbance, but the scatter coefficient (S) is probably the major variable in spatial measurements of scattering if there is little variation in myoglobin content (as would be expected in breast muscles from birds of a similar age).

For the spatial scanning method developed by Birth *et al.* (1978), sections of pork longissimus dorsi were cut at a thickness of 25 mm with muscle fibres at an uncontrolled angle (probably about 45°) to the laser beam. Illumination was at 632 nm and the photodetector scanned unilaterally (only to one side of the laser beam) beneath the muscle with a 2 mm-diameter measuring aperture. Over a certain range, the logarithm of the photodetector response was approximately linear with respect to the optical path length through the meat, which is how the slope of the intensity–distance relationship could be used as a measure of scattering. But when spatial scanning was tested for sorting turkey breasts on-line, some other factors became apparent (Swatland, 1991).

Following the established method, the length of the light path through the meat was calculated trigonometrically from the position of the photodetector and the depth of the meat sample and the photodetector response was transformed to a logarithm. The data shown in Fig. 15.11 are complete bilateral scans passing completely across the area of meat illuminated by the laser. In a bilateral scan, the magnitude of the hysteresis shows the optical asymmetry caused by muscle fibre arrangement distorting the scattering pattern. In the particular examples shown in Fig. 15.11, the scan with the green laser was

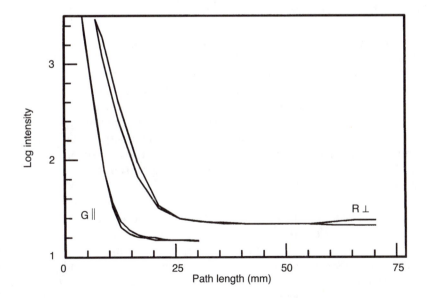

Fig. 15.11. Laser scanning of slices of turkey breast meat illuminated by a green laser parallel to and coaxial with the longitudinal axes of muscle fibres (G ‖) and by a red laser perpendicular to the muscle fibres (R⊥).

almost exactly symmetrical whereas the scan with the red laser shows slight asymmetry. The thickness of each sample is given by the minimum path length. The reason for using both red and green lasers is to obtain information on the myoglobin content.

Both the examples shown in Fig. 15.11 are composed of two segments. Nearest to the optical axis, where the light path through the meat is short, there is almost a linear slope in the log response of the photodetector, as expected. Further from the optical axis, however, where the light path through the meat is longer, the angle of the slope decreases and there is a segment that is almost horizontal, caused by a low level of highly scattered stray light. In the examples shown in Fig. 15.11, the junction between these two segments is a transitional curve where attenuated scattering of the incident illumination gives way to the low level of background illumination and there is no problem in finding the slope at short path lengths. But in data similar to those that might be expected on-line (without precise alignment of muscle fibres or accurate slice thickness), the relationship between photodetector response and optical path length may become curvilinear and more difficult to analyse. Other problems may be created by differences in sample thickness and muscle fibre orientation, but can be solved.

In conclusion, this potential method is in its infancy. It has never been used commercially and considerable investment would be needed to make it work. But if really high speed sorting of boned poultry meat was required, sorting by video analysis of laser scatter pattern might be the ideal method.

Fibreoptic Spectrophotometry

Fibreoptic spectrophotometry is a lot easier and more readily applicable than the previous method. In general, when using a fibreoptic spectrophotometer, it is essential to examine its construction to see what it is measuring. Given that muscle is composed of a scattering microstructure immersed in a fluid containing a strongly absorbing chromophore, myoglobin, a single sample of meat can yield different spectra, depending on how they are measured. As shown in Fig. 15.12, if the apparatus forces a long light path through the tissue, because illuminating and recording optical fibres are widely separated or have a wide angular divergence, then it will be more sensitive to myoglobin concentration than to the level of scattering. On the other hand, if illuminating and recording optical fibres are small, close and parallel, the light path through the meat will be minimal and the apparatus will be more sensitive to scattering directly at the interface than to myoglobin beyond the interface. Thus, a probe that has been optimized for the detection of scattering (as for PSE pork) should not be used for myoglobin concentration (as for veal grading), or vice versa. Apart from this, the technology is relatively straightforward and a variety of commercial equipment is obtainable or relatively easily assembled by an optical engineering company to produce spectra such as those shown in Fig. 15.12. Conventional chromaticity coordinates for colorimetry can be obtained from fibreoptic spectra by the weighted ordinate method but, as can

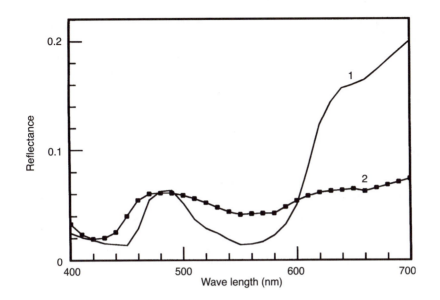

Fig. 15.12. Two spectra collected from the same meat sample by the same fibreoptic probe. The difference is that for spectrum 1, a long light path was forced through the tissue whereas, for spectrum 2, the path was short.

be seen from Fig. 15.12, it is important first to transform the spectrum to correct for the direct interface between the meat and the optical system (a conventional colorimeter has an air-space with a defined geometry between the optics and the sample).

Fibreoptic spectrophotometry is very much an area where the sensor technology is already adequate for most commercial on-line evaluation requirements of poultry meat quality, what is needed is the technology to launch the probe. The method can be almost instantaneous, by synchronizing the discharge of a xenon flash to the reading of a photodiode array spectrograph (Swatland, 1995a).

OPTOELECTRICAL SORTING FOR TURKEY PSE AND TEXTURE

Concepts

Electrical sorting of poultry meat has not developed since the initial observations by Ranken and Shrimpton (1968) and Aberle *et al.* (1971) mentioned earlier. Electrical testing is robust, relatively inexpensive and ideally suited for on-line sorting. So, for the sake of making the point, a small study was undertaken on turkey breast meat using some of the technology currently being investigated to improve PSE detection in pork. Turkey breasts were brought to the University of Guelph by a food processor because the meat was flaking apart after being boned and was obviously unsuitable for secondary processing. This condition has not yet been properly investigated (because it can be avoided easily by not growing turkeys too large), but appears at first sight to be a consequence of inadequate connective tissue development coupled with PSE (Swatland, 1995c). Thus, if the perimysium has already been outgrown by the myofibrils, then release of fluid by the myofibrils may then expand the volume of the interfibre space beyond its perimysial restraints, thus neatly separating all the fasciculi so that they gape open and fall apart when processed.

Technical Details

Two pairs of parallel 16-gauge hypodermic needles 3 mm apart penetrated through from both sides of samples so that the needle tips were 3 mm apart (Fig. 15.13). The needles were connected via programmable relays (HP 69730A, Hewlett-Packard, Palo Alto, California) to a modification of the two-electrode AC bridge circuit of Burger and van Dongen (1960) so that impedance could be examined at different directions through the meat. The AC test current was generated from a digital function generator (HP 33120A) and passed to both sides of a bridge circuit based on two balanced resistors (500 W). The reference current was monitored from an analogue to digital (A : D) converter (HP 69715A with 69790B 4k memory card), with a matching converter for the test current through the meat balanced against a programmable resistance and capacitance. A : D converters were programmed by the armed-card interrupt method, using a first-in, first-out (FIFO) buffer with stack pointers and were triggered externally from a pulse train generator (HP 69735A) which, in turn, was triggered from the digital function generator. Thus, the start of the data collection window was latched to the start of a single sine wave. The programmable resistance was based on a binary series of resistors engaged through mercury-wetted relays with a resolution of 2 ohms and a range of 16 kW. The programmable capacitance was based on an incremental series of capacitors with a resolution of 0.2 mF and a range of 26.6 mF. Resistors were in parallel with capacitors.

After finding the initial phase angle, the bridge was balanced using the programmable resistance until the test signal had the same amplitude as the reference, then the bridge was balanced for capacitance until the phase angle of the sample was close to that of the reference. Balancing of resistance followed by capacitance was repeated until no further change occurred. The digital function generator was operated in single cycle bursts to minimize exposure of the meat to the test current. With only one complete sine wave in the measuring window, amplitudes and phase angles were found by taking the mean voltage:time coordinates of the maximum and minimum values. The frequency was very low (100 Hz), relative to that found in most commercial apparatus for PSE pork, following the suggestion by Whitman et al. (1996) that low frequencies are more sensitive than high frequencies for PSE detection. However, the pioneer work of Ranken and Shrimpton (1968) on poultry used a relatively low frequency (50 Hz). In theory, the initial phase angle contains all the information required but the impedance of the A : D converters may impose rudely on the theory so, for a prototype, it is nice to balance the bridge to be sure of what is really happening.

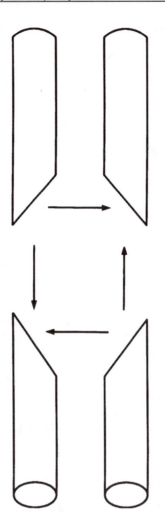

Fig. 15.13. Parallel needle configuration used for combined optical and electrical measurements of meat. Each stainless-steel hypodermic needle contains an optical fibre allowing electrical impedance and optical transmittance measurements to be made in different directions relative to the muscle fibre arrangement of the meat.

Results

Electrical impedance may be measured as a phase angle, which is determined by an interaction of sample capacitance and reactance. Thus, in Fig. 15.14, the test current through the sample lags behind that of the reference. Results are shown in Table 15.2. Thus, if one was an engineer viewing this as a pilot study to select an electrical circuit to sort turkey breasts automatically for a commercial client, one would take the highest t-statistic for separating normal from flaky breasts (which was t = 12 for the lateral phase angle). Hence, a rapid measurement laterally between two pairs of parallel needles would be the best

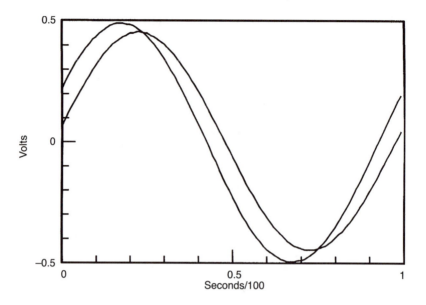

Fig. 15.14. Electrical impedance measured laterally between two electrodes in a sample of flaky turkey breast meat, showing the current through the sample lagging behind that of the reference.

Table 15.2. Selecting a configuration of electrodes and measurements to separate turkey breasts with a normal texture from those with a flaky texture.

Direction and property	Normal mean ± SD	Flaky mean ± SD
Coaxial phase angle, radians	0.21 ± 0.01[a]	0.14 ± 0.01
Coaxial capacitance, μF	2.37 ± 0.15	1.92 ± 0.56
Coaxial resistance, Ω	695 ± 43[a]	556 ± 97
Lateral phase angle, radians	0.24 ± 0.01[a]	0.17 ± 0.01
Lateral capacitance, μF	3.01 ± 0.06	2.73 ± 0.65
Lateral resistance, Ω	714 ± 103[a]	485 ± 82

[a]$P < 0.01$, 2-tails, $n = 18$.

way to sort on-line. Of the two determinants of the phase angle, resistance (electrolyte conductivity) appeared to contain the required information, whereas capacitance had a high variance. Obviously, one would undertake a lot more research for a real-life application rather than for a demonstration case study to present at a conference.

If one wished to go a step further in achieving reliability, an obvious possibility is to include optical fibres inside the hypodermic needles. Light could then be passed from one needle to another, either coaxially between opposing needles or laterally between parallel needles to monitor light scattering. But which wavelengths contain the required information? In this demonstration case study, plotting the t-statistic as a function of wavelength shows forward transmittance from one needle to its opposing coaxial partner

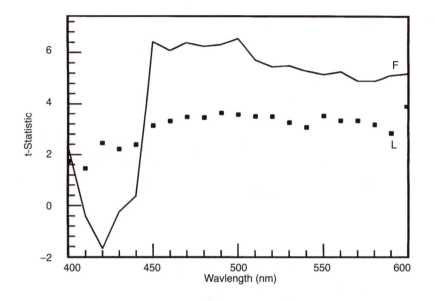

Fig. 15.15. Spectral distribution of the t-statistic for separating normal from flaky turkey breasts measured by forward transmittance (F) and lateral transmittance (L) between needles.

gives reasonable results at > 450 nm (Fig. 15.15). Lateral transmittance is not adversely affected by the Soret absorbance band at 420 nm, as is forward transmittance. But, across the remainder of the spectrum examined, lateral transmittance is less reliable than forward transmittance for separating normal from flaky breasts. A bonus to incorporating the optical measurement is that it is independent of the electrical measurement and is far less likely to require a temperature correction, as is an electrical measurement (temperature has a major effect on electrolyte conductivity). Sorting decisions made from the inputs of two independent predictors can usually be programmed to be more reliable than for a single input. Multiple wavelengths could be used, as in the widely used near-infrared methods of food product sorting, but the penalty would be a lack of robustness from one situation to another.

CONCLUSIONS

Many of the commercially important attributes of poultry meat such as tenderness, colour of muscle and fat, water-holding capacity and suitability for further processing can be measured rapidly and non-destructively. Simple straightforward methods already exist, such as electrical impedance, fibreoptic spectrophotometry and video image analysis and many other possibilities await development, such as laser scattering and optomechanical needle penetrometry. Poultry meat examples show that needle probes have much to offer because they can be used simultaneously for many different types of measurements:

- dynamic rheological analysis
- electrical impedance
- UV fluorometry
- visible light spectrophotometry
- NIR transmittance
- ellipsometry with polarized light.

Use of multiple needles also allows data to be collected in a multidirectional matrix. Thus, on-line evaluation of poultry meat quality already is technically feasible and could provide feedback information to primary producers, as well as feed-forward information for niche marketing and the optimization of secondary processing. Meat quality could be measured in every bird produced to achieve total quality management.

REFERENCES

Aberle, E.D., Stadelman, W.J., Zachariah, G.L. and Haugh, C.G. (1971) Impedance of turkey muscle: relation to post mortem metabolites and tenderness. *Poultry Science* 50, 743–746.

Ahn, D.U. and Maurer, A.J. (1990) Poultry meat color: pH and the heme-complex forming reaction. *Poultry Science* 69, 2040–2050.

Arafa, A.S. and Chen, T.C. (1978) Biophysical and organoleptic evaluation of hot-packaged cut-up broiler meats. *Poultry Science* 57, 1567–1572.

Barbut, S. (1996) Estimates and detection of the PSE problem in young turkey breast meat. *Canadian Journal of Animal Science* 76, 455–457.

Bendall, J.R. and Wismer-Pedersen, J. (1962) Some properties of the fibrillar proteins of normal and watery pork muscle. *Journal of Food Science* 27, 144–159.

Berdagué, J-L. and Talou, T. (1993) Examples d'application aux produits carnés des senseurs de gaz à semi-conducteurs. *Sciences des Aliments* 13, 141–148.

Billmeyer, F.W. and Saltzman, M. (1981) *Principles of Color Technology,* 2nd edn. John Wiley, New York.

Birth, G.S., Davis, C.E. and Townsend, W.E. (1978) The scatter coefficient as a measure of pork quality. *Journal of Animal Science* 46, 639–645.

Burger, H.C. and van Dongen, R. (1960) Specific electric resistance of body tissues. *Physics in Medicine and Biology* 5, 431–447.

Cartwright, A.L. (1991) Adipose cellularity in *Gallus domesticus*: investigations to control body composition in growing chickens. *Journal of Nutrition* 121, 1486–1497.

Chen, Y.R. (1992) Nondestructive technique for detecting diseased poultry carcasses. *Society of Photo-Optical Instrumentation Engineers* 1796, 310–321.

Chen, Y.R. and Massie, D.R. (1993) Visible/near-infrared reflectance and interactance spectroscopy for detection of abnormal poultry carcasses. *Transaction of the American Society of Agricultural Engineers* 36, 863–869.

Claus, J.R., Shaw, D.E. and Marcy, J.A. (1994) Pink color development in turkey meat as affected by nicotinamide, cooking temperature, chilling rate, and storage time. *Journal of Food Science* 59, 1283–1285.

Conway, J.M., Norris, K.H. and Bodwell, C.E. (1984) A new approach for the estimation of body composition: infrared interactance. *American Journal of Clinical Nutrition* 40, 1123–1130.

Cox, N.A., Juven, B.J., Thomson, J.E., Mercuri, A.J. and Chew, V. (1975) Spoilage odors in poultry meat produced by pigmented and nonpigmented *Pseudomonas. Poultry Science* 54, 2001–2006.

Cunningham, F.E. and Froning, G.W. (1972) A review of factors affecting emulsifying characteristics of poultry meat. *Poultry Science* 51, 1714–1720.

De Fremery, D. (1966) Some aspects of postmortem changes in poultry muscle. In: Briskey, E.J., Cassens, R.G. and Trautman, J.C. (eds) *The Physiology and Biochemistry of Muscle as a Food.* University of Wisconsin Press, Madison, Wisconsin, pp. 181–212.

Dickinson, T.A., White, J., Kauer, J.S. and Walt, D.R. (1996) A chemical-detecting system based on a cross-reactive optical sensor array. *Nature* 382, 697–700.

Dunn, A.A., Kilpatrick, D.J. and Gault, N.F.S. (1993) Influence of ultimate pH, sarcomere length and cooking loss on the textural variability of cooked *M. pectoralis major* from free range and standard broilers. *British Poultry Science* 34, 663–675.

Dunn, A.A., Kilpatrick, D.J. and Gault, N.F.S. (1995) Contribution of rigor shortening and cold shortening to variability in the texture of *Pectoralis major* muscle from commercially-processed broilers. *British Poultry Science* 36, 401–413.

Fischer, C., Hamm, R. and Honikel, K.O. (1979) Changes in solubility and enzymic activity of muscle glycogen phosphorylase in PSE-muscles. *Meat Science* 3, 11–19.

Fletcher, D.L. and Thomason, D.M. (1980) The influence of environmental and processing conditions on the physical carcass quality factors associated with oily bird syndrome. *Poultry Science* 59, 731–736.

Fritjers, J.E.R. (1976) Evaluation of a texture profile for cooked chicken breast meat by principal component analysis. *Poultry Science* 55, 229–234.

Froning, G.W. (1972) Autoxidation of crystallized and crude turkey meat myoglobin. *Poultry Science* 51, 1940–1943.

Froning, G.W., Babji, A.S. and Mather, F.B. (1978) The effect of preslaughter temperature, stress, struggle and anesthetization on color and textural characteristics of turkey muscle. *Poultry Science* 57, 630–633.

Grey, T.C., Griffiths, N.M., Jones, J.M. and Robinson, D. (1986) A study of some factors influencing the tenderness of turkey breast meat. *Lebensmittel-Wissenschaft und Technolgie* 19, 412–414.

Hamm, R. (1960) Biochemistry of meat hydration. *Advances in Food Research* 10, 355–436.

Heath, J.L. and Thomas, O.P. (1973) The xanthophyll content and color of broiler skin after scalding. *Poultry Science* 52, 967–971.

Jacquemond, V., Oetliker, H., Rougier, O. and Takeda, K. (1996) Picrotoxin potentiates contraction while inhibiting Ca current but increasing birefringence signal in frog skeletal muscle fibers. *Japanese Journal of Physiology* 46, 99–104.

Jones, J.M. (1977) Quick detection now for 'Oregon disease'. *Poultry Industry* July, p. 15.

Julian, R.J. (1993) Ascites in poultry. *Avian Pathology* 22, 419–454.

Liu, A., Nishimura, T. and Takahashi, K. (1994a) Structural weakening of intramuscular connective tissue during post mortem ageing of chicken semitendinosus muscle. *Meat Science* 39, 135–142.

Liu, A., Nishimura, T. and Takahashi, K. (1994b) Structural changes in endomysium and perimysium during post-mortem aging of chicken semitendinosus muscle – contribution of structural weakening of intramuscular connective tissue to meat tenderization. *Meat Science* 38, 315–328.

MacNaughtan, A.F. (1978) A histological study of post mortem changes in the skeletal muscle of the fowl (*Gallus domesticus*). II. The cytoarchitecture. *Journal of Anatomy* 126, 7–20.

Martin Jones, H., Baskin, R.J. and Yeh, Y. (1991) The molecular origin of birefringence in skeletal muscle. Contribution of myosin subfragment S-1. *Biophysical Journal* 60, 1217–1228.

McCurdy, R.D., S. Barbut, S. and Quinton, M. (1996) Seasonal effect on pale soft exudative (PSE) occurrence in young turkey breast meat. *Food Research International* 29, 363–366.

Millar, S., Wilson, R., Moss, B.W. and Ledward, D.A. (1994) Oxymyoglobin formation in meat and poultry. *Meat Science* 36, 397–406.

Mugler, D.J., Mitchell, J.D. and Adams, A.W. (1970) Factors affecting turkey meat color. *Poultry Science* 49, 1510–1513.

Nakamura, R., Sekoguchi, S. and Sato, Y. (1975) The contribution of intramuscular collagen to the tenderness of meat from chickens with different ages. *Poultry Science* 54, 1604–1612.

Norris, K.H. (1984) Reflectance spectroscopy. In: Stewark, K.K. and Whitaker, J.R. (eds) *Modern Methods of Food Analysis.* AVI Press, Westport, Connecticut, pp. 167–186.

Offer, G., Knight, P., Jeacocke, R., Almond, R., Cousins, T., Elsey, J., Parsons, N., Sharp, A., Starr, R. and Purslow, P. (1989) The structural basis of the water-holding, appearance and toughness of meat and meat products. *Food Microstructure* 8, 151–170.

Ranken, M.D. and Shrimpton, D.H. (1968) Non-destructive method of assessing the toughness of individual turkeys. *Journal of the Science of Food and Agriculture* 19, 611–614.

Santé, V.S., Lebert, A., Le Pottier, G. and Ouali, A. (1996) Comparison between two statistical models for prediction of turkey breast meat colour. *Meat Science* 43, 283–290.

Siller, W.G. (1985) Deep pectoral myopathy: a penalty of successful selection for muscle growth. *Poultry Science* 64, 1591–1595.

Stabursvik, E., Fretheim, K. and Frøystein, T. (1984) Myosin denaturation in pale, soft, exudative (PSE) porcine muscle tissue as studied by differential scanning calorimetry. *Journal of the Science of Food and Agriculture* 35, 240–244.

Stone, H.A., Collins, W.M. and Urban, W.E. (1971) Evaluation of carotenoid concentration in chicken tissues. *Poultry Science* 50, 675–681.

Swatland, H.J. (1989) Birefringence of beef and pork muscle fibers measured by scanning and ellipsometry with a computer-assisted polarizing microscope. *Journal of Computer-Assisted Microscopy* 1, 249–262.

Swatland, H.J. (1990) A note on the growth of connective tissues binding turkey muscle fibers together. *Canadian Institute of Food Science and Technology Journal* 23, 239–241.

Swatland, H.J. (1991) Spatial and spectrophotometric measurements of light scattering in turkey breast meat using lasers and a xenon arc. *Canadian Institute of Food Science and Technology Journal* 24, 27–31.

Swatland, H.J. (1994) *Structure and Development of Meat Animals and Poultry.* Technomic Publishing, Lancaster, Pennsylvania.

Swatland, H.J. (1995a) *On-line Evaluation of Meat.* Technomic Publishing, Lancaster, Pennsylvania.

Swatland, H.J. (1995b) Reversible pH effect on pork paleness in a model system. *Journal of Food Science* 60, 988–995.

Swatland, H.J. (1995c) Physiology of growth and development. In: Hunton, P. (ed.) *Poultry Production.* Elsevier, Amsterdam, pp. 23–51.

Swatland, H.J. (1995d) Prediction of physical properties of turkey meat from ultraviolet fluorescence measured through a hypodermic needle. *Archiv für Tierzucht* 38, 437–444.

Swatland, H.J. (1996) Effect of stretching pre-rigor muscle on the backscattering of polarized near-infrared. *Food Research International* 29, 445–449.

Swatland, H.J. and Barbut, S. (1991) Fluorimetry via a quartz-glass rod for predicting the skin content and processing characteristics of poultry meat slurry. *International Journal of Food Science and Technology* 26, 373–380.

Swatland, H.J. and Barbut, S. (1995) Optical prediction of processing characteristics of turkey meat using UV fluorescence and NIR birefringence. *Food Research International* 28, 227–232.

Swatland, H.J. and Lutte, G.H. (1984) Optical characteristics of deep pectoral myopathy in turkey carcasses. *Poultry Science* 63, 289–293.

Taylor, R.G., Geesink, G.H., Thompson, V.F., Koohmaraie, M. and Goll, D.E. (1995) Is Z-disk degradation responsible for postmortem tenderization. *Journal of Animal Science* 73, 1351–1367.

Trout, G.R. (1990) The rate of metmyoglobin formation in beef, pork, and turkey meat as influenced by pH, sodium chloride, and sodium tripolyphosphate. *Meat Science* 28, 203–210.

van Hoof, J. (1979) Influence of ante- and peri-mortem factors on biochemical and physical characteristics of turkey breast muscle. *Veterinary Quarterly* 1, 29–36.

Vanderstoep, J. and Richards, J.F. (1974) Post-mortem glycolytic and physical changes in turkey breast muscle. *Canadian Institute of Food Science and Technology Journal* 7, 120–124.

White, J., Kauer, J.S., Dickinson, T.A. and Walt, D.R. (1996) Rapid analyte recognition in a device based on optical sensors and the olfactory system. *Analytical Chemistry* 68, 2191–2202.

Whitman, T.A., Forrest, J.C., Morgan, M.T. and Okos, M.R. (1996) Electrical measurement for detecting early postmortem changes in porcine muscle. *Journal of Animal Science* 74, 80–90.

Wilson, B.W., Nieberg, P.S. and Buhr, R.J. (1990) Turkey muscle growth and focal myopathy. *Poultry Science* 69, 1553–1562.

Wood, D.F. and Richards, J.F. (1975) Effect of some antemortem stressors on postmortem aspects of chicken broiler pectoralis muscle. *Poultry Science* 54, 528–531.

Wu, W., Jerome, D. and Nagaraj, R. (1994) Increased redness in turkey breast muscle induced by Fusarial culture materials. *Poultry Science* 73, 331–335.

Yacowitz, H., Davies, R.E. and Jones, M.L. (1978) Direct instrumental measurement of skin color in broilers. *Poultry Science* 57, 443–448.

Yano, Y., Miyaguchi, N., Watanabe, M., Nakamura, T., Youdou, T., Miyai, J., Numat, M. and Asano, Y. (1996a) Monitoring of beef aging using a two-line flow injection analysis biosensor consisting of putrescine and xanthine electrodes. *Food Research International* 28, 611–617.

Yano, Y., Yokoyama, K. and Karube, I. (1996b) Evaluation of meat spoilage using a chemiluminescence–flow injection analysis system based on immobilized putrescine oxidase and a photodiode. *Lebensmittel-Wissenschaft und Technolgie* 29, 498–502.

Young, L.L. and Lyon, C.E. (1994) Effects of rigor state and addition of polyphosphate on the color of cooked turkey meat. *Poultry Science* 73, 1149–1152.

CHAPTER 16
Problems and solutions in deboning poultry meat

A. Sams

Department of Poultry Science, Texas A&M University, College Station, TX 77843-2472, USA

INTRODUCTION

The trend in consumption and production of poultry meat has progressed from whole carcasses, through cut-up parts, to boneless meat. This trend stems from the consumer's demand and willingness to pay for the convenience and minimal waste associated with boneless meat. However, along with the willingness to pay a premium price comes a demand for maximum quality and consistency. As a result, processors are under extreme pressure in the production of boneless breast meat for not only quality and uniformity, but also for efficiency. This chapter explores the limitations of the harvesting of boneless meat and the problems associated with them. Also, current and future technologies directed at reducing or eliminating these limitations are presented.

The limitations in the production of boneless meat are two main categories. Probably the most important from the consumer's standpoint are the sensory properties of the meat, particularly tenderness. This has been the focus of the majority of the research in meat harvesting. Also, appearance is an emerging consideration as more boneless, skinless meat is displayed in retail display. Second, meat yield is equally important to the processor because of both the high profit on the product and its impact on production efficiency.

SENSORY PROPERTIES

Rigor Mortis Development

For the purpose of understanding the death process and its effect on meat quality, the muscle can be thought of as an aggregate of individual muscle cells, with each of these cells undergoing its own response to the environment and death. As the animal dies due to loss of blood and the resulting anoxia, the muscle cells continue to respire, producing and consuming adenosine triphosphate (ATP), the primary currency of cellular energy. As cellular oxygen is depleted, the cell depends almost solely on anaerobic metabolism for the production of its needed ATP. As glycogen is depleted and lactic acid, the end product of anaerobic metabolism, accumulates, due to the lack of blood flow to remove it, sarcoplasmic pH decreases to a level that inhibits further glycolysis and ATP production ceases. However, ATP consumption continues, most importantly in the role of ATP as a plasticizer to dissociate actin and myosin, maintaining muscle extensibility. When the ATP concentration falls to a critical level [1 μmol g⁻¹ (Hamm, 1982)] and there is insufficient ATP to dissociate all of the actin and myosin, they begin to remain complexed as actomyosin and the onset phase of rigor mortis begins. These complexes continue to accumulate until the ATP concentration reaches about 0.1 μmol g⁻¹ at which rigor is developed. In this state, rigor mortis has developed, the muscle is not extensible (cannot 'relax') and becomes stiff.

The stiffness of a muscle in rigor mortis is a function of the extent of myofibrillar overlap of thick and thin filaments, which is determined by the strength of the opposing muscle groups (Cason *et al.*, 1997), the presence of skeletal attachments (Stewart *et al.*, 1984), the presence of external restraints (Papa and Fletcher, 1988) and temperature (Smith *et al.*, 1969; Lee and Rickansrud, 1978; Bilgili *et al.*, 1989; Dunn *et al.*, 1995). All these factors serve to prevent or increase myofibrillar overlap, sarcomere shortening and contraction that can occur during rigor mortis development. Opposing muscles, skeletal attachments and external restraints are all various forms of resistance to filament overlap and sarcomere shortening. Temperature has its primary effect through 'cold shortening', a phenomenon involving calcium leaking from the sarcoplasmic reticulum when ATP is present, initiating a contraction. Although 'heat shortening' is a possibility if prerigor meat is cooked, its effect on tenderness depends on the rate of heating and the condition of the meat before cooking (de Fremery and Pool, 1960; Khan, 1971; Lawrie, 1991). In addition to the effect of sarcomere shortening on toughness via filament overlap, it also increases water loss which can further increase toughness (Honikel *et al.*, 1968; Dunn *et al.*, 1993).

Tenderness

The impact of rigor mortis development on boneless poultry meat tenderness has been studied for many years. Lowe (1948) and de Fremery and Pool (1960) provided early reports that poultry meat harvested before the development of rigor mortis was objectionably tough. Therefore, the research objective became to determine the time course of rigor mortis development in an attempt to determine the earliest possible time at which the meat could be deboned without causing toughness. de Fremery and Pool (1960) measured the time course of rigor mortis development according to biochemical changes and the loss of extensibility and determined that the onset of rigor mortis occurred between 2.5 and 4 h post-mortem. Kijowski *et al.* (1982) reported that chicken breast muscle ATP concentration declined to its minimum value by 2 h post-mortem whereas lactic acid levels required between 4 and 8 h post-mortem to reach their ultimate plateau. Lyon *et al.* (1985) reported that breast muscle pH reached its ultimate level (5.59) by 2 h post-mortem and that meat deboned after 4 h of refrigerated post-mortem ageing was not significantly toughened. Dawson *et al.* (1987) reported that meat deboned after 3.3 h post-mortem was not significantly toughened. Together, these reports suggest that different metabolic indices have different abilities to predict rigor mortis development and resulting meat tenderness. This was later reinforced by Stewart *et al.* (1984) and Sams and Janky (1986) who reported that the relationship between muscle pH at the time of excision is not significantly ($P > 0.05$) correlated to the tenderness of the resulting meat.

Stewart *et al.* (1984), Lyon *et al.* (1985) and Dawson *et al.* (1987) all reported that at some time between 2 and 4 h post-mortem was the critical period after which deboning did not cause toughening. This was taken by the poultry industry as a working indication of rigor mortis completion and it adopted recommendations to store intact carcasses at refrigerated temperatures ($< 4°C$) for at least 4 h prior to deboning. For logistical reasons, such as shift changes, many processors store the carcasses or breast halves for 8–12 h. It should be noted that this minimum ageing time evolved as the time needed to prevent any statistically detectable change in shear value. This is not to say that it is the minimum time needed to produce meat that would be considered 'tender' to consumers. It is also important to note that there is variation around a mean shear value that can cause a considerable percentage of the fillets to be tough, despite a mean that would indicate acceptable tenderness (Young, 1997). It may therefore be necessary to report shear data as frequency distributions rather than simple means with a pooled variance.

Although most of the research on ageing poultry meat has been done using shear value as an indication of tenderness, there have also been reports on the sensory responses. However, the results of these studies have been generally consistent with those using shear values (Simpson and Goodwin, 1974; Lyon and Lyon, 1990a, b, 1991). This work has been instrumental in developing target shear values that would be considered tender by consumers. Because shear values are easier to measure for routine quality control uses, they are usually the method of choice provided some appropriate target is available. A 10-blade Allo-Kramer shear compression value of 8 kg g^{-1} has been widely used as the threshold between tough and tender broiler breast meat. However, Sams and Hirschler (1994) and other cooperative research between ours and five other laboratories suggest that identical meat preparation and shearing procedures can produce quite different shear results. To address this issue, Lyon and Lyon (1990a, b, 1991) used several shearing methods and reported ranges of shear values that corresponded to the various sensory tenderness responses. It is therefore important to a processor desiring a particular level of tenderness to establish the level for the target consumers using consistent methodology. Furthermore, the tough/tender threshold differs between people, cultures and geographic regions of the world. In some parts of the world, broiler breast meat that is aged under refrigeration before deboning is considered too tender/soft by consumers. Slightly toughening the meat by abbreviating the ageing period is an easy way to toughen the meat.

Appearance

Although texture is the primary sensory attribute affected by accelerated harvesting of broiler breast meat, other characteristics such as appearance also need to be considered. The visibility of breast meat has greatly increased with the skin removed and with its use in loaf/roll-type delicatessen items. Two common appearance problems are haemorrhages, with the associated yield losses from trimming, and cellular-based discoloration (paleness) that is generalized throughout the muscle. The haemorrhaging problem is much greater in Europe and is thought to be primarily due to high electrical stunning amperages before slaughter (Veerkamp and de Vries, 1983; Gregory and Wilkins, 1989a, b, 1993). Unfortunately, such amperages are required for poultry slaughter in some countries. Innovative stunning methods, such as high frequency stunning (Gregory et al., 1991; Gregory and Wilkins, 1993), constant current stunning (Rawles et al., 1995a, b) and gas stunning (Raj et al., 1990) are being studied to reduce this problem.

As for the generalized, cellular-based discoloration, the use of electrical stunning has been reported to lighten (van Hoof, 1979) and darken (Ngoka and Froning, 1982) poultry meat. Electrical stunning amperage (Papinaho and Fletcher, 1995), electrical stunning duration (Young et al., 1996), gas stunning with CO_2 or argon (Raj et al., 1990, 1997; Kang and Sams, 1995; Sams and Dzuik, 1995) or ageing prior to harvest (Owens and Sams, 1997) do not seem to affect fresh broiler meat colour. However, meat colour lightens with preslaughter heat stress (McKee and Sams, 1997), inadequate chilling (McKee and Sams, 1998) and ageing after harvest (Sams and Dzuik, 1995).

MEAT YIELD

Although ageing is practically a universal practice among poultry processors producing boneless meat, there is little documentation regarding its effect on product yield and, therefore, the cost of the practice. In an effort to determine this cost for the purpose of providing justification for its elimination, we have recently conducted a survey of the cost of ageing in a commercial plant (Hirschler and Sams, 1998). The results of this survey indicated that deboning breast fillets at 2 h post-mortem would increase meat yield by 3.4% compared to deboning at 11 h post-mortem (9 h of ageing), but only if the deboning was manual. This gain in meat yield was due to a combination of reduced drip loss occurring during ageing and a softening of the muscle during ageing that caused it to tear on harvesting. This tearing left some residual meat on the skeleton during deboning. The mechanism for the softening of muscle tissue probably involves post-mortem myofibrillar proteolysis (Etherington et al., 1987; Birkhold and Sams, 1995; Walker et al., 1995; McKee et al., 1997) or weakening of the connective tissue network (Stanton and Light, 1987, 1988; Nishimura et al., 1995).

The cost analysis of the ageing period indicated that, although labor was a substantial cost, drip loss and reduced meat yield were the largest expenses that could be saved by eliminating the ageing period before deboning. As an example, the test plant processed 1.3 million broilers per week. The labour cost that could be saved by the elimination of ageing was approximately US$ 210,000 annually. It was determined that the cooler space was inconsequential as it was small relative to the overall space in the plant and would be readily used for another purpose. This also negated the energy savings from eliminating ageing. However, it was estimated that using the processing volume, bird size and meat yields measured in the study, the plant would produce an additional 45,000 kg of boneless breast meat per week. At US$ 2.2 kg^{-1}, this added yield would multiply to US$ 5,200,000 in additional revenue for this single plant each year. Clearly, ageing is an expensive process with the majority of the costs being associated with the loss in meat yield, not labor and energy. The additional revenue gained should justify any capital outlay needed for implementing technologies to eliminate ageing.

TECHNIQUES TO ACCELERATE MEAT HARVESTING

The extreme costs of ageing meat on the carcass prior to harvest have made the reduction/elimination of this processing step the target of much research. Many techniques have been evaluated over the years, all directed at the primary limitation to reducing ageing. These technologies either accelerate rigor mortis development, to prevent the toughness that would result from harvesting too early, or attempt to tenderize the meat that was toughened by deboning without sufficient ageing. Yet another technique simply attempts to reduce some of the costs involved in the ageing process. Although some of these technologies are in various stages of commercial implementation, ageing is still practised by most processors producing boneless meat.

Electrical Stimulation to Prevent Toughness

Post-mortem electrical stimulation (ES) of meat carcasses was first commercially used by the red meat industry. This technique pulses electricity through a carcass immediately after death, causing generalized muscle contractions throughout the carcass. These contractions serve to exercise the muscles using up stored energy and can therefore affect the rate of rigor mortis development. Cross (1979) reviewed three theories by which post-mortem ES may tenderize meat. First, ES accelerates ATP depletion, resulting in the prevention of cold shortening and improved tenderness. Secondly, ES hastens the decline of post-mortem pH while muscle temperatures are still high, enhancing the possible action of endogenous proteases responsible for tenderization during the ageing process. Finally, ES tenderizes meat by inducing physical disruption of muscle fibres.

Many methods of using ES with poultry, with varying degrees of effectiveness, have been reported in the literature and were reviewed by Li et al. (1993). ES systems that use 'low' amperages of 0–200 mA per bird induce contractions, exercise the muscle and accelerate rigor mortis development. Although rigor is accelerated and the toughening of the resulting meat is significantly reduced, it is not reduced to a sufficient degree to allow the elimination of ageing. These systems only allow some abbreviation of the ageing period and the meat is tough or only 'slightly tender' (Thompson et al., 1987; Lyon et al., 1989; Sams, 1990; Lyon and Dickens, 1993). These systems are in commercial use in the USA but are usually used in combination with other techniques such as extended chilling.

ES systems using 'high' amperages of 350–500 mA per bird induce such forceful contractions that the muscle not only exercises, but tears itself. Birkhold and Sams (1995) presented transmission electron micrographs of ES-treated muscle in which the myofilaments were torn and contracture bands had formed. This physical disruption tenderizes the meat and the rigor mortis acceleration from the exercising prevents toughening. The combination of these two mechanisms has generally made high amperage ES more effective at reducing the need for the ageing period. Whereas low amperage ES results in statistically significant reduction in toughness, high amperage ES results in sufficient reduction in the toughening to produce meat with a shear value that would be considered 'slightly to moderately tender' to consumers (< 8 kg g^{-1}) (Birkhold et al., 1992; Birkhold and Sams, 1993). Both low and high amperage electrical stimulation systems have been commercially implemented to some degree and a commercially available high amperage ES device was recently introduced by a USA manufacturer.

Although most of the published research on ES has been conducted using immersion chilling, we recently evaluated its effect when using a simulated air-chilling system (Skarovsky and Sams, 1997 unpublished data). Because air chilling can have slower muscle cooling rates, there is a potential for the accelerated metabolism to deplete ATP and/or create a low pH/high temperature environment which may increase heat shortening of sarcomeres and proteolytic activity, all of which may affect tenderness. The results suggested that, when followed by air chilling, high amperage ES accelerated post-mortem metabolism, reducing the need for ageing by up to 50%, but increased drip loss.

Gas Stunning to Prevent Toughness

Gas stunning has been reported to affect harvested meat in two ways. First, it reduces the incidence of haemorrhaging on the surface of the pectoralis and therefore improves the appearance of the fillet (Raj et al., 1990; Hirschler and Sams, 1993; Kang and Sams, 1995). However, stunning with CO_2 or argon has been shown to have no effect on the more generalized, cellular-based colour measured by L-value (Raj et al., 1990; 1997; Sams and Dzuik, 1995). Second, gas stunning has been reported to cause anoxia, accelerating post-mortem pH decline and rigor mortis development and reducing the ageing needed before harvesting fillets (Raj and Gregory, 1991; Raj et al., 1991; 1997; Raj, 1994). These effects are observed when using an atmosphere of less than 2% oxygen with air displacement by either argon (Ar) or a mixture of Ar and CO_2. However, it appears as though using high concentrations of CO_2 to create this anoxia prevents the metabolic acceleration, probably because of the anaesthetic effect of the CO_2 (Sams and Dzuik, 1995; Kang and Sams, 1995). However, research suggests that the benefit from gas stunning largely depends on electric stunning to which it is compared (Craig and Fletcher, 1995). The higher amperage (90–120 mA per bird) electric stunning used in Europe causes more carcass damage and slows rigor mortis development. The lower amperage (10–30 mA per bird) electric stunning used in the USA causes very little damage (if done properly) and has little if any delaying effect on rigor mortis development.

Chemical and Physical Methods of Tenderization

Instead of attempting to accelerate metabolism to reduce the need for ageing, other studies have attempted to correct the toughness developed when meat was harvested without sufficient ageing. Lyon and Hamm (1986) harvested broiler breast fillets within 40 min of death and treated them with blade tenderization and a combination of NaCl and polyphosphates. Their results indicated that the treatments involving the phosphates produced meat with a tenderness equivalent to ageing 24 h before harvest. However, such extensive treatments may not be acceptable for markets demanding minimally pro- cessed fillets. Restraining the wings during rigor mortis development to reduce sarcomere shortening also has been reported to reduce the toughening associated with early-harvested fillets (Birkhold et al., 1992; Birkhold and Sams, 1993; Lyon and Dickens, 1993), but not to a sufficient degree to produce acceptably tender meat and thereby completely eliminate the need for ageing. A final physical method was the use of a belt flattener to apply pressure to the fillets and reduce their height (Lyon et al., 1992). Flattening reduced shear values but not enough to cause the fillets to be tender.

Extended Ageing after Harvesting

Because of the extremely rapid pace and variations in poultry meat pro- cessing, the industry generally operates under the minimum guideline of 4–6 h of ageing before deboning. As previously stated, this is to prevent toughening. The resolution of rigor mortis, the physical and biochemical degradation of the muscle ultrastructure responsible for toughness, was not considered in developing this guideline because processors cannot always predict the destiny of their product. McKee et al. (1997) reported that if meat was deboned immediately after chilling without any ageing and then stored for 71 h at 2°C, it achieved shear value of 8 kg g^{-1} or less, a tenderness level considered 'slightly to moderately tender' by consumers (Lyon and Lyon, 1990b). However, in addition to uncertain product destiny, processors in the USA are increasingly demanding 'maximum' tenderness and not simply 'acceptable' tenderness. This may not be the case in some other countries where the population prefers slightly tougher meat.

Extended Chilling to Reduce Ageing Costs

A final approach to reducing the cost of ageing meat on the carcass prior to harvesting is to extend the chilling time to include the ageing period. This process, called extended chilling, would eliminate the labour involved in transferring the carcasses into a separate area/container. If done with immersion chilling, extended chilling would reduce the drip loss associated with ageing. However, excessive evaporative loss can already be a problem for air chilling and extending the chilling time would only increase this loss. Another limitation of extended chilling is the additional plant and chiller space needed to contain four or more hours of production. Also, although drip loss may be reduced with extended immersion chilling, it would not reduce the loss in meat yield resulting from muscle softening occurring during ageing.

REFERENCES

Bilgili, S.F., Egbert, W.R. and Huffman, D.L. (1989) Effect of postmortem aging temperature on sarcomere length and tenderness of broiler *pectoralis major. Poultry Science* 68, 1588–1591.

Birkhold, S.G. and Sams, A.R. (1993) Fragmentation, tenderness and post-mortem metabolism of early-harvested broiler breast fillets from carcasses treated with electrical stimulation and muscle tensioning. *Poultry Science* 72, 577–582.

Birkhold, S.G. and Sams, A.R. (1995) Comparative ultrastructure of *pectoralis* fibers from electrically stimulated and muscle-tensioned broiler carcasses. *Poultry Science* 74, 194–200.

Birkhold, S.G., Janky, D.M. and Sams, A.R. (1992) Tenderization of early-harvested broiler breast fillets by high-voltage post-mortem electrical stimulation and muscle tensioning. *Poultry Science* 71, 2106–2112.

Cason, J.A., Lyon, C.E. and Papa, C.M. (1997) Effect of muscle opposition during rigor on development of broiler breast meat tenderness. *Poultry Science* 76, 785–787.

Craig, E.W. and D.L. Fletcher (1995) A comparison of European (EC) and US electrical stunning systems of broiler carcass and meat quality. *Poultry Science* 74 (Suppl. 1), 30.

Cross, H.R. (1979) Effects of electrical stimulation on meat tissue and muscle properties: a review. *Journal of Food Science* 44, 509–512, 514, 523.

Dawson, P.L., Janky, D.M., Dukes, M.G., Thompson, L.D. and Woodward, S.A. (1987) Effect of post-mortem boning time during simulated commercial processing on the tenderness of broiler breast meat. *Poultry Science* 66, 1331–1333.

de Fremery, R. and Pool, M.F. (1960) Biochemistry of chicken muscle as related to rigor mortis and tenderization. *Food Research* 25, 73–87.

de Fremery, R. and Pool, M.F. (1963) The influence of post-mortem glycolysis on poultry tenderness. *Journal of Food Science* 28, 173–176.

Dunn, A.A., Kilpatrick, D.J. and Gault, N.F.S. (1993) Effect of *post-mortem* temperature on chicken *M. pectoralis major*: muscle shortening and cooked meat tenderness. *British Poultry Science* 34, 689–697.

Dunn, A.A., Kilpatrick, D.J. and Gault, N.F.S. (1995) Contribution of *rigor* shortening and cold shortening to variability in the texture of *Pectoralis major* muscle from commercially-processed broilers. *British Poultry Science* 36, 401–413.

Dzuik, C.S. and Sams, A.R. (1996) Rigor mortis, toughness and color development in breast fillets from broilers treated with argon-induced anoxia and post-mortem electrical stimulation. *Poultry Science* 75, 21.

Etherington, D.J., Taylor, M.A.J. and Dransfield, E. (1987) Conditioning of meat from different species. Relationship between tenderising and the levels of cathepsin B, cathepsin L, calpain I, calpain II and β-glucuronidase. *Meat Science* 20, 1–18.

Gregory, N.G. and Wilkins, L.J. (1989a) Effect of ventricular fibrillation at stunning and ineffective bleeding on carcass quality defects in broiler chickens. *British Poultry Science* 30, 825–829.

Gregory, N.G. and Wilkins, L.J. (1989b) Effect of stunning current on carcass quality in chickens. *Veterinary Record* 124, 530–532.

Gregory, N.G. and Wilkins, L.J. (1993) Causes of downgrading. *Broiler Industry* 56 (4), 42–45.

Gregory, N.G., Wilkins, L.J. and Wotton, S.B. (1991) Effect of electrical stunning frequency on ventricular fibrillation, downgrading and broken bones in broilers, hens and quails. *British Veterinary Journal* 147, 71–77.

Hamm, R. (1982) Post mortem changes in muscle with regard to processing of hot-boned beef. *Food Technology* 36 (11), 105–115.

Hirschler, E.M. and Sams, A.R. (1993) Comparison of carbon dioxide and electricity for the preslaughter stunning of broilers. *Poultry Science* 72, 143.

Hirschler, E.M. and Sams, A.R. (1998) Commercial-scale electrical stimulation of poultry: the effects on tenderness, breast meat yield and production costs. *Journal of Applied Poultry Research* 7, 99–103.

Honikel, K.O., Kim, C.J., Hamm, R. and Roncales, P. (1968) Sarcomere shortening of prerigor muscles and its influence on drip loss. *Meat Science* 16, 267–282.

Kang, I.S. and Sams, A.R. (1995) Rigor mortis development and meat quality in broilers stunned with electricity, stunned with carbon dioxide, or killed with carbon dioxide. *Poultry Science* 74, 79.

Khan, A.W. (1971) Effect of temperature during postmortem glycolysis and dephosphorylation of high energy phosphates on poultry meat tenderness. *Journal of Food Science* 36, 120–121.

Kijowski, J., Niewiarowicz, A. and Kujawska-Biernat, B. (1982) Biochemical and technological characteristics of hot chicken meat. *Journal of Food Technology* 17, 553–560.

Lawrie, R. (1991) Meat Science, 5th edn. Pergammon Press, Elmsford, NY, pp. 206–207.

Lee, Y.B. and Rickansrud, D.A. (1978) Effect of temperature on shortening in chicken muscle. *Journal of Food Science* 43, 1614–1615

Li, Y., Siebenmorgen, T.J. and Griffin, C.L. (1993) Electrical stimulation in poultry: a review and evaluation. *Poultry Science* 72, 7–22.

Lowe, B. (1948) Factors affecting the palatability of poultry with emphasis on the histological post-mortem changes. *Advances in Food Research* 1, 203–256.

Lyon, C.E. and Dickens, J.A. (1993) Effects of electric treatments and wing restraints on the rate of post-mortem biochemical changes and objective texture of broiler *pectoralis major* muscles deboned after chilling. *Poultry Science* 72, 1577–1583.

Lyon, B.G. and Hamm, D. (1986) Effects of mechanical tenderization with sodium chloride and polyphosphates on sensory attributes and shear values of hot-stripped broiler breast meat. *Poultry Science* 65, 1702–1707.

Lyon, B.G. and Lyon, C.E. (1990a) Texture profile of broiler *pectoralis major* as influenced by post-mortem deboning time and heat method. *Poultry Science* 69, 329–340.

Lyon, C.E. and Lyon, B.G. (1990b). The relationship of objective shear values and sensory tests to changes in tenderness of broiler breast meat. *Poultry Science* 69, 1420–1427.

Lyon, B.G. and Lyon, C.E. (1991) Shear value ranges by Instron Warner–Bratzler and single-blade Allo-Kramer devices that correspond to sensory tenderness. *Poultry Science* 70, 188–191.

Lyon, C.E., Hamm, D. and Thomson, J.E. (1985) pH and tenderness of broiler breast meat deboned at various times after chilling. *Poultry Science* 64, 307–310.

Lyon, C.E., Davis, C.E., Dickens, J.A., Papa, C.M. and Reagan, J.O. (1989) Effects of electrical stimulation on the post-mortem biochemical changes and objective texture of broiler *pectoralis* muscle. *Poultry Science* 68, 249–257.

Lyon, C.E., Silvers, S.H. and Robach, M.C. (1992) Effects of a physical treatment applied immediately after chilling on the structure of muscle fiber and the texture of cooked broiler breast meat. *Journal of Applied Poultry Research* 1, 300–304.

McKee, S.R. and Sams, A.R. (1997) The effect of seasonal heat stress on rigor development and the incidence of pale, exudative turkey meat. *Poultry Science* 76, 1616–1622.

McKee, S.R. and Sams, A.R. (1998) Development at elevated temperatures induces pale exudative turkey meat characteristics. *Poultry Science* 77, 169–174.

McKee, S.R., Hirschler, E.M. and Sams, A.R. (1997) Physical and biochemical effects associated with tenderization of broiler breast fillets during aging after pre-rigor deboning. *Journal of Food Science* 62, 959–962.

Ngoka, D.A. and Froning, G.W. (1982) Effect of free struggle and preslaughter excitement on color of turkey breast muscles. *Poultry Science* 61, 2291–2293.

Nishimura, T., Hattori, A. and Takahashi, K. (1995) Structural weakening of intra-muscular connective tissue during conditioning of beef. *Meat Science* 39, 127–133.

Owens, C.M. and Sams, A.R. (1997) Muscle metabolism and meat quality of pectoralis from turkeys treated with postmortem electrical stimulation. *Poultry Science* 76, 1047–1052.

Papa, C.M. and Fletcher, D.L. (1988) Effect of wing restraint on postmortem muscle shortening and the textural quality of broiler breast meat. *Poultry Science* 67, 275–279.

Papinaho, P.A. and Fletcher, D.L. (1995) Effect of stunning amperage on broiler breast muscle rigor development and meat quality. *Poultry Science* 74, 1527–1532.

Raj, A.B.M. (1994) Effect of stunning method, carcase chilling temperature and filleting time on the texture of turkey breast meat. *British Poultry Science* 35, 77–89.

Raj, A.B.M. and Gregory, N.G. (1991) Effect of argon stunning, rapid filleting and early filleting on texture of broiler breast meat. *British Poultry Science* 32, 741–746.

Raj, A.B.M., Grey, T.C., Audsley, A.R. and Gregory, N.G. (1990) Effect of electrical and gaseous stunning on the carcass and meat quality of broilers. *British Poultry Science* 31, 725–733.

Raj, A.B.M., Grey, T.C. and Gregory, N.G. (1991) Effect of early filleting on the texture of breast muscle of broilers stunned with argon-induced anoxia. *British Poultry Science* 32, 319–325.

Raj, A.B.M., Wilkins, L.J., Richardson, R.I., Johnson, S.P. and Wotton, S.B. (1997) Carcase and meat quality in broilers either killed with a gas mixture or stunned with an electric current under commercial processing conditions. *British Poultry Science* 38, 169–174.

Rawles, D., Marcy, J. and Hulet, M. (1995a) Constant current stunning of market weight broilers. *Journal of Applied Poultry Research* 4, 109–116.

Rawles, D., Marcy, J. and Hulet, M. (1995b) Constant current stunning of market weight turkeys. *Journal of Applied Poultry Research* 4, 117–126.

Sams, A.R. (1990) Electrical stimulation and high temperature conditioning of broiler carcasses. *Poultry Science* 69, 1781–1786.

Sams, A.R. and Dzuik, C.S. (1995) Gas stunning and post-mortem electrical stimulation of broiler chickens. In: Briz, C.P. (ed.) *Proceedings of the XIIth European Symposium on the Quality of Poultry Meat.* Zaragosa, Spain, pp. 307–314.

Sams, A.R. and Hirschler, E.M. (1994) A reevaluation of the toughness/tenderness threshold shear value as affected by cooking method, deboning time and laboratory. *Poultry Science* 73 (Suppl. 1), 159.

Sams, A.R. and Janky, D.M. (1986) The influence of brine-chilling on tenderness of hot-boned chill-boned and age-boned broiler breast fillets. *Poultry Science* 65, 1316–1321.

Simpson, M.D. and Goodwin, T.L. (1974) Comparison between shear values and taste panel scores for predicting tenderness of broilers. *Poultry Science* 53, 2042–2046.

Smith, M.C. Jr, Judge, M.D.and Stadelman, W.J. (1969) A 'cold shortening' effect in avian muscle. *Journal of Food Science* 34, 42–46.

Stanton, C. and Light, N. (1987) The effects of conditioning on meat collagen: part 1. evidence for gross *in situ* proteolysis. *Meat Science* 21, 249–265.

Stanton, C. and Light, N. (1988) The effects of conditioning on meat collagen: part 2. direct biochemical evidence for proteolytic damage in insoluble perimysial collagen after conditioning. *Meat Science* 23, 179–199.

Stewart, M.K., Fletcher, D.L., Hamm, D. and Thomson, J.E. (1984) The influence of hot boning broiler breast muscle on pH decline and toughening. *Poultry Science* 63, 1935–1939.

Thompson, L.D., Janky, M.D. and Woodward, S.A. (1987) Tenderness and physical characteristics of broiler breast fillets harvested at various times from post-mortem electrically stimulated carcasses. *Poultry Science* 66, 1158–1167.

Veerkamp, C.H. and de Vries, A.W. (1983) Influence of electrical stunning on quality aspects of broilers. In: Eikelenboom, G. (ed.) *Stunning of Animals for Slaughter.* Martinus Nijhoff, Boston, MA, pp. 197–212.

Van Hoof, J. (1979) Influence of ante- and peri-mortem factors on biochemical and physical characteristics of turkey breast muscle. *Veterinary Quarterly* 1, 29–36.

Walker, L.T., Shackelford, S.D., Birkhold, S.G. and Sams, A.R. (1995) Biochemical and structural effects of rigor mortis-accelerating treatments in broiler *pectoralis*. *Poultry Science* 74, 176–186.

Young, L.L. (1997) Effect of post-chill deboning on tenderness of broiler breast fillets. *Journal of Applied Poultry Research* 6, 174–179.

Young, L.L., Northcutt, J.K. and Lyon, C.E. (1996) Effect of stunning time and polyphosphates on quality of cooked chicken breast meat. *Poultry Science* 75, 677–681.

CHAPTER 17
Sensory assessment of poultry meat quality

G.R. Nute
Division of Food Animal Science, School of Veterinary Science, University of Bristol, Langford, Bristol BS40 5DU, UK

INTRODUCTION

Sensory analysis of poultry meat encompasses many techniques that are applicable to other foodstuffs and uses people instead of, or in parallel with, instruments to analyse the characteristics of a food. In industry, sensory evaluation can be used in conjunction with product developers to identify problems with a product or to optimize a number of desirable characteristics of a prototype product or in the reformulation of products caused by supply problems.

The sensory attributes of a food will provide a number of stimuli that will involve the senses of sight, smell, taste, touch and hearing. Sight is used to assess the colour, size and shape of a food; smell and taste are used to detect aroma and flavour. Touch, using tactile senses such as mouthfeel, can be used to sense the feel of a food which can include hardness, texture characteristics, viscosity etc. Finally, hearing can be used when dealing with coated poultry products where the crunchiness of the outer covering could be of importance. All of these qualities can have an influence on the quality of a food and can be assessed by sensory panels.

SENSORY PANELS

Companies may use in-house panels made up of staff members available within the company. It is important that members of the panel are screened for their basic taste acuity and colour vision and their ability to describe the characteristics of a food product. Motivation is most important and assessors must be reliable and attend all panel sessions. Missing values cause many problems in sensory analysis, substitution of an assessor just to make up the numbers invalidates the opportunity to analyse individual assessor perform- ance and their contribution to the panel results. As part of reinforcing motivation it is a good idea to give a presentation of the results found in sensory experiments. This typically takes the form of giving assessors access to copies of the scientific publications that include the sensory information provided by the panel as a whole.

It is necessary that line managers support the concept of the sensory panel and view them as a necessary part of the production process in much the same way as you might support the need to provide instruments to measure colour or texture etc. There will be occasions when it will not be possible to convene a full panel on a regular basis and if this becomes a common occurrence, thought should be given to the idea of employing part-time sensory assessors (Nally, 1987).

This has the advantage in that they turn up for the sessions and could prove to be a more cost-effective method of obtaining sensory information. It also has the advantage that because they are employed from outside the organization they will not have knowledge of the ongoing research projects and will therefore not have preconceived ideas of the products or research aims.

To conduct effective sensory panels, the assessors need to be free of distractions and the tests should be carried out in a special room in which there is controlled lighting and good ventilation. Assessors should be seated at separate booths and should not be able to communicate with each other during the assessments. There are many design briefs of what constitutes a sensory laboratory and examples are given by Meilgaard *et al.* (1991) and in International Standards BS7183 / ISO8589 (1989).

PRESENTATION OF SAMPLES

Samples of food should be uniform in size and at the same temperature of serving. They should be coded by a random three-digit number and presented in clean odour-free containers. If more than one sample is to be assessed, then care is needed to ensure that the assessors do not receive the samples in the same order, since this will introduce a bias. Assessors are typically instructed to rinse their mouth out with water between each sample to remove traces of the previous sample from their mouth although in the assessment of chicken, palate cleansers, such as bread, water biscuits (crackers) can be used.

In relation to the preparation of poultry meat for sensory evaluation, outlines of preparation are given by Mead (1987), and Jones and Griffiths (1981). Inevitably there will be differences in culinary procedures between countries which in many circumstances will affect eating quality, therefore, it is necessary for the conditions and final internal muscle temperature to be stated.

SENSORY TESTS

These can broadly be divided into 'difference tests', 'category tests', 'ranking', 'scaling tests' and 'profiling tests'.

Difference Tests

These are essentially tests where the assessor is presented with a choice, i.e. identify the odd sample, match the sample to the reference, classify these samples into two groups etc.

Paired comparison (BS5929: part 2, 1982, ISO 5495)

The paired comparison test is used to determine differences or preferences between two samples for a specified attribute, e.g. tougher or more tender, more chicken flavour. These differences may be directional or non-directional. A typical question in a directional test would be, 'Which sample is tougher?'. Here the method requires at least seven experts or 20 selected assessors. Again it is necessary to balance the order of presentation of samples A and B as shown in Table 17.1. A typical question for a non-directional test would be, 'Which of these two meat samples do you prefer?' Directional tests are one-sided (one-tailed tests) whereas non-directional tests are two-sided (two-tailed tests).

Van der Marel *et al.* (1989) used a forced choice non-directional preference test to investigate the influence of a lactic acid treatment on the sensory quality of fresh broiler chickens. Twelve broilers were submerged in 1% (v/v) lactic acid (15 s, pH 2.4, 15°C) at three times during processing, i.e. after defeathering, evisceration and air chilling. Controls were treated in a similar fashion using tap water. Carcasses were stored at 0°C for 2 days in trays. Samples of thigh and drumstick were grilled for 30 min (internal muscle temperature not stated), cut into 48 samples per group and served to 12 assessors. Each assessor received in random order one control and one treated thigh and drumstick over two sessions.

The test yielded 22 choices for the treated sample and 26 for the controls where using $P = 0.5$ the expected value would be 32 choices in a particular

Table 17.1. The order of presentation of samples in a paired comparison test.

Assessor	Directional test Presentation order		Non-directional preference test Presentation order	
	Set 1	Set 2	Set 1	Set 2
1	AB	BA	AB	AA
2	BA	BA	BB	BA
3	BA	AB	BA	AB
4	AB	AB	AB	BA
5	BA	AB	AA	BB
6	AB	BA	BB	AA
7	AB	AB	AB	BB
8	BA	BA	AA	AB
9	BA	AB	BB	AB
10	BA	BA	AA	BA

direction. Therefore it was concluded that the lactic acid treatment did not affect the eating quality of the chickens.

Triangular test (BS5929: part 3, 1984; ISO 4120-1983)

This test is used for revealing slight differences between samples and can also be used in selecting and training of assessors. Three coded samples are presented simultaneously, two are the same and one is different. Assessors are asked to select the odd sample. All six combinations are served (ABB, AAB, ABA, BAA, BBA, BAB), therefore some assessors will receive two samples of A and one of B, whereas some will receive two samples of B and one of A. If the number of assessors is not a multiple of six then it is necessary to present the six sets to each assessor on several occasions. The probability of selecting the correct odd sample by chance alone is 1/3. To analyse the test results, the number of correct replies is compared with those in the reference table and checked to see if the samples are significantly different. To ensure strict statistical validity the 'forced choice' option is used, i.e. assessors are not allowed to state 'no difference'.

Triangular tests are relatively easy to set up, but there are underlying problems that could introduce a bias if account is not taken of sources of variation that could occur as a result of bird to bird variation.

Dickens *et al.* (1994) in their study on the effect of acetic acid dips on cooked breast meat used triangular tests to ascertain whether a difference could be detected in those birds that had received an immersion in an acetic acid dip against controls. In each triad the two duplicate samples were from the same bird. Two methods of preparation were used, a boil in the bag preparation and an oven roast method. All assessments were conducted under red light to mask any appearance differences. Sixty triangles were presented in each cooking method and the results showed that acetic acid prechill water had no adverse effects on the sensory quality of the cooked meat.

Triangular tests are used to detect differences and not specific differences, i.e. 'select the odd sample on the basis of texture'. However, an extended triangular test may be used whereby assessors are asked to select the odd sample and then comment on their reason for selecting the odd sample. Only comments from those assessors who correctly identified the odd sample are taken into account. Triangular tests can also be used in training, selection or monitoring assessors performance in sensory tests.

The criteria for the tests are:

α is the probability of saying that a difference occurs when it does not.
   (probability of selecting an unacceptable assessor)
β is the probability of saying that no difference occurs, when it does.
   (probability of rejecting an acceptable assessor)
P_o is the expected proportion of correct decisions when the samples are identical.
   (maximum proportion of correct decisions ruled as an unacceptable assessor)
P_1 is the expected proportion of correct decisions when the odd sample is

detected (excluding guessing) on half of the total number of occasions.
(minimum proportion of correct decisions ruled as an acceptable assessor)

Figure 17.1 was constructed on the basis that:

$\alpha = 0.05$ $P_o = 0.33$
$\beta = 0.10$ $P_1 = 0.66$

- The chart is used by plotting the results of individual tests on a cumulative basis, e.g. 1 point is awarded for a correct identification, 0 for an incorrect identification.
- If the odd sample in the first test is correct, the point is plotted at co-ordinate 1,1.
- If the second test is correct, the point is plotted at coordinate 2,2.
- If the third test is incorrect, the point is plotted at coordinate 2,3.
- Tests are continued until the points fall either in the region of acceptance or the region of rejection when the tests are terminated.
- If the plot remains in the region of indecision, then testing is continued.

Duo-trio test (BS5929: part 8, 1992; ISO 10399, 1991)
The duo-trio test is an intermediate between the duo (paired) and the trio (triangular) test and is statistically less powerful than the triangle test. In this test the assessor receives one sample marked as a reference sample and two other coded samples and is asked which of the two samples matches the reference sample. The probability of selecting the correct sample by chance is 1/2. The presentation order for the duo-trio test is shown in Table 17.2. The

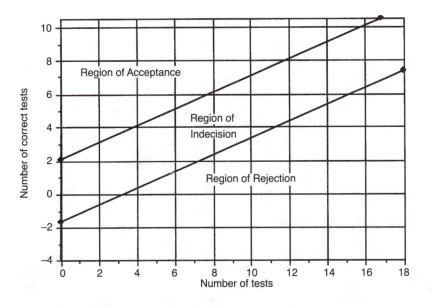

Fig. 17.1. Sequential approach for a triangular test.

Table 17.2. Order of presentation of samples for a duo-trio test.

Assessor	Constant reference technique sample A is the reference sample Presentation order	
	Set 1	Set 2
1	R AB	R BA
2	R BA	R BA
3	R AB	R AB
4	R BA	R AB
5	R AB	R AB
6	R BA	R AB
7	R AB	R BA
8	R BA	R BA
9	R AB	R AB
10	R BA	R AB
11	R AB	R BA
12	R BA	R BA

constant reference technique is most often used when one of the samples is very familiar or is a routinely assessed product.

An alternative method is the 'balanced reference technique' where the reference sample is alternated such that the four combinations are:

A (ref) AB
A (ref) BA
B (ref) AB
B (ref) BA

Janky and Salman (1986) used duo-trio tests to investigate whether there were differences in poultry meat from carcasses that had been water chilled or brine chilled. Chickens, after initial chilling, were cut in half and the portions were assigned to each of the two treatments, either packed in ice or blast frozen. Samples were battered, breaded and deep fried and then allowed to cool overnight. The batter and bread coating was removed and bite sized samples given to a panel of 20 to 25 assessors. Both light and dark meat were assessed in separate trials. It was concluded that panellists were able to distinguish differences between ice-packed and chill-packed products mainly on the basis of texture. Interestingly instrumental shear tests did not reveal this result, therefore there may have been influences other than texture that enabled panellists to distinguish between the samples.

'A' – 'not A' test (BS5929: part 5, 1988; ISO 8588, 1988)
This test is another variation on difference testing and is used for evaluating samples that have variations in appearance (when it is difficult to obtain strictly identical repeat samples), or it can be used as a perception test, to determine the sensitivity of an assessor to a stimulus.

Assessors are asked to taste sample A, the sample is then removed and replaced with an even number of 'A' and 'not A' samples (the numbers of 'A' and 'not A' samples need not be equal). The assessors do not know the number of 'A' and 'not A' samples in the sample set. The number of correct and incorrect responses are recorded for each sample and a contingency table constructed. The chi-squared test is used to determine whether 'A' is recognized in a different way to 'not A'. If equal numbers of 'A' and 'not A' are presented it is possible to use Tables where $p = 1/2$ to assess whether the number of correct identifications of both 'A' and 'not A' are significant. Note that the procedure is slightly different in American standards where assessors are given examples of both 'A' and 'not A'.

Consider the situation where, when using a decontaminant washing procedure, it is thought that the appearance of chicken carcasses may be altered. Assessors are presented with equal numbers of 'A' and 'not A'. Twenty assessors took part in the test and are given five samples of 'A' and five samples of 'not A'. The order of presentation is given in Table 17.3.

Having completed the test, the results are assembled into a 2 × 2 contingency table (Table 17.4). The chi-squared index is calculated using the expression:

$$\chi^2 = \sum_{ij} \frac{(E_0 - E_t)^2}{E_t}$$

where E_o is the observed number in box i,j (in which i is the number of the row and j is the number of the column) and E_t is the theoretical number in the same box given by the ratio of the product of the number from the row and the number from the column to the total number.

In this case the χ^2 index is 12.53 and the critical value 3.84 at 5% risk.

Table 17.3. Order of presentation of samples for the 'A' – 'not A' test.

Assessor	Sample presentation order
1 to 5	A A B B A B A B B A
6 to 10	B A B A A B A A B B
11 to 15	A B A B B A B B A A
16 to 20	B B A A B A B A A B

Table 17.4. A 2 × 2 contingency table for the 'A' – 'not A' test.

Sample identified as	Sample presented		Total
	'A'	'Not A'	
'A'	60	35	95
'Not A'	40	65	105
Total	100	100	200

Therefore, in this case there is a significant difference between 'A' and 'not A' and the conclusion would be that chickens that have undergone a decon-taminant washing procedure could be distinguished on the basis of appearance.

Ranking Tests (BS5929: part 6, 1989; ISO 8587, 1988)

Ranking tests can be used to put samples in order of some predetermined sensory stimulus, e.g. off odour. Ranking tests have the advantage that more than two samples can be compared at the same time, whereas, only two samples can be compared in difference tests. However, the disadvantage is that inexact results can be obtained if the differences are very small or the samples themselves have wide variations between them.

Assessors evaluate a number of samples in random order and are asked to place them in rank order based on a specified criterion, e.g. off odour. Assessors are instructed to avoid tied rankings where possible. Results are then collated and the rank sums for individual samples calculated. For an overall comparison of all the samples the Friedman value F is calculated using the following formula:

$$F = \frac{12}{JP(P+1)} \ (R_1^2 + R_2^2 + \ldots R_P^2) - 3J(P+1)$$

where J is the number of assessors, P is the number of samples, and R_1, R_2 are the rank sums given to P samples for J assessors. If F is equal to or greater than the critical value corresponding to the number of assessors, the number of samples and the selected level of significance, it can be concluded that there is an overall difference between the samples. If an overall difference has been established between samples, the rank sums of each sample can be used to identify the significant differences between sample pairs as follows:

Let i and j be the samples with R_i and R_j their rank sums.
Using the normal approximation, the two samples are different if:
$| R_i - R_j | \geq 1.960 \ \sqrt{JP(P+1)/6}$ for 5% level of probability

Two from Five Test

This is a general difference test which can be more efficient statistically than the triangular test since the probability of correctly guessing the two odd samples is 1/10 compared to the triangular test and paired comparison which are 1/3 and 1/2, respectively. Unfortunately the two from five test can be affected by sensory fatigue and this should be taken into consideration before this procedure is selected.

Basically the test consists of presenting assessors with five samples where three of the samples are A and two are B or three are A and two are B. There are 20 possible combinations of two from five samples as shown in Table 17.5. If the number of assessors are less than twenty it is important to select at

Table 17.5. The 20 possible combinations of samples that can be presented to an assessor in a 'two from five' test.

AAABB	ABABA	BBBAA	BABAB
AABAB	BAABA	BBABA	ABBAB
ABAAB	ABBAA	BABBA	BAABB
BAAAB	BABAA	ABBBA	ABABB
AABBA	BBAAA	BBAAB	AABBB

random from these combinations ensuring that there are an equal number of combinations that contain 3 As and 3 Bs.

Difference testing is relatively easy to set up, but requires careful thought in its execution as assessors will regard the idea of selecting the odd samples as a game of chance. Consequently they will use any information they can gather to obtain what they see as the right answer. This means that appearance factors, e.g. shape of sample, colour etc., must be masked if they are not part of the property under test. Similarly with a hot sample there must be no difference in the temperature of the different products under test. Otherwise there will be a positive response in the test, but the wrong conclusion.

CATEGORY SCALES

Category scales are often used to rate a number of different stimuli, e.g. texture, flavour, juiciness, etc. They have the advantage that they are easy to use and can cover a number of attributes, as well as up to six samples in a session. For the test to be successful it is necessary to have good experimental design. The results are then analysed, using appropriate statistical techniques, for example analysis of variance to establish the differences between and within the samples or Kruskal Wallis one-way analysis of variance by ranks.

There are many applications in poultry research that have used category scales to investigate influences of production, processing methods that could affect eating quality. Griffiths *et al.* (1984) used a combination of *difference from control* intensity ratings for flavour evaluation and an eight point category texture scale for texture in their study of the effect of storage on uneviscerated turkeys. For flavour evaluation assessors were given a labelled control (frozen on day 1) and a test sample and were asked to rate the difference on a 5-point category scale where 0 = no difference and 4 = a large difference. Six samples were assessed on each occasion, one of which was a coded control (internal control). Results showed that flavour differences were very marked after 16 days storage and more so after 24 days storage. Assessors commented that at 16 days flavour terms such as 'strong', livery' and 'gamey' were detected. Storage time had no significant effect on texture .

Sonaiya *et al.* (1990) studied the influence of environmental temperature, dietary energy, age and sex on the eating quality of broilers in Nigeria. They used 7-point category scales for juiciness, tenderness, flavour and overall impression and showed that neither age (up to 54 days), sex, dietary energy nor environmental temperature had an effect on tenderness, but the flavour of meat from birds that were reared at high temperatures (cycling 21 to 30°C diurnally) was more intense than meat from birds reared at low temperatures (constant 21°C).

Self *et al.* (1990) used 8-point category scales in their study on the effects of pressure cooking and cooling (fast or slow) in vacuum on the eating quality of chicken breast. Juiciness decreased with increased pressure and reduced cooling rate.

Raj *et al.* (1992) used 8-point category scales covering the attributes of flavour, texture, juiciness and a hedonic scale of overall liking (liking scales as against acceptability scales imply that the data came from a small group of trained assessors and does not constitute consumer response) to investigate the influence of stunning method on eating quality of early filleted (2 hours) broiler breast. The assessments were done on cold meat and showed that the mean values for texture were significantly different at 4.08, 6.04 and 7.26 for electrically stunned, argon and control (electrically stunned followed by electrical stimulation and then filleted after overnight ageing), respectively.

Berge *et al.* (1997) in their study of meat quality traits in emus (*Dromaius novaehollandiae*) used 10-point category scales to evaluate tenderness, juiciness and flavour in eight different muscles of the emu when grilled to an internal temperature of 60°C. They found that m. iliofibularis and m. iloitibialis cranialis were the most tender and m. gastrocnemius medialis and m. fibularis longus the toughest. The age of the emus and its effect on tenderness was also studied and showed that older birds, 17 months and older, were tougher than younger birds. Juiciness and flavour were not affected by age.

Graphic or Line Scales

Salmon *et al.* (1988) used 15 cm unstructured line scales with anchor points at each end to resolve a conflict in cooking recommendations in cookbooks. Some suggested that turkeys should be cooked breast down whereas others stated they should be cooked breast up. Twenty turkeys were used in the trial. Turkeys were cooked to a standard internal muscle temperature of 85°C. Results showed that there was no difference in the eating quality of breast muscle but the dark meat had increased flavour and tenderness.

In another trial on cooking effects, Oltrogge and Prusa (1987) used variable-power microwave cooking to investigate influences of cooking on eating quality characteristics. Assessors scored attributes of tenderness, juiciness, mealiness and chicken flavour on 15 cm unstructured line scales labelled at each end with the extremes of each characteristic. They further indicated how each attribute was described. Tenderness was the force to compress the samples with the molars, mealiness was the ease of sample fragmentation during sustained chewing and juiciness was the amount of expressed fluid during chewing. Chicken flavour intensity was not defined. Chicken breasts were cooked to 82°C internal muscle temperature at either 100%, 80%, 60% or 40% power in a 600 W microwave. Results showed that cooking at 60% power produced the most tender chicken and this was also correlated with Instron compression values which were the lowest in this group. There were no significant differences in the other sensory attributes.

Caron *et al.* (1990), in their study of Japanese quail selected for body mass at 45 days, used 15 cm line scales with anchor points 1.5 cm from each end to assess flavour, juiciness and tenderness. They concluded that there was no effect of sex on eating quality but there were differences in juiciness and tenderness between some of the selection lines used.

A similar approach was used by Chambers *et al.* (1989) to compare the sensory properties between different stocks of broilers differing in growth and fatness. Both dark meat and white meat were assessed for flavour, juiciness, tenderness and overall acceptability. In this study, there were significant differences between panel days which were attributed to differences in carcasses within treatment. There were also large variations in sensory properties observed between judges which were attributed to tendencies among judges to use different parts or portions of the scale. These differences were accounted for in the statistical analysis by including a model term for assessors and effectively removing assessor effect from the analysis. Results showed that faster-growing modern broilers had meat that was either similar or had higher values for texture, juiciness etc. than the experimental strain broilers of similar age. Dark meat also showed a similar trend. Fatter carcasses had more flavour, were juicier and had more tender dark meat; the white meat was also juicier.

Whether to use category scales or line scales to measure 'gross' changes is a matter of choice and will depend on the type of panel and the training that has been done in setting up the panel. Lawless and Malone (1986) compared four types of rating scales, 9-point category, line marking, magnitude estimation and a hybrid of the category and line scale for their ability to discriminate differences among products, for variability, reliability and ease of use. Using consumers who by definition are untrained, it was shown that there was a modest advantage in using category scales in almost all the comparisons. However, all approaches were able to generate significant differences among the products tested.

Sensory Profile Methods (BS5929: part 4, 1986 and ISO 11035, 1994)

There are various ways of carrying out descriptive analysis of foods and there are two basic methods of profiling. In the fixed choice method, the assessors each develop a vocabulary to describe the food under test. One of the assessors acts as panel leader and their task is to discuss the words generated by the other assessors so that a consensus can be agreed. The agreed set of descriptors is then used to describe the food.

The free-choice method involves the assessors being given the likely range of samples during a number of training sessions to derive a profile that is unique to them. The assessors then use this profile to describe the foods in the experiment. In both these methods, it is important that the experiments are well designed statistically since if they are not it is unlikely that meaningful results will be obtained.

A fixed profile using the descriptors shown in Table 17.6 was developed for cold roast turkey breast. Over a number of training sessions assessors were presented with examples of turkey from the range of treatments under test, the identities of the treatments were unknown to the assessors.

The objective was to establish if there were texture differences in turkey breast meat from turkeys (22 weeks old) that had been either electrically stunned or anoxia stunned (argon-induced anoxia). This approach by Raj and Nute (1995) showed that there were differences in the characteristics of texture attributes caused by the stunning method. Using a multivariate approach, the first two principal components accounted for 59% of the total variation and the third, 10%. The first dimension was a contrast between tender, powdery, firm and fibrous samples and the second dimension a contrast of between dry and moist samples. The principal component scores, which represent sample plots based on all the descriptive terms used, showed that there were differences in texture between anoxia and electrically stunned turkeys. Comparing the loadings plot with the scores plot showed that anoxia stunned turkeys were more tender and powdery than electrically stunned turkeys, which were firmer on cutting and more fibrous on eating.

A more complex texture profile was developed by Lyon and Lyon (1990) in their study of post-mortem deboning time (5 min, 2 h, 6 h, 24 h) and two

Table 17.6. Line scales used in a sensory profile of cold turkey breast meat. Each line was 100 mm in length where the left hand anchor point is nil and the right anchor point extreme (after Raj and Nute, 1995).

Descriptor	Definitions
On cutting	Cut along the grain
Firmness	Perceived force required to cut the samples with a knife
Layers	Degree of disintegration on cutting
Moisture	Moistness visible on cutting
Initial mouthfeel	Press the sample gently against the palate
Dry	Dryness
Moisture	Moistness
Clammy	Possible dampness, slipperiness
On eating	
Tender	Texture, tough to tender
Moisture	Internal moisture in chewing
Slimy	Slippery feel
Fibres	Fibres evident during mastication
Stringy	Long fibres or groups of fibres
Sticky	Adhesiveness to teeth on chewing the sample
Residue	
Pulpy	Moist bulky feel
Crumby	Non-cohesive particles, either soft, moist or dry
Powdery	Dry fine particles

cooking methods (water cooked in heat-and-seal bags and micowave cooking) on broiler breast meat. The texture profile consisted of 17 attributes (marked on 10 cm line scales) that were arranged in four stages that represented stages in the mastication process. At each stage assessors were given instructions of how the assessment should be determined as shown in Table 17.7.

The results from this study showed that for all sensory attributes except residual particles there were significant differences between the 5 min and 2 h treatments and the 6 h and 24 h treatments. By texture profile analysis the microwave meat was more cohesive and chewy than waterbath prepared meat.

A similar profile by the same authors (Lyon and Lyon, 1993) but with an extra three sensory texture terms (Stage 1, wetness; Stage 2, rate of break-down; Stage 3, persistence of moisture release) investigated the effect of deboning time and cooking method on the texture characteristics of broiler meat. The results showed that after factor analysis of the sensory data, the first two factors explained 84% of the variation. Factor one (64%) was essentially concerned with mechanical and geometrical characteristics (hardness, chewiness, fibrousness and particle size) and separated samples on the basis of post-mortem deboning time, whereas factor two (20%) was concerned with moisture characteristics and discriminated samples on the basis of cooking method.

Lyon and Lyon (1997) used the above texture profile to explore the relationship between a sensory descriptive profile and shear values (Warner-Bratzler and Allo-Kramer) in deboned poultry meat. Chicken breasts that were deboned at 2, 6, and 24 h were prepared as this would provide a range of texture characteristics. The sensory descriptive terms were split into five clusters after undergoing cluster analyses. Cluster 1 was related to mechanical characteristics of texture; cluster 2 was related to moisture; cluster 3 was related to chewdown characteristics of meat; clusters 4 and 5 were related to saliva and residual characteristics. There were clear differences in texture between 2 h, 6 h and 24 h fillets. The mechanical characteristics, excluding breakdown, in

Table 17.7. Stages in the process of assessing broiler breast meat during mastication (after Lyon and Lyon, 1990).

Stage 1	Place the sample between molars. Compress slowly, for three cycles without biting through the sample. Assess the attribute, springiness
Stage 2	Place the sample between molars. Bite through the sample, not more than six cycles using the rate of one chew per second. Assess the attributes, initial cohesiveness, hardness, initial juiciness
Stage 3	Place the sample between the molars. Chew at the rate of one chew per second and at 15 to 25 chews assess the attributes below. Hardness, cohesiveness of mass, saliva produced, particle size and shape, fibrousness, chewiness, chew count, bolus size, bolus wetness.
Stage 4	Evaluate the following at the point the sample is swallowed. Ease of swallow, residual particles, toothpack, mouth coating.

cluster 1 were highly related to both shear values produced by Warner-Bratzler and Allo-Kramer, $r > 0.75$. The overall conclusion was that meat texture is highly complex and instrumental methods will provide only one dimension of texture, that which is involved in mechanical breakdown. Sensory perception of texture also includes many other aspects that as yet cannot be related to instrumental methods. Therefore instrumental measurements of texture should be looked at together with sensory descriptive profiles to provide a fuller picture of the texture characteristics of poultry meat.

Probably one of the most challenging areas of sensory analysis is concerned with flavour. In the red meat area it is known that texture will dominate the overall judgement of meat and only when the meat is tender does flavour play an important role (Dransfield et al., 1984).

Much of the work on flavour is related to the identification of off-flavours or taints. Land (1980) reviewed the many flavours and taints found in poultry meat and game birds. He made the important point that flavour and taints are perceived via the stimulation of olfactory cells in the nose and gustatory cells in the mouth by the chemicals present in the food. However, the flavour or taint is measured in the human as a response not necessarily as the concentrations of specific chemical present in the food. He stated that much of the sensory work on flavour was flawed as it involved the use of hedonic data which caused the misinterpretation of results or produced misleading information as the wrong methodology was applied. However, studies on the systematic evaluation of chicken flavour by a trained descriptive sensory panel are comparatively rare.

Lyon (1987) used chicken patties as a vehicle to develop descriptive terms for profiling the taste and aroma of fresh and reheated chicken meat. Initially, panellists were allowed free choice to describe the character notes perceived and this resulted in an initial set of 45 terms. These terms were used to describe the flavour of freshly cooked patties and patties reheated after 1, 3 and 5 days. Multiple analysis of variance (Manova) showed that differences in test samples existed in the overall data set of 45 terms. Further examination of the panellists' individual use of the terms reduced the list to 31 adjectives. Factor analysis was then applied as a means of grouping terms together according to the newly created factors. Of the 31 terms, eight factors were extracted that explained 77% of the variation in the data. These were further reduced after discussions with panellists and further factor analysis, plus verification of the redundant terms by variable cluster analysis and stepwise discriminate analysis to the 12 terms and definitions shown in Table 17.8. This profile was used to study the changes in broiler tissues (breast, thigh, skin) due to cooking, storage (1, 2, 3 and 5 days) and reheating (Lyon, 1993). Each storage time was compared with a freshly cooked control. Changes were mapped using factor analysis. Stored breast muscles were significantly different from control at each storage time for all descriptors except meaty and liver, organy. Thigh muscles were also significantly different from controls except for bitter and metallic descriptors. In skin, which was evaluated by aroma only, significant differences between control and stored were noted except for the terms, meaty and liver, organy.

Table 17.8. Terms used for profiling the taste and aroma of fresh and reheated chicken meat (after Lyon, 1987).

Descriptive term	Definition
	Aromatic, taste sensation associated with:
Chickeny	Cooked white chicken muscle
Meaty	Cooked dark chicken muscle
Brothy	Chicken stock
Liver, organy	Liver, serum or blood vessels
Browned	Roasted, grilled or broiled chicken patties (not seared, blackened or burned)
Burned	Excessive heating or browning (scorched, seared, charred)
Cardboard, musty	Cardboard, paper, mould or mildew: described as nutty, stale
Warmed-over	Reheated meat; not newly cooked nor rancid, painty
Rancid, painty	Oxidized fat and linseed oil
	Primary taste associated with:
Sweet	Sucrose, sugar
Bitter	Quinine or caffeine
	Feeling factor on tongue associated with:
Metallic	iron or copper ions

In all profile studies it is generally helpful if the definitions used by the assessors are published together with an exact description of the cooking procedure and endpoint temperatures used. This enables workers to compare their work in relation to other published profiles.

Descriptive analysis depends on obtaining objective descriptions in terms of perceived sensory attributes, therefore language will play an important role in determining the accuracy of a set of descriptions. However, this is often given scant attention despite its importance (Civille and Lawless, 1986).

Training is often time consuming and expensive, therefore it is of considerable advantage if existing profiles are accurately described and published so that other workers in the field can use them as a starting point for their studies. However, there is no guarantee that the words will be used by a new panel in the same way.

CONCLUSION

Sensory analysis is an important analytical tool in obtaining hard evidence of how a food, in this case poultry, is perceived by humans.

There are very different sensory procedures that are used to obtain sensory information, but they all have one thing in common, that is, the requirement that the assessors have been screened for their basic sensory ability. Without this any results obtained will be open to question.

It is a powerful tool in establishing how different diets, processing, packaging, storage time etc. affect poultry quality. Sensory analysis is concerned with objective findings and it is not to be confused with consumer testing which is mainly concerned with preference.

REFERENCES

Berge, P., Lepetit, J., Renerre, M. and Touraille, C. (1997) Meat quality traits in emu (*Dromaius novaehollandiae*) as affected by muscle type and animal age. *Meat Science* 45, 209–221.

BSI Design of test rooms for sensory analysis of food. BS7183 (1989) British Standards Institution, Milton Keynes, UK.

BSI Sensory analysis of food. Part 2. Paired comparison test. BS5929 (1982) British Standards Institution, Milton Keynes, UK.

BSI Sensory analysis of food. Part 3. Triangle test. BS5929 (1984) British Standards Institution, Milton Keynes, UK.

BSI Sensory analysis of food. Part 4. Flavour profile methods. BS5929 (1985) British Standards Institution, Milton Keynes, UK.

BSI Sensory analysis of food. Part 6. Ranking. BS5929 (1989) British Standards Institution, Milton Keynes, UK.

BSI Sensory analysis of food. Part 8. Duo-trio test. BS5929 (1992) British Standards Institution, Milton Keynes, UK.

Caron, N., Monvielle, F., Desmarais, M. and Poste, L.M. (1990) Mass selection for 45 day body weight in Japanese quail: selection response, carcass composition, cooking properties, and sensory characteristics. *Poultry Science* 69, 1037–1045.

Chambers, J.R., Fortin, A., Mackie, D.A. and Lamond, E. (1989) Comparison of sensory properties of meat from broilers of modern stocks and experimental strains differing in growth and fatness. *Canadian Institute of Food Science and Technology Journal* 4, 353–358.

Civille, G.V and Lawless, H.T. (1986) The importance of language in describing perceptions. *Journal of Sensory Studies* 3/4, 203–215.

Dickens, J.A., Lyon, B.G., Whittemore, A.D. and Lyon, C.E. (1994) The effect of an acetic acid dip on carcass appearance, microbiological quality and cooked breast meat texture and flavour. *Poultry Science* 73, 576–581.

Dransfield, E., Nute, G.R., Roberts, T.A., Boccard, R., Touraille, C., Buchter, L., Casteels, M., Cosentino, E., Hood, D.E., Joseph, R.L., Schon, I. and Paardekooper, E.J.C. (1984) Beef quality assessed at European research centres. *Meat Science* 10, 1–20.

Griffiths, N.M., Mead, G.C., Jones, J.M. and Grey, T.C. (1984) Effect of storage on meat quality in uneviscerated turkeys held at 4°C. *British Poultry Science* 25, 259–266.

International Standard (ISO 11035) (1994) Sensory analysis. Identification and selection of descriptors for establishing a sensory profile by a multidimensional approach. International Organisation for Standardisation, Geneva, Switzerland.

Janky, D.M. and Salman, H.K. (1986) Influence of chill packaging and brine chilling on physical and sensory characteristics of broiler meat. *Poultry Science* 65, 1934–1938.

Jones, J.M. and Griffiths, N.M. (1981) The assessment of the eating quality of chicken meat. In: Quality of poultry meat, *Proceedings of the Fifth European Symposium on Poultry Meat Quality.* Apeldon 17–23 May, pp. 248–253.

Land, D.G. (1980) Flavours and taint in poultry meat and game birds. In: *Meat Quality in Poultry and Game Birds.* British Poultry Science Ltd, Edinburgh, UK, pp. 17–30.

Lawless, H.T and Malone, G.J. (1986) The discriminative efficiency of common scaling methods. *Journal of Sensory Studies* 1, 85–98.

Lyon, B.G. (1987) Development of chicken flavour descriptive attribute terms aided by multivariate statistical procedures. *Journal of Sensory Studies* 2, 55–67.

Lyon, B.G. (1993) Sensory profile changes in broiler tissues due to cooking, storage and reheating. *Poultry Science* 72, 1981–1988.

Lyon, B.G. and Lyon, C.E. (1990) Texture profile of broiler pectoralis major as influenced by post-mortem deboning time and heat method. *Poultry Science* 69, 329–340.

Lyon, B.G and Lyon, C.E. (1993) Effects of water-cooking in heat sealed bags versus conveyor belt grilling on yield, moisture and texture of broiler breast meat. *Poultry Science* 2, 2157–2165.

Lyon, B.G. and Lyon, C.E. (1997) Sensory descriptive profile relationships to shear values of deboned poultry. *Journal of Food Science* 62, 885–897.

Mead, G.C. (1987) Recommendations for a standardised method of sensory analysis for broilers. A Report of Working Group 5 – Poultry Meat Quality – of the European Federation of WPSA branches. *Worlds Poultry Science Journal* 43, 64–68.

Meilgaard, M.C., Civille, G.V. and Carr, B.T. (1991) Controls for test room, product and panel. In: *Sensory Evaluation Techniques*. CRC Press, Boca Raton, USA, pp. 23–36.

Nally, C.L. (1987) Implementation of consumer taste panels. *Journal of Sensory Studies* 2, 77–83.

Oltrogge, M.H. and Prusa, K.J. (1987) Research note: sensory analysis and Instron measurements of variable power microwave heated baking hen breasts. *Poultry Science* 66, 1548–1551.

Raj, A.B.M. and Nute, G.R. (1995) Effect of stunning method and filleting time on sensory profile of turkey breast meat. *British Poultry Science* 36, 221–227.

Raj, A.B.M., Nute, G.R., Wotton, S.B. and Baker, A. (1992) Sensory evaluation of breast fillets from argon-stunned and electrically stimulated broiler carcasses processed under commercial conditions. *British Poultry Science* 33, 963–971.

Salmon, R.E., Stevens, V.I., Poste, L.M., Agar, V. and Butler, G. (1988) Research note: Effect of roasting breast up or breast down and dietary canola meal on the sensory quality of turkeys. *Poultry Science* 67, 680–683.

Self, K.P., Nute, G.R., Burfoot, D. and Moncrieff, C.B. (1990) Effect of pressure cooking and pressure rate change during cooling in vacuum on chicken breast quality and yield. *Journal of Food Science* 6, 1531–1551.

Sonaiya, E.B., Ristic, M. and Klein, F.W. (1990) Effect of environmental temperature, dietary energy, age and sex on broiler carcass portions and palatability. *British Poultry Science* 31, 121–128.

Van Der Marel, G.M., De Vries, A.W., Van Logtestijn, J.G. and Mossel, D.A.A. (1989) Effect of lactic acid treatment during processing on the sensory quality and lactic acid content of fresh broiler chickens. *International Journal of Food Science and Technology* 24, 11–16.

CHAPTER *18*
Functional properties of muscle proteins in processed poultry products

A.B. Smyth[2], E. O'Neill[2] and D.M. Smith[1]
[1]Department of Food Science and Human Nutrition, Michigan State University, East Lansing, MI 48824-1224, USA; [2]Department of Food Chemistry, University College, Cork, Ireland

INTRODUCTION

Proteins are the principal structural and functional components in many food systems. Kinsella (1976) defined protein functionality as any physicochemical property which affects the processing and behaviour of proteins in food systems as judged by the quality attributes of the final product. More recently, functionality has been defined as the behavioural features of a food identifiable by human senses as relevant to quality (Dickinson and McClements, 1996).

Protein functionality is influenced by structural features and molecular properties of proteins (e.g. hydrophobicity, surface charge, sulphydryl content, molecular weight, conformational stability and association/dissociation behaviour). Furthermore, processing conditions, environmental factors (e.g. pH, ionic strength) and interactions with other components affect the functional behaviour of proteins in food systems (Kinsella, 1976).

Functional properties determine the usefulness of a protein and its impact on final product quality. The functional properties required of a protein or a mixture of proteins varies with the particular food system in question and the stage of processing. In further processed poultry products, water binding, fat binding, solubility, viscosity and emulsification, are the principal functional properties required in raw meat products (Smith, 1988). Heat-induced gelation, water binding and fat binding are some of the important functional properties in cooked meat products. By understanding the mechanism and the key factors which influence muscle protein functionality, it may be possible to manipulate product formulation and processing conditions to improve the quality of existing further-processed poultry products and to produce new products.

This chapter will provide an overview of the functional requirements of processed poultry meat products and the properties muscle proteins impart to these food systems. The chapter will conclude with a focused discussion on the mechanism of action of myosin in processed poultry products.

INTERACTIONS OF MUSCLE PROTEINS IN MEAT BATTERS

Meat batters formed during the preparation of comminuted poultry products, such as sausages, bologna and frankfurters, can be described as complex multiphasic systems consisting of solubilized muscle proteins, muscle fibres, fat cells, fat droplets, water, salt and other ingredients (Gordon and Barbut, 1992a). Two theories have been proposed to explain fat stabilization in meat batters. The first, referred to as the emulsion theory, is based on the formation of an interfacial protein film around the fat globules that stabilizes the fat phase during processing. The other, referred to as the physical entrapment theory, postulates that the fat particles in meat batters are physically entrapped within the highly viscous protein matrix prior to heating and then within a gel matrix after thermal processing (Morrissey *et al.*, 1987; Gordon and Barbut, 1992a).

The Emulsion Theory

A classical emulsion consists of two immiscible liquid phases, one of which is dispersed in the form of a colloidal suspension (Dickinson, 1992). Emulsions are thermodynamically unstable because the free energy of the dispersion is higher than that of the separated liquid phases. Proteins are amphiphilic molecules and are used in many food systems as emulsion stabilizers. They have the ability to adsorb at interfaces, form continuous protein films surrounding lipid droplets and reduce interfacial tension (Dickinson, 1992).

Meat batters have traditionally been viewed as emulsion-type systems (Schut, 1976) even though they do not possess all the properties of a classical oil-in-water emulsion. Except for finely comminuted products, fat droplets in meat batters are generally greater than 1 μm and are beyond the colloidal size range of oil droplets found in true emulsions (Dickinson, 1992). At several stages during processing, temperatures are low enough that the fat is partially crystallized and not liquid as in a true emulsion. Also, in many coarse-cut products, fat is still primarily contained within intact fat cells. Nonetheless, raw meat batters have some characteristics which resemble an emulsion and thus the term meat emulsion is still used to describe these systems.

The microstructure of raw meat batters varies depending on the selection of raw ingredients, processing equipment and comminution temperature and time (Smith, 1988). Photomicrographs of raw and cooked batters show a proteinaceous membrane surrounding the lipid particles (Borchert *et al.*, 1967; Gordon and Barbut, 1990). However, not all fat particles are of uniform size or uniformly surrounded by a protein film. Furthermore, the properties of the interfacial protein films in emulsions are greatly affected by the physicochemical properties of the emulsifying protein, the environmental conditions and the method of emulsion formation (Morrissey *et al.*, 1987; Dickinson, 1992).

The myofibrillar proteins play an important role in interfacial film formation in meat batters. Timed emulsification studies showed that myosin is rapidly taken up at the fat–aqueous interface followed by actomyosin, troponin, tropomyosin and actin (Galluzzo and Regenstein, 1978a, b). In model systems, myosin forms finely divided, viscous emulsions which are considered more stable than the coarse thin emulsions produced by actin. Photomicrographs show that myosin-stabilized emulsions consist of small globules of uniform size which show little change on cooking. Actin-stabilized emulsions are composed of larger globules of a greater size range, which often undergo coalescence on cooking (Tsai *et al.*, 1972; Galluzzo and Regenstein, 1978a). Emulsions stabilized by actomyosin are not as fine as myosin emulsions and seem to have some characteristics of both actin and myosin emulsions. In a more recent study, Gordon and Barbut (1992b) confirmed that myosin and actomyosin are the major proteins involved in interfacial film formation in meat batters.

Transmission electron micrographs produced by Gordon and Barbut (1990) provide evidence for the multilayer nature of the protein film of some meat batters. Borchert *et al.* (1967) showed that small holes or pores exist in the interfacial protein film of cooked meat products. Jones and Mandigo (1982) found a large number of pores in the protein film surrounding large fat globules and several smaller fat droplets in the vicinity of these pores. The myofibrillar proteins involved in interfacial protein film formation begin to denature at about 43–45°C (Wang *et al.*, 1990; Xiong, 1992). Therefore, the film becomes semi-rigid during thermal processing of meat batters to 60–70°C. Jones and Mandigo (1982) postulated that the pores in the film act as pressure release valves that allow expansion of fat during cooking without disrupting the interfacial protein film. Based on evidence provided by scanning electron micrographs of cooked meat batters, Gordon and Barbut (1990) suggested that fat pushes through the film at points of weakness and forms spherical stable appendages. These break off to form smaller, round globules with the same type of film as the parent globule. However, there is not enough protein left at the breakpoint of the initial droplet to properly seal the gap and hence pores or indentations form. The authors observed several small uniform pockets of exuded fat in stable batters. In contrast, large fat exudations which are more likely to form fat channels and facilitate fat coalescence were observed in unstable batters.

It is to noteworthy that coarse-cut sausage products, such as salami, seldom experience 'fatting out' problems. This is probably due to the lack of extensive rupture of fat cells, which allows the intact fat cell membranes to prevent fat coalescence.

Physical Entrapment Theory

The physical entrapment theory proposes that the fat phase in meat batters is stabilized by physical entrapment within a viscous protein matrix prior to heating and within a three-dimensional protein gel matrix after heating (Morrissey *et al.*, 1987; Gordon and Barbut, 1992a). During the preparation of meat batters, muscle is comminuted in the presence of added salt and water. This causes disruption of the muscle tissue, facilitates protein solubilization and swelling of muscle fibres, leading to increases in the viscosity of the mix. The viscosity developed in the continuous phase of a raw batter helps to stabilize the dispersed fat by physically retarding coalescence. During thermal processing, myofibrillar proteins in the continuous phase undergo con- formational changes leading to the formation of a three-dimensional gel matrix which physically entraps water and the fat particles (Morrissey *et al.*, 1987; Gordon and Barbut, 1992a).

Gordon and Barbut (1990) observed that many fat globules were bound to the continuous protein matrix via the interfacial protein film. Studies using transmission electron microscopy have illustrated that there was continuity between the protein film around fat globules and the surrounding protein gel matrix at several points on their circumference (Gordon and Barbut, 1990). It is therefore logical to assume that cooking increases the immobilization of globules due to network formation between the protein film and the protein gel matrix within the continuous phase, thereby further stabilizing these globules and preventing coalescence. Gordon and Barbut (1990) suggested that the lacy structures often seen on the surface of fat globules in scanning electron micrographs are remnants of the thread-like connections between the matrix proteins and the interfacial protein film.

During thermal processing, poultry fat is liquefied between about 13 and 33°C (Findlay and Barbut, 1990). Although the thermal transition of myosin from sol-to-gel begins at about 50°C, maximum gel strength is not reached until 60°C or above (Wu *et al.*, 1991; Wang and Smith, 1994b). Therefore, fat liquefaction occurs before optimal gel strength is achieved. Thus, the protein film surrounding the fat droplets and high viscosity of the continuous phase may help stabilize meat batters, at least during the early stages of cooking (Barbut, 1995).

Smith (1988) suggested that both emulsification and physical entrapment may be important in certain processed products; an interfacial protein film may stabilize fat droplets of highly comminuted products during pumping and holding of raw product, whereas physical entrapment may be more important in coarse-cut sausages prior to cooking and in all further-processed poultry products during and after cooking. The relative contribution of each factor also depends on environmental factors (e.g. pH and ionic strength), physical state of the fat phase (e.g. fat particle size, the melting point of the fat), the temperature history of the lean phase and processing conditions (e.g. final chopping temperature) (Schut, 1976; Gordon and Barbut, 1992a). Although the relative importance of these two mechanisms to fat stabilization in meat batters is not yet clearly understood, current evidence strongly favours the physical entrapment model as the primary mechanism of meat batter stabilization in processed poultry products.

MYOFIBRILLAR PROTEINS

It is well established that in muscle, the myofibrillar proteins are primarily responsible for the functional properties of both raw and cooked further-processed poultry meat products. Furthermore, of the myofibrillar proteins, myosin is the most important functional protein (Samejima *et al.*, 1969, 1982; Yasui *et al.*, 1980). In raw products, solubilized myosin plays a role in the increased viscosity observed during chopping and is a major component of the interfacial protein film seen around fat droplets (Barbut, 1995). Myosin is the only myofibrillar protein to form a gel during heating, so it is largely responsible for producing the characteristic texture, appearance and stability of cooked products. The other myofibrillar proteins, such as actin, can modify the functional properties of myosin in both raw and cooked systems (Wang and Smith, 1994b, 1995).

The role of myosin in the stability of raw meat batters is understood only on an empirical basis. Barbut (1995) has prepared an excellent review on this subject. More work is needed to uncover the molecular mechanisms responsible for comminuted meat batter stability. Many product failures caused by 'emulsion breakdown' occur during commercial production of comminuted poultry products due to our incomplete understanding of the chemistry of proteins in raw batters.

The heat-induced gelation process of myosin appears to be the single most important step in the production of a consistently uniform and high quality processed poultry product. Recent work has focused on determining the molecular mechanisms that occur during thermal processing of poultry products. Consequently, the remainder of this chapter reviews the biochemical and functional properties of poultry muscle myosin during gel matrix formation. These findings should ultimately lead to a greater understanding of changes occurring within a meat batter during cooking and contribute to better control of the manufacturing process.

BIOCHEMICAL PROPERTIES OF SKELETAL MUSCLE MYOSIN

Muscle proteins are generally classified into three groups: sarcoplasmic proteins, stroma proteins and myofibrillar proteins. The myofibrillar proteins are the largest fraction of proteins in skeletal muscle tissue, constituting 52–56% of total muscle proteins and are composed of up to 20 distinct proteins. They are subclassified into three groups based on their functions: contractile proteins, regulatory proteins and cytoskeletal or scaffold proteins (Goll, 1977). Myofibrillar or salt-soluble proteins have frequently been defined as those muscle proteins insoluble in water but soluble in 0.6–1.0 M salt. However, some of the cytoskeletal proteins are large molecules and are insoluble (Goll, 1977).

Myosin and actin are the principal contractile proteins, accounting for 45% and 20% of the total myofibrillar proteins, respectively (Pearson and Young, 1989). Myosin has three important intrinsic properties which allow it to play a key role in muscle contraction. First, at physiological ionic strength and pH, 200–400 myosin molecules aggregate spontaneously to form filaments (Bendall, 1973). Secondly, myosin possesses ATPase activity which provides the energy required to drive muscle contraction. Thirdly, myosin binds to F-actin and hence is involved in cross-bridge formation between thick and thin filaments during muscle contraction. The ability of myosin to form filaments and to bind with actin has a large influence on the functional properties of myosin. The regulatory myofibrillar proteins, troponin and tropomyosin control the actin–myosin interaction during muscle contraction and relaxation. The cytoskeletal or scaffold proteins (e.g. C-protein, α-actinin, titin, desmin and nebulin) support and maintain the highly organized structure of the sarcomere (Pearson and Young, 1989). In postrigor meat, myosin, F-actin, tropomyosin and troponin form a complex referred to as natural actomyosin. Synthetic actomyosin can be produced in the laboratory when pure myosin and actin are mixed *in vitro.* This complex has a high viscosity and when solubilized during comminution, is largely responsible for the increased viscosity of the meat batter.

Myosin has two globular heads attached at one end of a long helical tail (Bailey, 1982) (Fig. 18.1). Due to the complex structure of myosin it has biochemical properties of both globular and fibrous proteins. Myosin has an isoelectric point of 5.3 which reflects its high content of aspartic and glutamic acid residues (Harrington, 1979; Pearson and Young, 1989). Native myosin has no disulphide bonds. Chicken myosin, like other skeletal myosins, contains 43 sulphydryl groups, one of which is buried inside the native molecule (Smyth, 1996). Rabbit skeletal myosin has a molecular mass of 521 kDa (Yates and Greaser, 1983).

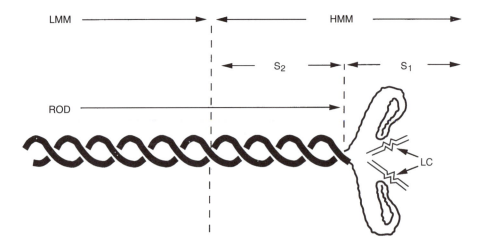

Fig. 18.1. Schematic diagram of the myosin molecule; HMM, heavy meromyosin; LC light chains; LMM light meromyosin; S2 subfragment 2; S1 subfragment 1.

Skeletal muscle myosin consists of six polypeptide chains (Lowey *et al.*, 1969). Two of these chains are referred to as myosin heavy chains, each with a molecular mass of 200–220 kDa. Approximately half of each myosin heavy chain starting at the C-terminal is α-helical in conformation. The helical regions of the myosin heavy chains wind around each other in a right-handed twist forming a double-stranded super coiled-coil (Lowey *et al.*, 1969). This part of the myosin molecule is involved in filament assembly and is referred to as the tail or rod portion of myosin. The interactions between the helices are governed by the packing of the side chains, those of one helix fitting into gaps between those of the other (McLachlan and Karn, 1982). The primary sequence of the rod has a heptapeptide repeating pattern (a-b-c-d-e-f-g) of coiled-coil structures where residues a and d are hydrophobic and form the interfaces between the α-helices in the folded protein. The helix surface is highly charged, with acidic and basic residues clustered mainly in the outer positions (b, c and f) (McLachlan and Karn, 1982).

At the N-terminal end of each myosin heavy chain a globular head region exists which possesses both enzymatic activity and actin binding ability. Associated with each globular head are two pairs of light chains (LC). There are two chemical classes of LC, designated essential or non-essential for ATPase activity. The non-essential LC are called DTNB LC (molecular mass ~18 kDa), since they are dissociated from the myosin molecule by the sulphydryl reagent 5,5′-dithiobis(2-nitrobenzoate) (Weeds and Lowey, 1971). The DTNB LC are not essential for ATPase activity, but affect the calcium-binding ability of myosin. They can be phosphorylated by a specific myosin LC kinase and are also referred to as regulatory LC or LC-2 (Adelstein and Eisenberg, 1980). Treatment of myosin with alkali solution (pH 11) causes dissociation of the remaining two non-phosphorylated LC which are referred to as the alkali LC and are essential for ATPase activity. These LC are designated alkali LC-1 (~ 22 kDa) and alkali LC-3 (~16 kDa). LC-1 and LC-3 have common amino acid sequences over their C-terminal 142 residues. The size difference is caused by an additional 41 amino acids present at the N-terminal end of LC-1 (Frank and Weeds, 1974). Both LC-1 and LC-3 contain one sulphydryl group, whereas each LC-2 contains two sulphydryl groups (Gazith *et al.*, 1970). The LC pattern in myosin from different muscle sources varies considerably. Poultry myosin extracted from vertebrate skeletal muscles with a fast twitch response (e.g. m. pectoralis) contain LC-1, LC-2 and LC-3, whereas myosin in slow twitch muscle (e.g. gastrocnemius) contains LC-1 and LC-2 (Liu and Foegeding, 1996).

Sequence homologies (percentage of identical amino acids) in myosin are greater between chicken embryonic m. pectoralis and rabbit skeletal myosin than between chicken cardiac and chicken gizzard myosin. This suggests that the amino acid substitutions in myosin reflect the type of muscle fibre (e.g. skeletal versus smooth) rather than species differences (Hayashida *et al.*, 1991; Komine *et al.*, 1991).

Much information on the structure and function of myosin has been gained by studying fragments obtained after treating the molecule with proteolytic enzymes, such as papain, trypsin and chymotrypsin (Lowey *et al.*, 1969). There are two main proteinase-sensitive regions in myosin. A region in the tail which lacks α-helical conformation is susceptible to proteolysis by trypsin. Trypsin cleaves the molecule into a heavy meromyosin fragment (HMM) (350 kDa), containing both globular heads and a portion of the helical tail. The remaining fragment is almost 100% α-helical and is known as light meromyosin (LMM) (150 kDa). Under controlled conditions, HMM can be cleaved into two additional subfragments at a second susceptible proteolytic region called the 'hinge,' producing the two globular heads, each termed subfragment-1 (S-1); (molecular mass 120 kDa) and the short helical region of HMM, known as subfragment-2 (S-2). The molecular mass of S-2 can vary from 35 kDa (short S-2) to 100 kDa (long S-2) depending on the experimental conditions used to isolate it (Sutoh *et al.*, 1978; Margossian and Lowey, 1982). Papain can also cleave the myosin molecule at the 'hinge' region producing S-1 and the entire tail/rod region, which can then be split into LMM and S-2 using trypsin (Lowey *et al.*, 1969). Borejdo (1983) showed that the surface hydrophobicity of myosin is confined to the head region. There are 1.34 surface hydrophobic sites per mole of myosin or per mole of double-headed HMM, indicating that S-1 may play a critical role in the functionality of myosin.

PROTEIN GELATION

A gel has been defined as a soft, solid-like material composed primarily of liquid and at least one other component (e.g. protein) that does not flow under its own weight on a time scale of seconds (Almdal *et al.*, 1993). Polymer–polymer and polymer–solvent interactions occur in an ordered manner, resulting in the immobilization of large amounts of liquid by a small amount of protein (Ferry, 1948; Clark, 1992).

Several general theories have been proposed to explain the mechanism of protein gelation. Ferry (1948) postulated that the gelation of proteins occurs in two stages and involves the initial denaturation of native proteins, which then associate to form a three-dimensional network. The Flory–Stockmayer model describes gelation as a sudden event that occurs when the degree of cross-linking between smaller aggregates of denatured protein reaches a critical threshold, called the gel point, at which the aggregates cross-link throughout the percolation lattice (Flory, 1941; Stockmayer, 1943, 1944). Once the gel point is reached the viscosity increases rapidly to infinity, along with the average molecular weight of the aggregates. At this point, the solid or elastic character of the system changes from zero to an increasing finite value (Clark, 1992).

Thus, the two-step process of Ferry (1948) can be expanded to include more completely aspects of other models by dividing gelation into a series of steps leading to the final gel structure (Foegeding and Hamann, 1992) (Fig. 18.2). In this model, proteins denature or partially unfold. Small aggregates of protein are formed leading to a progressively more viscous solution. Once the gel point is reached, a continuous gel network is formed which exhibits properties of a viscoelastic solid.

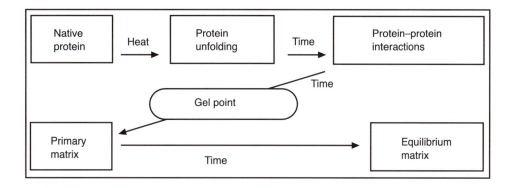

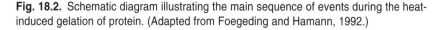

Fig. 18.2. Schematic diagram illustrating the main sequence of events during the heat-induced gelation of protein. (Adapted from Foegeding and Hamann, 1992.)

Disulphide bonds, hydrogen bonds, hydrophobic interactions and electrostatic forces are involved in gel formation. Furthermore, factors affecting the balance between these forces, for example pH, ionic strength and temperature, will alter the type of gel formed and its rheological properties. Knowledge of the forces involved allows identification of the key factors influencing gelation of a particular protein and allows manipulation of the environmental conditions to obtain the desired gel properties.

The structure and physicochemical properties of the gel matrix depend on the relative rates of denaturation and aggregation (Ferry, 1948). The slower the rate of protein aggregation relative to the rate of unfolding, the better the denatured chains orient themselves and thus the finer the gel network. When the rate of protein aggregation is greater than that of unfolding, coarse, less-organized gel structures or coagulums are formed (Hermansson, 1978). When attractive forces dominate, extensive protein aggregation occurs, which leads to the formation of a coagulum, or an opaque gel, which exhibits a high degree of syneresis. When repulsive forces dominate, gel formation does not occur because there is insufficient attraction between protein molecules. Translucent gels, with high water-holding capacity, are formed under environmental conditions which favour a suitable balance between attractive and repulsive forces (Clark and Lee-Tuffnell, 1986).

GELATION PROPERTIES OF POULTRY MYOSIN

The gelation mechanism of rabbit skeletal myosin is the most widely studied muscle protein gel system. However, discrete differences in the primary and secondary structure of myosin extracted from different muscle sources results in subtle changes in the protein gelation mechanism, therefore, the remainder of this discussion will be focused on the gelation properties of poultry muscle myosin. Two main steps in the thermal gelation of poultry muscle myosin will be presented: (i) denaturation of the native protein molecules, followed by (ii) aggregation of the partially unfolded myosin molecules, which results in the formation of a self-supporting protein gel network.

Denaturation of Myosin

Myosin is a multidomain protein and exhibits complex denaturation behaviour during heating (Privalov and Gill, 1988). Using high resolution differential scanning calorimetry, Smyth *et al.* (1996) found that broiler breast muscle (m. pectoralis) myosin in 0.6 M NaCl, 50 mM sodium phosphate buffer, pH 6.5, when heated at 1°C min^{-1}, began to denature at 37°C. The endotherm of myosin showed two peaks at 47.5 and 54°C and two shoulders at 57.4 and 63.1°C (Fig. 18.3). Wright *et al.* (1977) also using differential scanning calorimetry observed one to three temperature transitions for rabbit skeletal myosin depending on the conditions of pH and ionic strength used to suspend the protein. At pH 7.0 and at low ionic strength (0.048 M KCl), they observed one temperature transition at 55°C, whereas at pH 6.0 and high ionic strength (1 M KCl) three temperature transitions at 42, 49.5 and 60.5°C were recorded. Bertazzon and Tsong (1989) reported that rabbit myosin had transition temperatures of 43, 46, 49 and 54°C in 0.5 M KCl, 20 mM potassium phosphate buffer, pH 7.0 using microcalorimetric techniques. These results demonstrate that the heat-induced denaturation of myosin is directly influenced by species, muscle type, buffer conditions and heating rate, and illustrates that conclusions regarding the mechanism of myosin gelation are best when myosin is extracted from the same muscle source and when analysed under identical experimental conditions. To overcome some of these

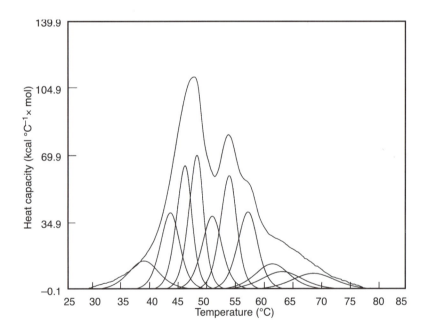

Fig. 18.3. Heat capacity profile and deconvoluted peaks of broiler pectoralis major myosin in 0.6 M NaCl, 50 mM Na phosphate buffer, pH 6.5, heated at 1°C min^{-1}. (From Smyth *et al.*, 1996 with permission.)

problems, several researchers have studied the gelation of myosin (1%, w/w) extracted from chicken breast muscle (m. pectoralis) when heated at 1°C min⁻¹ in a 0.6 M NaCl, 50 mM sodium phosphate buffer, pH 6.5 (Wang and Smith, 1994a, b; Wang and Smith, 1995; Smyth et al., 1996). Some key findings from these studies are summarized below.

Chicken breast myosin contains at least 10 domains unfolding between about 39 and 70°C (Fig. 18.3) (Wang and Smith, 1994a; Smyth et al., 1996). Domains are independent, cooperative units found within folded protein molecules and each domain exhibits a distinct thermal stability. Some of the myosin subfragments have been reported to have more than one domain; for example, myosin rod, LMM and S-2 extracted from rabbit skeletal muscle contain six, five and three domains, respectively (Lopez-Lacomba et al., 1989; Bertazzon and Tsong, 1990). Smyth et al. (1996) compared the temperature transitions of purified chicken myosin subfragments against the temperature transitions of the domains within the intact myosin molecule. The authors were able to postulate the order in which different regions of the myosin molecule unfold on heating. They found that a region of LMM was first to unfold at 39°C, followed by the hinge region in the myosin rod and a domain of S-2 at 46°C. Subfragment-1 and alkali LC unfolded at 48°C. The DTNB LC unfolded at 57°C, followed by several domains on the myosin rod, including another region of S-2. More work is needed to positively identify the order in which myosin unfolds, but these findings can be used to help interpret myosin aggregation and gelation profiles.

Conformational changes in broiler breast muscle myosin due to heating have been evaluated using Fourier transform infrared spectroscopy (Wang and Smith, 1994b). No changes in secondary structure were observed when myosin was heated isothermally at 45°C for 30 min, although the rod region of myosin begins to unfold in this temperature range. Purified myosin rod is thermally reversible, that is, in dilute solutions it will refold into its native conformation after heating (Arteaga and Nakai, 1992). When the myosin solutions were cooled before analysis, the rod may have refolded so that no changes in secondary structure were observed. These findings agree with those found in a similar study using turkey breast myosin (Arteaga and Nakai, 1992).

Lepock et al. (1992) reported that denaturation of a reversible protein often becomes irreversible once it aggregates with other proteins. Thus, at higher temperatures, interactions between the rod and other regions of myosin resulted in irreversible conformational changes to the molecule. Wang and Smith (1994b) reported a decrease in the α-helical and β-sheet content of myosin when heated isothermally at temperatures greater than or equal to 55°C. New intermolecular β-sheet structures appeared at 55°C that increased in intensity when myosin solutions were isothermally heated at 65 and 75°C. This increase in intermolecular β-sheet did not correlate with the increase in gel firmness observed using small strain testing, suggesting that other chemical bonds are involved in gel matrix formation.

Aggregation of Myosin

Using turbidity measurements, Smyth *et al.* (1996) analysed the aggregation profiles of myosin and seven of its subfragments. Broiler breast myosin aggregated rapidly from 50 to 54°C, followed by a plateau from 55 to 60°C. Myosin then aggregated more slowly between 60 and 70°C. The results obtained from the protein–protein interactions of the myosin subfragments demonstrated that LMM and S-1 aggregated at temperatures less than or equal to 55°C, whereas S-2 aggregated from 60 to 75°C. The rod aggregated continuously between 25 and 85°C. The myosin LC did not aggregate, but when associated with the myosin heavy chain increased the stability of the myosin molecule during heating. These results indicate that LMM and S-1 play a critical role in the initial stages of network formation, whereas S-2 is involved in the final phase of gel matrix formation.

Gelation of Myosin

Small strain dynamic rheological testing was used to monitor structure formation during the gelation of chicken breast muscle myosin. Wang and Smith (1994a) showed that myosin network formation began at 53.5°C. Myosin gel structure increased rapidly from 53.5 to 59°C, followed by a slight decrease between 59 and 62°C (Fig. 18.4). On the basis of the denaturation and

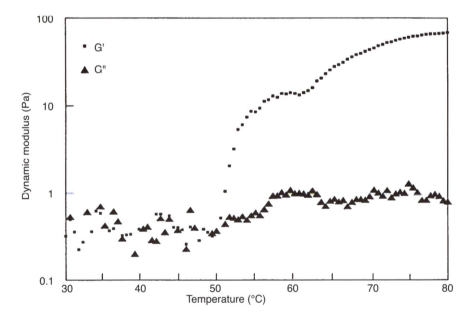

Fig 18.4. Rheogram showing storage (G′) and loss (G ″) moduli of broiler breast muscle myosin (10 mg ml⁻¹) in 0.6 M NaCl, 50 mM Na phosphate buffer, pH 6.5, heated at 1°C min⁻¹. (From Wang and Smith, 1994a with permission.)

aggregation studies on the myosin subfragments, it is possible to conclude that the decrease observed in network formation between 59 and 62°C represents the point at which the rate of bond disruption as a result of thermal denaturation of some of the domains within the rod, or more specifically domains within S-2, surpasses that of bond formation due to protein aggregation in S-1 and the domains within LMM. At temperatures between 62 and 75°C a further increase in network formation was recorded. This increase in structure formation coincides with the temperature at which complete denaturation of the myosin molecule was observed and can be attributed to aggregation of the domains within S-2 and any remaining domains in the rod (Smyth *et al.*, 1996). Several researchers have concluded that conformational changes occurring in the supercoiled α-helical myosin rod at temperatures greater than 55°C are the most crucial, since myosin gels do not attain appreciable gel strength until this temperature is reached (Foegeding *et al.*, 1986; Morrissey *et al.*, 1987; O'Neill *et al.*, 1993). Heating to temperatures greater than 75°C did not result in any further increase in the gel network structure, as all the myosin domains had unfolded (Wang and Smith, 1994a; Smyth, 1996).

However, it is important to reiterate that both the temperature and the order at which the domains within a protein molecule unfold and subsequently aggregate are determined by environmental conditions (Potekhin and Privalov, 1982). Thus, changing extrinsic factors will alter the intrinsic properties of the protein gelation mechanism and alter the properties of the resulting protein gel. For example, the thermally induced unfolding of S-l was found to be less sensitive to pH changes and more sensitive to changes in heating rate than the rod (Bertazzon and Tsong, 1989).

The role played by disulphide bonds and the temperature at which they are formed during the gelation of chicken myosin has not been widely studied. Native chicken myosin contains 43 thiol groups and no disulphide bonds (Smyth, 1996), therefore it is likely that oxidation of the thiol groups to disulphide bonds occurs during heating (Roussel and Cheftel, 1990). To evaluate the role of disulphide bonds in the heat-induced gelation of chicken breast myosin, Smyth (1996) prepared gels in the presence and absence of the reducing agent, dithiothreitol. When disulphide bond formation was inhibited, the aggregation and gelation onset temperatures increased by 3°C and 5°C, respectively. Furthermore, myosin gels formed with dithiothreitol were weaker than those prepared without the reducing agent. The microstructure of the gels formed without disulphide bonds was less uniform, had larger pores, and had less cross-linking than those gels formed in the presence of disulphide bonds. The results of this study suggested that although disulphide bond formation is not a prerequisite for the gelation of chicken breast muscle myosin, intermolecular disulphide bonds are formed during the heat-induced gelation process at temperatures above 48°C and contribute to the firmness and integrity of the gel matrix.

Similarly, Itoh *et al.* (1979a, b, c) and Niwa *et al.* (1982) demonstrated that disulphide bond formation played an important role in gel network formation by carp actomyosin and fish muscle myosin, respectively, at temperatures as low as 40°C. Sano *et al.* (1994) showed that the total number of reactive thiol groups in carp actomyosin started to increase at 20–30°C, suggesting that thiol groups were exposed as a result of heat-induced denaturation. As the temperature was increased from 30 to 50°C, the number of reactive thiol groups decreased considerably, indicating that the exposed thiol groups were oxidized to disulphide bonds in this temperature range.

FACTORS INFLUENCING MYOSIN GELATION

Myosin Polymorphism

The effect of fibre type of the muscle from which myosin is extracted on gel properties is not entirely clear, although pH has a large influence on the final gel. Distinct differences in the thermally induced denaturation and aggregation profiles of white and red muscle chicken myosin have been reported (Liu *et al.*, 1996). Using differential scanning calorimetry, Liu *et al.* (1996) reported that chicken m. pectoralis (breast, white muscle fibre) myosin undergoes the first thermal transition at 48.1°C, whereas the first thermal transitions of iliotibialis (thigh, red muscle fibre) and gastrocnemius (red muscle fibre, type 1) myosin were at 49.5 and 49.3°C, respectively, in 0.6 M NaCl, 0.05 M sodium phosphate buffer, pH 6.0. Myosin from m. pectoralis had a higher calorimetric enthalpy than either iliotibialis or gastrocnemius myosin. Using isothermal heating experiments, Liu *et al.* (1996) found that only m. pectoralis myosin aggregated on heating at 45°C. iliotibialis and gastrocnemius myosins did not start to aggregate until heated isothermally at 50°C. At 50°C and above, gastrocnemius myosin formed the most turbid aggregates on heating.

Asghar *et al.* (1984) reported that myosin extracted from chicken pectoralis profundus (white muscle fibre, type 1 lb) (in 0.6 M NaCl, pH 6.0) formed more rigid gels than myosin from gastrocnemius (red muscle fibre, type 1) at 65°C from pH 5.5 to 6.75. Similarly, Morita *et al.* (1987) reported that broiler breast myosin formed more rigid gels than myosin from leg muscle at 65°C at pH 5.1 to 6.0. Liu and Foegeding (1996) examined the rigidity of myosin gels prepared from chicken pectoralis, iliotibialis and gastrocnemius muscles (pH 6.0) during heating and after cooling using small strain rheological techniques. Pectoralis myosin began to gel at a lower temperature and had a higher storage modulus at 75°C than gels prepared using myosin from red muscles. However, on cooling to 25°C, the storage moduli of myosin gels prepared from the three muscles did not differ. No studies have examined the failure properties of poultry myosin gels prepared from muscles of different fibre type, as it is difficult to purify the large quantities of myosin needed for these studies.

Conflicting results have been reported when failure properties of red and white muscle protein gels prepared from myofibrils and salt-soluble protein have been compared, although gel properties have been found to vary greatly with pH. More research is needed to fully understand the interaction of protein isoform and pH on the gelation properties of myosin isolated from muscles of different fibre types.

Environmental Conditions

The influence of ionic strength and pH on the gelation properties of poultry myosin have not been widely documented. However, such interactions have been extensively studied using rabbit skeletal myosin. For this reason, general observations on the influence of ionic strength, pH and heating temperature on the gelation mechanism of rabbit skeletal myosin are reported here. Similar trends in the gelation of myosin isolated from chicken muscle (m. pectoralis) have been observed in our laboratory.

In an extensive study on the ultrastructure of rabbit myosin gels, Hermansson *et al.* (1986) observed that myosin can form two different types of gels on heating in the pH range 5.5–6.0, depending on the ionic strength of the buffer in which myosin is suspended. Fine-stranded gel structures are formed at low ionic strength (0.25 M KCl). These gels have a higher rigidity than the coarsely aggregated networks which are formed at high ionic strength (0.6 M KCl). Yamamoto *et al.* (1987) prepared rabbit skeletal muscle myosin filaments in 0.1 M KCl, pH 6.0, by both dialysis and rapid dilution. The average length and diameter of myosin filaments prepared by dialysis was greater than when prepared by dilution and the strength of myosin gels prepared by dialysis was much higher than by dilution at 65°C. In addition, a fine-stranded gel network structure was formed from dialysed myosin, but diluted myosin formed a rather coarse network structure when examined by scanning electron microscopy. These results suggest that the rheological properties of myosin gels formed at low ionic strength depend on the structure of the filaments formed before heating. Larger and thicker filaments form stronger heat-induced gels. Furthermore, the very good heat-induced gel-forming properties of myosin at low ionic strength diminish with storage time as a result of the loss of filament-forming properties (Ishioroshi *et al.*, 1979, 1980).

The optimum pH for the heat-induced gelation of rabbit skeletal myosin in 0.6 M KCl is 6.0 (Ishioroshi *et al.*, 1979; Yasui *et al.*, 1980). Gels produced at pH values greater than 6.0 are translucent, whereas those formed at pH values less than 6.0 are opaque and exhibited syneresis. The pH dependence of gel strength is mainly due to changes in protein–protein interactions, since protein conformation and charge distribution are affected by pH.

Role of Actin

By using differential scanning microcalorimetry, filamentous actin (F-actin) extracted from chicken breast muscle has been found to have a single transition at 75.5°C, with a calorimetric enthalpy of 143.4 ± 9.6 kcal mol^{-1} in 0.6 M NaCl, pH 6.5 (Wang and Smith, 1994a). When F-actin is heated, it coagulates, forming bead-like aggregates which exhibit none of the viscoelastic properties associated with myosin gels (Samejima *et al.*, 1969; Yasui *et al.*, 1979, 1980). Wang and Smith (1995) examined the denaturation profiles of chicken breast myosin alone and when mixed with different weight ratios of F-actin. In all cases, three temperature transitions were recorded. However, the initial denaturation temperature and the temperature at which the transitions occurred increased when myosin was in the presence of F-actin. Wang *et al.* (1996) suggested that the thermal stability of myosin is increased when F-actin binds to the S-1 region. This theory was substantiated further when the denaturation profiles of actomyosin in the presence of pyrophosphate, which dissociates actin from myosin, were similar to those of free myosin (Wang and Smith, 1995).

The different denaturation profiles of myosin and actomyosin suggest that the gel forming properties of these proteins when heated will not be the same. Wang and Smith (1995) reported that although the proteins underwent different viscoelastic transitions during heating from 30 to 80°C at 1°C min^{-1} in 0.6 M NaCl, pH 6.5, no difference in the extent of gel matrix development was observed at 80°C between the pure myosin gels and actomyosin gels, where the weight ratio of F-actin to myosin was 1:15. Similarly, F-actin exerted a synergistic effect on the heat-induced gelation of rabbit skeletal myosin in 0.6 M KCl, pH 7.0, and maximum gel strength was obtained when the myosin to actin molar ratio was 2.7:1 (which corresponds to 80% free myosin and 20% actomyosin). Further, addition of F-actin to myosin caused a decrease in rigidity similar to what would be observed when the gelling potential of myosin decreased as a result of diluting the concentration of the protein in a system where myosin is the only protein present (Yasui *et al.*, 1980). It has been suggested that the formation of a suitable but relatively small amount of actomyosin in the system may be a prerequisite for actin-induced improvement of rigidity of myosin gels and that it may act to form cross-links between free myosin molecules within the gel structure (Ishioroshi *et al.*, 1980; Yasui *et al.*, 1980). Thus, the gel strength of myosin–actin systems depends more on the ratio of free myosin to actomyosin than on the ratio of myosin to actin.

CONCLUSIONS

Understanding the functional properties that proteins can impart to a meat system at the molecular level should ultimately lead to a greater understanding of changes occurring within a meat batter during cooking and contribute to better control of the manufacturing process. Protein gelation is an important functional property of muscle proteins. Elucidating the mechanism of muscle protein gelation will help processors to manipulate product formulations and processing conditions to improve the quality of existing further-processed poultry products and to produce new products.

ACKNOWLEDGEMENT

This chapter is based in part on the doctoral dissertation of Anne B. Smyth.

REFERENCES

Adelstein, R.S. and Eisenberg, E. (1980) Regulation and kinetics of the actin–myosin ATP interaction. *Annual Reviews in Biochemistry* 49, 921–956.

Almdal, K., Hvidt, J.D. and Kramer, O. (1993) Towards a phenomenological definition of the term gel. *Polymers, Gels and Networks* 1, 5–8.

Arteaga, G.E. and Nakai, S. (1992) Thermal denaturation of turkey breast myosin under different conditions. Effect of temperature and pH, and reversibility of denaturation. *Meat Science* 3l, 191–200.

Asghar, A., Morita, J.T., Samejima K. and Yasui, T. (1984) Biochemical and functional characteristics of myosin from red and white muscles of chicken as influenced by nutritional stress. *Agricultural and Biological Chemistry* 48, 2217–2224.

Bailey, A.J. (1982) Muscle proteins and muscle structure. In: Fox, P.F. and Condon, J.J. (eds) *Food Proteins.* Applied Science Publishers, London, pp. 245–259.

Barbut, S. (1995) Importance of fat emulsification and protein matrix characteristics in meat batter stability. *Journal of Muscle Foods* 6, 161–177.

Bendall, J.R. (1973) Post-mortem changes in muscle. In: Bourne, G.H. (ed.) *Structure and Function of Muscle,* 2nd edn, Vol. 2. Academic Press, London, pp. 243–309.

Bertazzon, A. and Tsong, T.Y. (1989) High-resolution differential scanning calorimetric study of myosin, functional domains and supramolecular structures. *Biochemistry* 28, 9784–9790.

Bertazzon, A. and Tsong, T.Y. (1990) Study of effects of pH on the stability of domains in myosin rod by high resolution differential scanning calorimetry. *Biochemistry* 29, 6453–6459.

Borchert, L., Greaser, M.L., Brad, J.C., Cassens, R.G. and Briskey, E.J. (1967) Electron microscopy of a meat emulsion. *Journal of Food Science* 32, 419–421.

Borejdo, J. (1983) Mapping of hydrophobic sites on the surface of myosin and its fragments. *Biochemistry* 22, 1182–1187.

Clark, A.H. (1992) Gels and gelling. In: Schwartzberg, H.G. and Hartel, R.W. (eds) *Physical Chemistry of Foods.* Marcel Dekker, New York, pp. 263–305.

Clark, A.H. and Lee-Tuffnell, C.D. (1986) Gelation of globular proteins. In: Mitchell, J.R. and Ledward, D.A. (eds) *Functional Properties of Food Macromolecules.* Elsevier Applied Science Publishers, London, pp. 240–284.

Dickinson, E. (1992) *An Introduction to Food Colloids.* Oxford University Press, Oxford.

Dickinson, E. and McClements, D.J. (1996) *Advances in Food Colloids.* Blackie, Academic Press, New York.

Ferry, J.D. (1948) Protein gels. *Advances in Protein Chemistry* 4, 1–78.

Findlay, C.F. and Barbut, S. (1990) Differential scanning calorimetry of meat. In: Harwalkar, V.R. and Ma, C.Y. (eds) *Thermal Analysis of Foods.* Elsevier Applied Science Publishers, London, pp. 92–125.

Flory, P.J. (1941) Molecular size distribution in three dimensional polymers. I. Gelation. *Journal of the American Chemical Society* 63, 3083–3091.

Foegeding, E.A. and Hamann, D.D. (1992) Physicochemical aspects of muscle tissue behaviour. In: Schwartzberg, H.G. and Hartel, R.W. (eds) *Physical Chemistry of Foods.* Marcel Dekker, New York, pp. 423–441.

Foegeding, E.A., Allen, C.E. and Dayton, W.R. (1986) Effect of heating rate on thermally formed myosin, fibrinogen and albumin gels. *Journal of Food Science* 51, 104–108, 112.

Frank, G. and Weeds, A.G. (1974) The amino acid sequence of the alkali light chains of rabbit skeletal muscle myosin. *European Journal of Biochemistry* 44, 317–334.

Galluzzo, S.J. and Regenstein, J.M. (1978a) Role of chicken breast muscle proteins in meat emulsion formation: myosin, actin and synthetic actomyosin. *Journal of Food Science* 43, 1761–1765.

Galluzzo, S.J. and Regenstein, J.M. (1978b) Emulsion capacity and timed emulsification of chicken breast muscle myosin. *Journal of Food Science* 43, 1757–1760.

Gazith, J., Himmelfarb, S. and Harrington, W.F. (1970) Studies on the subunit structure of myosin. *Journal of Biological Chemistry* 245, 15–22.

Goll, D.E. (1977) Muscle proteins. In: Whitaker, J.R. and Tannenbaum, S.R. (eds) *Food Proteins*. AVI Publishing, Westport, Connecticut, pp. 121–174.

Gordon, A. and Barbut, S. (1990) The role of the interfacial protein film in meat bater stabilization. *Food Structure* 9, 77–90.

Gordon, A. and Barbut, S. (1992a) Mechanisms of meat batter stabilization: a review. *CRC Critical Reviews in Food Science and Nutrition* 32, 299–332.

Gordon, A. and Barbut, S. (1992b) The effect of chloride salts on protein extraction and interfacial protein film formation in meat batters. *Journal of the Science of Food and Agriculture* 58, 227–238.

Harrington, W.F. (1979) Contractile proteins of the myofibril. In: Neurath, H. and Hill, R.L. (eds) *The Proteins*. Academic Press, New York, pp. 245–409.

Hayashida, M., Maita, T. and Matsuda, G. (1991) The primary structure of skeletal muscle myosin heavy chain. 1. Sequence of the amino-terminal 23 kDa fragment. *Journal of Biochemistry* 110, 54–59.

Hermansson, A.M. (1978) Physico-chemical aspects of soy proteins structure formation. *Journal of Texture Studies* 9, 33–58.

Hermansson, A.M., Harbitz, O. and Langton, M. (1986) Formation of two types of gels from bovine myosin. *Journal of the Science of Food and Agriculture* 37, 69–84.

Ishioroshi, M., Samejima, K. and Yasui, T. (1979) Heat-induced gelation of myosin: factors of pH and salt concentration. *Journal of Food Science* 44, 1280–1283.

Ishioroshi, M., Samejima, K., Arie, Y. and Yasui, T. (1980) Effect of blocking the myosin-actin interaction in heat-induced gelation of myosin in the presence of actin. *Agricultural and Biological Chemistry* 44, 2185–2194.

Itoh, Y., Yoshinaka, R. and Ikeda, S. (1979a) Effects of cysteine and cystine on the gel formation of fish meats by heating. *Bulletin of the Japanese Society of the Science of Fisheries* 45, 341–345.

Itoh, Y., Yoshinaka, R. and Ikeda, S. (1979b) Behaviour of the sulfhydryl groups of carp actomyosin by heating. *Bulletin of the Japanese Society of the Science of Fisheries* 45, 1019–1022.

Itoh, Y., Yoshinaka, R. and Ikeda, S. (1979c) Effects of SH reagents on the gel formation of carp actomyosin on heating. *Bulletin of the Japanese Society of the Science of Fisheries* 45, 1023–1025.

Jones, K.W. and Mandigo, R.W. (1982) Effects of chopping temperature on the microstructure of meat emulsions. *Journal of Food Science* 47, 1930–1935.

Kinsella, J.E. (1976) Functional properties of proteins in foods: a survey. *CRC Critical Reviews in Food Science and Nutrition* 7, 219–280.

Komine, Y., Maita, T. and Matsuda, G. (1991) The primary structure of skeletal muscle myosin heavy chain. II. Sequence of the 50 kDa fragment of subfragment-1. *Journal of Biochemistry* 110, 60–67.

Lepock, J.R., Ritchie, K.P., Kolios, M.C., Rodhl, A.M., Heinz, K.A. and Kruuv, J. (1992) Influence of transition rates and scan rate on kinetic simulations of differential scanning calorimetry profiles of reversible and irreversible protein denaturation. *Biochemistry* 31, 12706–12712.

Liu, M.N. and Foegeding, E.A. (1996) Thermally induced gelation of chicken myosin isoforms. *Journal of Agricultural and Food Chemistry* 44, 1441–1446.

Liu, M.N., Foegeding, E.A., Wang, S.F., Smith, D.M. and Davidian, M. (1996) Denaturation and aggregation of chicken myosin isoforms. *Journal of Agricultural and Food Chemistry* 44, 1435–1440.

Lopez-Lacomba, J.L., Guzman, M., Cortijo, M., Mateo, P.L., Aguirre, R., Harvey, S.C. and Cheung, H.C. (1989) Differential scanning calorimetric study of the thermal unfolding of myosin rod, light meromyosin and subfragment 2. *Biopolymers* 28, 2143–2159.

Lowey, S., Slayter, H.S., Weeds, A. and Baker, H. (1969) Substructure of the myosin molecule. I. Sub-fragments of myosin byenzymatic degradation. *Journal of Molecular Biology* 42, 1–29.

Margossian, S.S. and Lowey, A. (1982) Preparation of muscle and its subfragment from rabbit skeletal muscle. *Methods in Enzymology* 85, 56–71.

McLachlan, A.D. and Karn, J. (1982) Periodic charge distribution in the myosin rod amino acid sequence match cross-bridge spacings in muscle. *Nature* 299, 226–231.

Morita, J.-I., Choe, I.-S., Yamamoto, K., Samejima, K. and Yasui, T. (1987) Heat-induced gelation of myosin from leg and breast muscles of chicken. *Agricultural and Biological Chemistry* 51, 2895–2900.

Morrissey, P.A., Mulvihill, D.M. and O'Neill, E. (1987) Functional properties of muscle foods, In: Hudson, B.J.F. (ed.) *Developments in Food Proteins.* Elsevier Applied Science, London, pp. 195–257.

Niwa, E., Matsubara, Y. and Hamada, L. (1982) Participation of disulphide bonding in the appearance of setting. *Bulletin of the Japanese Society of Fisheries* 48, 727–730.

O'Neill, E., Morrissey, P.A. and Mulvihill, D.M. (1993) Heat-induced gelation of actomyosin. *Meat Science* 33, 61–74.

Pearson, A.M. and Young, R.B. (1989) In: *Muscle and Meat Biochemistry.* Academic Press, San Diego.

Potekhin, S.A. and Privalov, P.L. (1982) Co-operative blocks in tropomyosin. *Journal of Molecular Biochemistry* 159, 519–535.

Privalov, P.L. and Gill, S.J. (1988) Stability of protein structure and hydrophobic interactions. *Advances in Protein Chemistry* 39, 191–239.

Roussel, H. and Cheftel, J.C. (1990) Mechanisms of gelation of sardine proteins: influence of thermal processing and of various additives on the texture and protein solubility of kamaboto gels. *International Journal of Food Science and Technology* 25, 260–280.

Samejima, K., Hashimdo, Y., Yasui, T. and Fukazawa, T. (1969) Heat gelling properties of myosin, actin, actomyosin and myosin subunits in a saline model system. *Journal of Food Science* 34, 242–245.

Samejima, K., Ishioroshi, M. and Yasui, T. (1982) Heat-induced gelling properties of actomyosin: effect of tropomyosin and troponin. *Agricultural and Biological Chemistry* 46, 535–540.

Sano, T., Ohno, T., Otsuka-Fuchino, H., Matsumoto, J.J. and Tsuychiya, T. (1994) Carp natural actomyosin: thermal denaturation mechanism. *Journal of Food Science* 59, 1002–1008.

Schut, J. (1976) Meat emulsions, In: Friberg, S. (ed.) *Food Emulsions.* Marcel Dekker, New York, pp. 385–458.

Smith, D.M. (1988) Meat proteins: functional properties of comminuted meat products. *Food Technology* 42 (4), 116–121.

Smyth, A.B. (1996) Heat-induced gelation properties of muscle proteins. Ph.D Dissertation. University College, Cork, Ireland.

Smyth, A.B., Smith, D.M., Vega-Warner, V. and O'Neill, E. (1996) Thermal denaturation and aggregation of chicken breast muscle myosin and subfragments. *Journal of Agricultural and Food Chemistry* 44, 996–1007.

Stockmayer, W.H. (1943) Theory of molecular size distribution and gel formation in branched-chain polymers. *Journal of Chemistry and Physics* 11, 45–55.

Stockmayer, W.H. (1944) Theory of molecular size distribution and gel formation in branched polymers. II. General cross linking. *Journal of Chemistry and Physics* 12, 125–131.

Sutoh, K., Sutoh, K., Karr, T. and Harrington, W. (1978) Isolation and physico-chemical properties of a high molecular weight subfragment-2 of myosin. *Journal of Molecular Biochemistry* 126, 1–22.

Tsai, R., Cassens, R.G. and Briskey, E.J. (1972) The emulsifying properties of purified muscle proteins. *Journal of Food Science* 37, 286–288.

Wang, S.F. and Smith, D.M. (1994a) Heat-induced denaturation and rheological properties of chicken breast myosin and F-actin in the presence and absence of pyrophosphate. *Journal of Agricultural and Food Chemistry* 42, 2665–2670.

Wang, S.F. and Smith, D.M. (1994b) Dynamic rheological properties and secondary structure of chicken breast myosin as influenced by isothermal heating. *Journal of Agricultural and Food Chemistry* 42, 1434–1439.

Wang, S.F. and Smith, D.M. (1995) Gelation of chicken breast muscle actomyosin as influenced by weight ratios of actin to myosin. *Journal of Agricultural and Food Chemistry* 43, 331–336.

Wang, S.F., Smith, D.M. and Steffe, J.F. (1990) Effect of pH on the dynamic rheological properties of chicken breast salt-soluble proteins during heat-induced gelation. *Poultry Science* 69, 220–227.

Wang, S.F., Smyth, A.B. and Smith, D.M. (1996) Gelation properties of myosin: role of subfragments and actin. In: Parris, N., Kato, A., Creamer, L.K. and Pearce, J. (eds) *Macromolecular Interactions in Food Technology.* American Chemical Society, Washington, DC, pp. 124–133.

Weeds, A.G. and Lowey, S. (1971) Substructure of the myosin molecule. 11. The light chains of myosin. *Journal of Molecular Biochemistry* 61, 701–725.

Wright, D.J., Leach, I.B. and Wilding, P. (1977) Differential scanning calorimetric studies of muscle and its constituent protein. *Journal of the Science of Food and Agriculture* 28, 557–564.

Wu, J.Q., Hamann, D.D. and Foegeding, E.A. (1991) Myosin gelation kinetic study based on rheological measurements. *Journal of Agricultural and Food Chemistry* 39, 229–236.

Xiong, Y.L. (1992) Thermally induced interactions and gelation of combined myofibrillar protein from white and red broiler muscles. *Journal of Food Science* 57, 581–585.

Yamamoto, K., Samejima, K. and Yasui, T. (1987) The structure of myosin filaments and the properties of heat-induced gels in the absence of C-protein. *Agricultural and Biological Chemistry* 51, 197–203.

Yasui, T., Ishioroshi, M., Nakano, H. and Samejima, K. (1979) Changes in shear modulus, ultrastructure and spin–spin relaxation times of water associated with heat induced gelation of myosin. *Journal of Food Science* 44, 1201–1204.

Yates, L.D. and Greaser, M.L. (1983) Quantitative determination of myosin and actin in rabbit skeletal muscle. *Journal of Molecular Biochemistry* 168, 123–141.

Yasui, T., Ishioroshi, M. and Samejima, K. (1980) Heat-induced gelation of myosin in the presence of actin. *Journal of Food Biochemistry* 4, 61–78.

CHAPTER 19
The role of processed products in the poultry meat industry

R. Mandava[1] and H. Hoogenkamp[2]

[1]Nestle R&D Centre, P.O. Box 520, S-26725 Bjuv, Sweden; [2]Protein Technologies International, Checkerboard Square, St Louis, MO 63164-00011, USA

ROLE OF POULTRY IN WORLD MEAT PRODUCTION AND CONSUMPTION

Although the chicken was domesticated in India around 2000 BC and since that time its meat has been the main source of animal protein in that country, the growth and consumption of poultry meat in other parts of world had been very slow and not very extensive for many years. However, in the past two or three decades, poultry meat of which chicken contributes nearly 80% has been the most successful meat not only in the Western world but in other regions as well.

Table 19.1 shows that from 1987 to 1997 there was an annual increase of about 3.2% in total world meat production. When compared to the growth of pork (2.5%) and beef (0.9%), poultry meat however had an amazing growth rate of 8.3%. In the last 10 years, more than 50% of the total increase in meat production came from poultry meat. In the same period beef was relegated from second to third place and chicken became second only to pork in total meat production. It will not be long before poultry meat replaces pork as the number one meat when one considers consumer preferences for poultry compared to pork in countries like China, with a population of more than one billion.

This strong growth in poultry meat production occurred in all regions of the world except in the former Soviet Union and Eastern Europe which had negative growth. This decline was probably due to the fall of government-controlled enterprises. Highest growth occurred in Asia followed by South America and North America. At present, USA and China together contribute slightly more than 50% of the overall world poultry meat production.

As for production, the highest growth in poultry meat consumption occurred in Asia (Table 19.2) followed by South America and Africa. Table 19.3 gives a comprehensive view of poultry and red meat consumption in the USA over the last 30 years. These data show two trends: (i) from 1960 to 1985 red

Table 19.1. World production of meats ('000 tonnes).

	1987	1997[a]	Average annual growth (%)
Poultry	28,739	52,478	8.3
Pork	59,094	73,800	2.5
Beef	43,668	47,488	0.9
Mutton	5,565	6,749	2
Total	137,066	180,515	3.2

Source: USDA/FAS. [a]Estimated.

Table 19.2. Poultry meat production and consumption in different regions of the world ('000 tonnes).

	Production		Consumption	
	Volume 1997[a]	% change vs. 1987	Volume 1997[a]	% change vs. 1987
North America	17,324	88.8	14,944	51.2
Asia	15,835	487.5	16,808	449.0
EU	8,040	40.8	7,241	34.3
South America	6,382	108.4	6,109	108.74
Africa	1,220	61.5	1,295	69.9
Middle East	1,215	21.1	1,428	12.3
Former USSR	992	−22.6	1,078	−40.0
Eastern Europe	960	−68.3	972	−2.0
Oceania	510	22.9	498	20.3
Total	52478	79.4	50,373	81.4

Source: USDA/FAS. [a]Estimated.

Table 19.3. Per capita consumption of red meat and poultry meat in the USA (kg).

Year	Red meat	Poultry meat	Total
1960	58.5	15.2	73.7
1965	59.6	18.1	77.7
1970	64.8	21.6	86.4
1975	60.6	21.7	82.3
1980	60.8	27.1	87.9
1985	59.5	31.2	90.7
1990	55.1	37.3	92.4
1995	53.3	38.5	91.8
1996[a]	51.9	39.5	91.4
1997[a]	50.7	41.1	91.8

Source: National Broiler Council, USA. [a]Estimated.

meat consumption remained stable whereas poultry meat consumption increased gradually, thereby contributing to the overall increase in the meat consumption, and (ii) from 1990 onwards there was no increase in overall meat consumption but poultry meat consumption still increased at the expense of red meat. All the estimates indicate that poultry meat consumption will continue to increase and the main reasons for the phenomenal success of poultry meat are as follows.

1. Animal efficiency – it takes only 2 kg of feed to produce 1 kg of broiler meat compared to 9–10 kg for pork and 12–13 kg for beef.
2. No adverse religious or cultural aspect – poultry meat is accepted by all cultures and religions of the world.
3. Health aspect – poultry meat being low in fat and high in protein is associated with better health.
4. Sensory quality – neutral in taste and flavour, good appearance especially white colour and excellent texture.
5. Cost advantage – low prices compared to the other meats.
6. Product versatility – development and availability of various further-processed products.

It is further-processed products that will play a major role in future increases in consumption of poultry meat in developed countries.

GROWTH OF FURTHER-PROCESSED POULTRY

For all the meats, there has been a marked increase on the part of the processed meat segment because of consumer demand for convenience and variety in the meat portion of the diet. This increase has been much more significant for poultry meat. Also, unlike pork and beef which have long been used for further processing, poultry processing is rather new.

The marketing of broilers in the USA over the past three decades is shown in Table 19.4. In 1960, only 2% of all broiler meat was further processed, whereas this proportion had increased to 37% in 1996. Estimates for 1997 and 1998 also show a continuation of this trend. Table 19.5 gives poultry meat marketing data for different regions of the world. Although the processed poultry segment has been increasing and is already an important segment of poultry meat business in North America, figures for the entire world show that processed poultry represents only 13%. Similarly, Table 19.6 shows that in many countries, especially in populated countries like China, India and Indonesia, processed poultry is only a small part of the poultry meat industry. However, this will change rapidly as convenience and variety become important in these countries too. The rapid rise of Western food service units in these countries will further accelerate the growth of processed poultry.

Market volumes of various segments of further-processed chicken in the UK are shown in Tables 19.7–19.10. The total volume of further-processed chicken increased from 92,410 tonnes in 1995 to 105,901 in 1996 showing an annual increase of 14.6% (Table 19.7). However, almost all of this increase came

Table 19.4. Marketing of broilers in the USA (%).

Year	Whole-bird	Cut-up parts	Further processed
1960	83	15	2
1965	78	19	3
1970	70	26	4
1975	61	32	7
1980	50	40	10
1985	29	53	17
1990	18	56	26
1995	11	53	36
1996[a]	10	53	37
1997[a]	10	52	38
1998[a]	9.5	51	39.5

Source: National Broiler Council, USA. [a]Estimated.

Table 19.5. Marketing of poultry meat worldwide in 1995 (%).

Region	Whole-bird	Cut-up parts	Further processed
North America	20	50	30
EU	55	25	20
Asia	48	34	18
South America	76	19	5
Africa	50	45	5
Middle East	90	8	2
Former USSR	84	12	4
Eastern Europe	61	25	14
Oceania	38	40	22
World	58	29	13

Source: USDA/FAS.

from the frozen segment. Although chilled products did not decrease in terms of total volume, the share of chilled products in total value-added products decreased from 40.9% to 35.7%. The decrease in chilled product segment came from all product groups with the biggest decrease occurring in meal centre followed by coated portions and marinated-uncooked portions (Table 19.8). However, in the frozen segment, there was an increase in all product groups with the biggest increase coming from meal centre.

When frozen and chilled segments are combined, all the product groups except marinated-uncooked products had an increase with the biggest increase coming from meal centre and burger product groups (Table 19.9). Marinated-uncooked products had a significant decrease from 1995 to 1996 and this decrease came from the chilled segment. This shows that processors wanted to move away from the uncooked–chilled segment because of safety issues involved. Coated portions and ready meals are by far the biggest product groups within the further-processed chicken category (Table 19.10).

The food service market segment is becoming more important for the

Table 19.6. Share of further-processed poultry (%) in important countries for 1995.

Country	Whole-bird	Cut-up parts	Further processed
Korea	41	4	55
UK	35	15	50
Canada	15	45	40
Japan	0	63	37
USA	11	53	36
China	30	60	10
India	80	15	5
Indonesia	85	10	5
Italy	55	27	18
Spain	80	15	5
Brazil	60	35	5
Argentina	91	5	4
Chile	78	16	6
Russia	84	12	4
South Africa	50	45	5

Source: USDA/FAS.

Table 19.7. Further-processed chicken products in the UK – frozen vs chilled.

	1995		1996		% Change in volume 1995–1996
	Volume (tonnes)	%	Volume (tonnes)	%	
Chilled	37,765	40.87	37,792	35.68	0.07
Frozen	54,645	59.13	68,109	64.32	24.63
Total	92,410	100.00	105,901	100.00	14.60

Source: British Chicken Information Service.

Table 19.8. Share of chilled and frozen segments in different product categories of further-processed chicken in the UK.

	1995		1996	
	% Chilled	% Frozen	% Chilled	% Frozen
Ready meals	24.60	75.40	22.97	77.13
Meal centre	71.35	28.65	59.90	40.10
Coated portions	50.93	49.17	45.23	54.77
Coated snacks	15.25	84.75	14.43	85.57
Marinated – uncooked	73.28	26.72	68.78	31.22
Marinated – cooked	100.00	0.00	100.00	0.00
Burgers	10.88	89.12	7.80	92.20

Source: British Chicken Information Service.

Table 19.9. Different categories of further-processed chicken products in the UK: change (%) from 1995 to 1996.

	Chilled	Frozen	Total
Ready meals	14.89	25.73	23.06
Meal centre	15.25	92.20	37.28
Coated portions	−9.86	13.33	1.48
Coated snacks	14.23	21.80	20.68
Marinated – uncooked	−19.30	0.50	−14.01
Marinated – cooked	13.72	–	13.72
Burgers	−1.60	41.91	37.25

Source: British Chicken Information Service.

Table 19.10. Different product categories in further-processed chicken in the UK.

	1995		1996	
	Volume (tonnes)	% of total	Volume (tonnes)	% of total
Ready meals	25,299	27.38	31,135	29.40
Meal centre	7,408	8.02	10,170	9.60
Coated portions	28,744	31.10	29,171	27.54
Coated snacks	15,073	16.31	18,191	17.18
Marinated – uncooked	7,376	7.98	6,343	5.99
Marinated – cooked	3,353	3.63	3,813	3.60
Burgers	5,157	5.58	7,078	6.68
Total	92,410	100.00	105,901	100.00

Source: British Chicken Information Service.

poultry meat market. Most of the increase in food service comes from fast food outlets who have been adding a number of chicken products to their menus – fried chicken, nuggets, chicken salads and filled sandwiches, etc. In the USA, the food service segment had gradually increased from 25% in 1970 to 44% in 1997 whereas the retail market segment had decreased from 75% in 1970 to 56% in 1997 (Table 19.11). The importance of the food service market segment for the poultry meat business in different regions of the world is shown in Table 19.12. In most important regions like North America, EU and Asia, the food service segment is 25–35% of total market and all the forecasts predict this trend will continue in the future as the Western fast food chains open more and more outlets.

TRENDS IN FURTHER-PROCESSED POULTRY

The trends in processed poultry meat products are different in different regions of the world. Trends such as precooked and low-fat products are very significant in North America, especially in the USA where safety and health are key issues in new meat product development (Table 19.13). Similarly,

Table 19.11. Broiler marketing in the USA – retail and food service segments (%).

	1970	1980	1990	1995	1996[a]	1997[a]
Retail	75	71	59	58	57	56
Food service	25	29	41	42	43	44

Source: National Broiler Council, USA. [a]Estimated.

Table 19.12. Marketing of poultry meat worldwide in 1995: breakdown by end market (%).

Region	Retail	Food service	Export
North America	48	35	17
EU	68	25	7
Asia	56	34	10
South America	64	28	8
Africa	50	50	0
Middle East	NA	NA	NA
Former USSR	93	7	0
Eastern Europe	85	10	5
Oceania	67	32	1
World	66	27	7

NA, not available.
Source: USDA/FAS.

Table 19.13. Processed poultry trends in the world: key issues.

	N. America	EU	Asia	S. America	Oceania	Others
Meal ingredient	•	–	••	–	–	–
Precooked	••	•	•	–	•	–
Low-fat	••	•	–	–	–	–
Flavour variation	••	••	•	•	•	•
Snacks	••	••	–	–	–	–
Spice combination	–	–	••	–	–	–
Chilled ready	•	••	•	–	–	–
Children	•	••	–	•	–	–
Food service	••	••	••	•	•	•

–, non-significant; •, significant; ••, very significant.
Source: Protein Technologies International, USA.

flavour variation and snacks are very significant in North America and Europe where consumers want variety and convenience. However, these are not very significant trends in other parts of the world. Table 19.13 also shows that food service is significant or very significant in all parts of the world. Table 19.14 shows that some product groups such as sausages, nuggets and fried chicken are significant in all parts of the world whereas other product groups, like chicken balls, are significant in Asia only. Similarly, meal kits are significant in North America and Asia but not in other regions.

Table 19.14. Processed poultry trends in the world: specific product categories.

	N. America	EU	Asia	S. America	Oceania	Others
Burgers	•	••	•	–	–	–
Chicken balls	–	–	••	–	–	–
Nuggets	••	•	•	•	•	–
Sausage	••	••	•	•	•	•
Marinated	••	••	••	•	•	–
Ready meals	••	••	•	–	•	–
Meal kits	•	–	•	–	–	–
Individually quick frozen products	••	•	•	•	–	–
Fried chicken	••	•	•	•	•	•

–, non-significant; •, significant; ••, very significant.
Source: Protein Technologies International, USA.

An in-depth analysis of the new product launches in 1996 in two of the most important markets for processed poultry – USA and UK – is shown in Table 19.15. In both these markets, chilled products outnumber frozen products. In the USA, products that mimic the traditional red meat products like sausage, ham, bacon and burger are still an important part (27%) of the new product launches where as in the UK they represent a very small portion (7.5%). Marinated products are by far the most numerous new product launches in the USA whereas they come close second to coated products in the UK. The other main difference is the virtual non-existence of pastry-based poultry products in the USA. However, these products are important in the UK.

Some of the special claims observed in these new product launches were of course related to health, the culinary aspect and special cooking, e.g. fat-free/low-fat, gourmet-style, char-grilled and rotisserie-style, etc. There have also been new flavours introduced in the last few years into various coated, marinated and prepared dishes. Introduction of yeast flavours (marmite-type) that are mixed together with the coating systems is one such example. The introduction of marinades that are traditionally associated with some other foods is becoming popular, for example pesto sauce marinated, cooked chicken. Similarly, the introduction of exotic flavours such as korma in traditional dishes such as chicken-kiev is becoming common. The introduction of formed products resembling sports equipment, e.g. baseball, football or basketball shaped products and popular cartoon characters is becoming very common. These product launches are planned to coincide with the season opening of these events or the release of cartoon movies.

Another major trend, especially in the USA, is the introduction of meal components or culinary aids such as marinated, cooked and diced/sliced poultry which the consumer could use in variety of meals/dishes at home. Another important trend is the introduction of home meal replacement (HMR) or comfort foods. These foods are packed in special containers and working people only have a minimal involvement in preparing a traditional looking meal in little time.

Table 19.15. New product launches in further-processed poultry in the USA and the UK for 1996.

	USA	UK
Total	136	107
Chilled	84	61
Frozen	49	42
Shelf-stable	3	4
Sausages	20	2
Hams	7	0
Bacon	0	2
Burgers	6	1
Salami-type	3	3
Marinated	31	26
Coated (including filled/stuffed)	15	32
Sliced breasts	14	4
Breasts/escalops in sauce	15	16
Pastry/pies	0	10
Meal components	11	2
Others (meat loaf, mignons, etc.)	14	9

Source: The IIS International New Product data base, UK.

RECENT INNOVATIVE DEVELOPMENTS IN FURTHER-PROCESSED POULTRY

Coated Products

Battered and breaded or coated systems have two clear benefits. The first is in their versatility. Virtually every trend in processed food can be adopted via the use of an appropriate coating system. The other benefit is their familiarity. The concept of coatings is well understood. They act as an excellent carrier for the introduction of new flavour and texture ideas. As consumers demand more variety in all types of food continues, there is an extra pressure on the food industry to come up with new and exciting products. Coating systems manufacturers are reacting to that pressure by introducing innovative ideas/ concepts.

One of the recent concepts is the use of non-traditional ingredients for coating different food products, especially poultry products. For example, the use of potato pieces instead of bread crumbs provides a new perspective in appearance, taste and texture. Similarly, the use of maize crispies provides distinctive visual and eating characteristics and the introduction of textured coaters – a novel combination of batter and bread crumbs – brings a novel appearance and taste. They are also ideal carriers for different flavours. Another new concept is to mix various ingredients, such as dried herbs and vegetables together with bread crumbs, to provide not only a variety of texture and taste but also to give a health concept.

Batters with extra adhesive properties are available for special products such as cordon bleu where product height and leakage may be a concern. Similarly, special batters are designed to maintain perfect performance and compensate for moisture migration in chilled products throughout shelf-life. The introduction of toasted crumbs makes it possible not only to enhance appearance and crispiness but also to deliver optimum performance in chilled products, i.e. to compensate for moisture migration thereby maintaining crispy texture and maintaining colour stability, even when exposed to harsh lighting conditions in stores.

Although coated products are well appreciated by many people for their versatility in taste and texture, most of them are not low in calories and fat. As consumers are becoming more health conscious and adopting healthier eating habits, coated systems specially for low-fat coated products are being developed. Two of the innovative systems in this area are the Fry Shield system from Kerry Ingredients, Ireland and No Fry system from Morton Foods, UK.

Fry Shield is a system developed to reduce oil absorption by coated products which undergo the deep fat frying process. It involves a reaction between a calcium-ion source and a calcium-reactive pectin, resulting in the formation of a calcium pectate film. This film acts as a barrier to oil absorption. The sequence of events in the process is shown in Fig. 19.1. The substrate is coated as usual and then dipped in pectin solution by submersion for only 3–5 s. The product may then be prefried, raw breaded or fully cooked. Upon reconstitution, the products exhibit a fat reduction of 20–50% depending on the type of substrate, coating systems and frying.

The No Fry system uses modified predust, batter and bread crumbs to coat the substrate. After coating, products are sprayed with an emulsion of oil, water, proteins and flavour compounds (Fig. 19.2). The amount of emulsion sprayed depends on the required fat content in the final product. The products are then heated using an infrared oven at 900°C for 40–60 s. This heating process is supposed to mimic the heating dynamics of a conventional frying

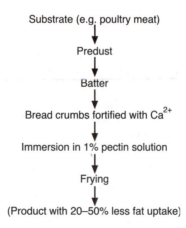

Substrate (e.g. poultry meat)

↓

Predust

↓

Batter

↓

Bread crumbs fortified with Ca^{2+}

↓

Immersion in 1% pectin solution

↓

Frying

↓

(Product with 20–50% less fat uptake)

Fig 19.1. Fry Shield™ process to reduce fat uptake in coated products.

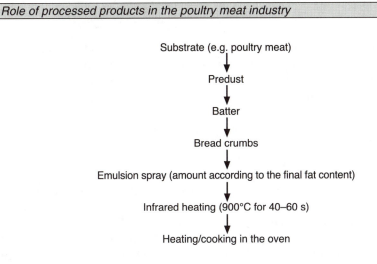

Substrate (e.g. poultry meat)
↓
Predust
↓
Batter
↓
Bread crumbs
↓
Emulsion spray (amount according to the final fat content)
↓
Infrared heating (900°C for 40–60 s)
↓
Heating/cooking in the oven

Fig. 19.2. The No Fry™ process to reduce fat uptake in coated products.

process. The heat emitter, in the infrared oven, is made of stainless steel instead of the glass that is normally used in infrared heaters.

Gourmet Sausages

It was not very long ago that sausage processors considered poultry sausages to be oddities. But as the low-fat craze coupled with worries about red meat came along, sausage processors took a close look and realized that both chicken and turkey meat were viable alternatives in this important market. Today, virtually all major sausage processors have at least one poultry sausage in their sausage-line. However, whereas some major processors were just trying to use poultry meat as an alternative to red meat, especially to lower the fat content and cost, other, smaller processors in the USA have become very innovative with poultry sausages. These processors, with help from some creative chefs, started experimenting with ingredients that are not tradition-ally associated with sausages. This resulted in the introduction of new lines of sausage known as gourmet sausages. These sausages are manufactured using good quality low-fat meat, exotic ingredients, that carry both taste and texture, fresh herbs and spices. Some examples are:

1. Thai sausage made with chicken, fresh ginger, fresh lemon grass, fresh cilantro, lime, green curry paste and white wine;
2. Caribbean sausage made with chicken, habenero pepper, coconut, corn and rum;
3. Tandoori sausage made with chicken, plain yoghurt and tandoori spices;
4. Tuscan sausage made with chicken, sun-dried tomatoes and fresh herbs such as rosemary;
5. Other sausages have been developed with fresh fruit pieces such as apple, cranberries and oranges.

Because of the enormous success of these sausages in trend-setting regions such as California, most of the major sausage processors in the USA have recently started embracing this concept, making these products available throughout the country.

Cooking Systems

Conventional convection ovens, operated with hot air and steam, are still widely used for cooking individual pieces of poultry meat. However, these ovens occupy a very large floor space and heat penetration is slow when products are thick. A recent innovation, the Hot Air Spiral Oven from Koppens, The Netherlands, overcomes these problems. In this oven, the path of the conveyor belt forms a double spiral thereby giving a large belt width on a relatively small floor space. The adjustable speed belt carries the products through the oven with feed and discharge of the product taking place at the same level.

In the oven, steam is injected into the hood and mixed with hot air. This mix circulates continuously around the products so that they are fully cooked. The fully insulated oven is divided into two zones in which the air temperature can be regulated independently. This enables cooking of products in the first zone with a high relative humidity, so as to limit cooking losses, and finish the cooking and browning in the second zone with low humidity. This kind of convection cooking technology allows the product to be optimally cooked first before applying the coating systems followed by flash-frying to set the coating systems. Cooking before flash-frying is supposed to reduce the oil uptake in the finished product.

Another innovative cooking system that has been introduced specially for meat products is the Radio-Frequency (RF) cooker from APV, Denmark. The fundamental principle of RF cooking is to expose the product to an electro-magnetic field at 13.56 MHz. Heat is generated throughout the material by the rapid reversal of polarization of individual molecules. With RF heating, heat transfer is much faster throughout the product compared to conventional heating.

The pretreated product is received in the buffer reservoir where it is sucked by a vacuum pump and transported into the RF chamber which is shaped in accordance with the desired product shape (square, round, rectangular and triangular) and heated to the required temperature. The RF chamber is made up of acid-proof stainless steel and teflon. The whole process takes about two to three minutes depending on the size and type of product. After the heat process, the product is ready for a large variety of treatments: flow packing, cooling, slicing, dicing, and grinding, etc. The system is specially useful to produce ham-like products which are traditionally filled in casings or moulds and cooked in a steam chamber for a long period of time. However, other types of meat products such as cooked and diced meat could also be produced at faster speeds and less energy costs as the RF heating is supposed to consume only about half the energy required for conventional cooking systems.

Freezing Systems

As discussed earlier in this chapter, the frozen segment of further-processed poultry is very important and will continue to do well. The recent growth could be attributed to many factors including safety issues with the chilled foods, processors' adeptness at creating new frozen foods, especially individually quick frozen (IQF) products, and also constant renovations and innovations in freezing systems. There have been a few developments recently in freezing systems, two of which are briefly described below.

Supercontact product surface freezer from York Food Systems, USA, is an efficient mechanical freezing system which produces rapid crust freezing through a highly effective contact heat transfer. Food products are carried on a thin continuous film (plastic) conveyor over a low temperature plate filled with recirculating refrigerant (–40°C). Upon contact, the bottom surface of the product begins to freeze instantly to set its shape. With a firm bottom surface, the product has enough integrity to be transferred to either a spiral or tunnel freezer where it can be deep frozen to –18°C. After usage, the film can be replaced easily and cheaply. Supercontact freezer solves the problem of soft products like chicken breasts sticking to wire mesh conveyor belts and also eliminates mesh marks. Another advantage is that the Supercontact freezer gives up to a 50% reduction in dehydration compared to conventional mechanical freezing systems. In addition, the freezer is self-defrosting as the frost build-up is continuously removed by the film conveyor.

Another innovative development in freezing equipment comes from Frigoscandia, Sweden. They have developed a compact and versatile freezer called PRIMO™ which is suitable for small- to medium-scale processors (100–500 kg h⁻¹). This is also useful for large-scale processors when they are looking for smaller increases in their production and do not want to invest in a big volume freezer. This freezer needs just 10 m² of floor space and could easily be plugged into standard ammonia refrigeration systems in the plant. It is useful for both batch and in-line freezing. The belt in the freezer can be run with or without agitation. Therefore, it is possible to run IQF products where belt agitation is required and single- or conveyor-frozen products.

CONCLUSIONS

The growth of poultry meat that we have seen in the last two decades will no doubt continue. One industry analyst summed it up very well when he said 'I have been saying for years that poultry can not maintain this kind of growth, and every year the industry seems to prove me wrong again'. Most of this growth in developed countries will probably come at the expense of red meat, especially beef.

Processed poultry meat products are a very important part of the poultry meat business in countries like the USA and the UK and it will not be very long before this trend is followed in other countries. In the developed countries, convenience and variety will still be the driving forces for the growth of processed poultry products. In developing countries, Western fast food chains will play a major role for the popularity and growth of processed poultry meat.

Ethnic or exotic flavours and tastes will still play a major role in any new food product development as more and more people are travelling to different parts of the world and being exposed to various tastes and flavours. This will reflect strongly in many of the further-processed poultry products. Another area that will see an increased activity is 'meal ingredients' or 'culinary aids' which the consumer uses to create the main meal. There are many people who want to prepare at least part of their own meal. However, they do not have the time or culinary skills to prepare the meat part of the meal.

Poultry meat will play an important role in the development of 'functional' or 'health' foods. Although vegetarianism is becoming popular, it is hard to imagine that meat will disappear completely. Many people who are interested in the 'health food' life style are also interested in having meat in moderate quantities. However, they like to see that this meat is low in fat and is not associated with any health problems. Poultry meat has already created this impression by being low in fat and white in colour.

Lastly, there will be some new developments in microwaveable products, especially coated, fried and baked or roasted poultry products. The main reason for the failure of these products has been the lack of crispiness or surface browning. However, recent advances in susceptor technology and innovations in packaging seem to solve these problems to a certain extent. This trend is already reflected by the recent introduction of microwaveable chicken pies that are packed in a special microwaveable paper-board tray with susceptor coating. Hopefully, it will not be too long before we see a poultry product that could be perfectly grilled or roasted in a microwave oven.

PART V
Abstracts

ABSTRACT
Retail requirements of meat

J.C. Hall
John Rannoch Ltd, Haughley Park, Stowmarket, Suffolk IP14 3JZ, UK

This paper is my interpretation of how I feel the British retailer is responding to changing consumer views on meat and the processing of poultry to prepare whole birds, portions and added-value products.

Although producers are all too well aware of the requirement to produce to higher standards of housing, husbandry and hygiene, they are also continuing to operate in a highly geared and very competitive market where value is a most critical factor. However, for the processor who is keen to develop a partnership with the major retailers, there is a chance to grasp and promote the future of British poultry meat retailing and use processing technology to upgrade the quality and uniformity of the poultry meat available to consumers.

In 1976, when the first EEC legislation came into force and the UK industry was required to upgrade its hygiene standards, there was concern as to the cost and doubt about any benefits. However, the result was that the poultry industry was then able to promote its upgraded processing facilities with considerable effect, one major benefit being the extension of keeping quality. The introduction of robotic carousel machines enabled processors to perform repetitive functions to good standards, allowed the labour to be used more usefully on added-value product or saved the cost totally.

The results are: poultry meat sold to consumers at prices which have remained virtually unchanged for 30 years; poultry meat becoming the base raw material for a massive spectrum of new added-value products. These products may be manufactured either by the poultry industry or by other food processors who, having exceeded the market for red meat and pork four years ago, will buy-in industry expertise and product knowing it is the number one meat choice of the consumer.

We have an educated and questioning consumer base. The epitaph of the problems in the beef industry will be the doubt in the consumer's mind to take comment at face value. We will now need to prove to all consumer bodies that the product is both safe, nutritious and meets the expectations of a consumer who is far better travelled and more sophisticated than even ten years ago.

Processing accuracy and repeatability will take a front seat and we must analyse and assess what actions are needed at all stages of the bird life and treatment after slaughter, to ensure the meat is to a high and consistent standard in terms of flavour, succulence and texture. Product life has moved from a chill life of five days, to ten or twelve days. At the same time the products must deliver uniform eating quality at all stages in the product life.

The processing requirements of the retailer to maintain and improve the product presentation has moved on a great deal and there are many aspects to be considered from live bird rearing and handling to upgraded tenderness and succulence in a chicken Tikka meal.

ABSTRACT

From meat inspection to consumer protection: a long way to go

J.H.G. Goebbels

Veterinary Health Inspectorate, Ministry of Health, P.O. Box 5406 NL-2280 HK, Rijswijk, The Netherlands

Meat inspection has not changed fundamentally in the last 50 years. It is still based on an organoleptic inspection of each individual animal. On the other hand the husbandry of animals, the meat industry and eating habits have been changed and therefore meat inspection cannot be considered any more as the appropriate way to protect consumers. This is supported by facts; in the Netherlands there are 700,000 cases of gastroenteritis each year caused by food of animal origin (mainly poultry products) and this costs 300 million guilders. Therefore, it is absolutely necessary that a new approach to consumer protection is found.

Governments should institute a food safety policy. By using risk assessment, risk management and risk communication, food safety policy can be translated into Food Safety Objectives (FSOs). The FSOs are the appropriate level of protection of consumers that a government considers necessary and achievable, and that any food operator should be made accountable for achieving.

Governments must establish FSOs. The FSOs can be, for example, pathogen reduction, zero tolerance or obligations for processing (F_o value in the canning industry). The government will only control, by several means, whether the FSO is achieved and approves the systems used by the industry. The industry is free to choose the systems which will be used to meet the FSO. This is a continuous process and not static as is present meat inspection.

Meat inspection will be just one of the tools (systems) which can be used just like any other systems, e.g. Hazard Analysis Critical Control Point (HACCP), GMP, etc. Meat inspection must never be counterproductive to the FSO. This means that handling in meat inspection must not cause contamination, which would be worse than the benefit of the detection of the abnormality. The role of HACCP will change from a more descriptive system to a system which will help to achieve FSOs. The goal of using HACCP must be to meet the FSO and then HACCP will be a real tool to protect the consumer. The outcome is the FSO and the tools to achieve it are the integrated quality systems.

© CAB *International* 1999.
Poultry Meat Science (eds R.I. Richardson and G.C. Mead)

A system based on FSO has great advantages.

1. Food Safety is no longer vague but clearly defined in the FSO.
2. Consumers, Government and Industry must work together;

- consumers must accept that zero risk does not exist;
- government must take responsibility by establishing the FSO;
- industry has the responsibility of achieving the FSO.

3. FSO makes a judgement easier about the equivalence of the level of consumer protection. It is transparent and based on science. The systems which are used in different countries to achieve the FSO can be different but the outcome must be the same.
4. The role of meat inspection will not be as dominant as it used to be. If the FSO is to reduce salmonella, meat inspection will probably be counter-productive.
5. Food industry safety assurances will be more in line with other industries, e.g. the car industry.
6. It will be a clearly defined responsibility of government and industry.
7. Food safety based on FSO is transparent and therefore more reliable for the consumer.

The move from the old meat inspection system to an integrated control system of the whole production chain, which is based on FSO, will not be an easy one. Nevertheless, we must go that way because, at the moment, safe food means nothing to the consumer. If we wait any longer to establish a new system, which protects the consumer better, then the present meat inspection will lose all credibility.

PART VI
Poster abstracts

POSTER ABSTRACT
Effect of broiler housing system on feeding and drinking behaviour

P.D. Fortomaris, A.S. Tserveni-Gousi and A.L. Yannakopoulos

Department of Animal Production, Veterinary School, Aristotle University, 54006 Thessaloniki, Greece

It is well known that designers of poultry facilities can benefit from a knowledge of poultry behaviour. Feeding and drinking behaviour of poultry, mostly physiological behaviour activities, may be modified by the housing system. Sykes (1983) observed that broilers may be considered to be more 'nibbler' than 'meal-eaters'. To analyse the behavioural changes we compared the feeding and drinking behaviour of broilers housed in different systems.

The frequency and duration of water and feed consumption was observed in Cobb broilers housed in cages and deep litter in stocking densities of 370 and 665 cm² per bird, respectively. Feeding and drinking space were similar between the two housing systems. The birds were observed visually at 28, 35 and 42 days of age, using the Focal Animal Sampling and All Occurrences methods (Lehner, 1992). Eight birds were observed for 30 min each per system. Identification was made by using different colours and care was taken to eliminate the disturbance of birds by the presence of the observers.

The results (Table 1) show that the housing system affected the duration and frequency of their feeding and drinking activities.

Broilers in cages performed 49.3% and 60.7% less feeding and drinking activities compared to broilers on the floor. The feeding and drinking frequency was also less in caged broilers than those on the floor (26.3% and 33.8%, respectively). The results support the conclusion that drinking activities are generally associated with feeding ones and that they are affected by the housing system.

Table 1. Effect of housing system on feeding and drinking behaviour of broilers (mean values/system).

	Feeding		Drinking	
System	Duration (min)	Frequency	Duration (min)	Frequency
Cages	0.77	1.33	4.62	1.92
Floor	1.96	2.01	9.11	2.59

© CAB *International* 1999.
Poultry Meat Science (eds R.I. Richardson and G.C. Mead)

REFERENCES

Lehner, P.N. (1992) Sampling methods in behaviour research. *Poultry Science* 71, 643–649.

Sykes, A.H. (1983) Food intake and its control. In: *Physiology and Biochemistry of the Domestic Fowl*, Vol.4, Academic Press, London, pp. 1–27.

POSTER ABSTRACT

The relative effects of concussion and electrical stunning on meat quality in broilers

E.Ö. Göksoy, I. Parkman, J. McKinstry, L.J. Wilkins and M.H. Anil

Division of Food Animal Science, School of Veterinary Science, University of Bristol, Langford, Bristol BS40 5DU, UK

Electrical stunning of poultry has long been held by the industry as a major cause of external downgrading and quality defects. An experiment was designed to compare the effects of electrical waterbath stunning and non-penetrative concussive stunning on a range of quality parameters. A total of 165 birds were assigned to one of four stunning treatments: (i) electrical, 80 mA, 50 Hz, AC, waterbath stunning which did not induce cardiac arrest; (ii) electrical, 80 mA, 50 Hz, AC, waterbath stunning which did induce cardiac arrest; (iii) non-penetrative concussive stunning with restraint; (iv) non-penetrative concussive stunning without restraint. Birds stunned electrically had a higher incidence of broken scapulas, coracoids, furculums and haemorrhages associated with them than concussion-stunned birds. They were also found to have a higher incidence of haemorrhages not associated with a broken bone. Both concussion stunned treatments had a higher incidence of red wing tips and shoulder haemorrhages. When pH was measured at 10 min post-mortem concussively stunned birds had a significantly ($P < 0.005$) lower pH than those stunned electrically. Electrically stunned non-cardiac arrested birds had a significantly ($P < 0.005$) faster rate of blood loss. Meat harvested from concussion stunned birds (3 h post-mortem) was found to be significantly more tender ($P < 0.005$) than that from birds stunned electrically. These preliminary results indicate that mechanical stunning has potential benefits for early portioning and reduced defects than conventional electrical stunning.

POSTER ABSTRACT
A novel stunning system for the slaughter of poultry

L. Hewitt
Division of Food Animal Science, School of Veterinary Science, University of Bristol, Langford, Bristol BS40 5DU, UK

Neck dislocation is used for about 80% of birds killed on-farm. Gregory and Wotton (1990) demonstrated that this method may not concuss chickens, and thus induce immediate unconsciousness, as required by UK legislation. Decapitation of poultry is also permitted under current legislation as it is believed to cause an immediate loss of consciousness. In the AVMA guidelines (1978) it states that decapitation is not an acceptable way of euthanizing laboratory rodents. This was supported by more recent research by N.G. Gregory and S.B. Wotton (unpublished data) who found that, in chickens, brain activity continued for as long as 30 s after severance of the head. This indicates that alternative stunning systems are required for the slaughter of poultry on-farm. Percussive stunning systems offer an alternative which, when operated correctly, result in a stun/kill.

A prototype gun has been developed to deliver a percussive blow to the head of broilers. The gun has been adapted from a pneumatically powered nail gun by the addition of a barrel and plastic percussive head. One hundred broilers (live weight 1.5–3.5 kg) were randomly allocated to five treatment groups. The ability of the gun to produce a concussed state was examined at different air pressures and, consequently, velocities. Birds were shackled and restrained by lightly holding the comb or the beak and the muzzle of the gun was applied to the back of the head and fired. Welfare assessment involved observation of the signs of an effective stun and signs of recovery.

All the birds showed signs of an effective stun and 83% of the birds were killed by the treatment. The remaining birds showed signs of recovery, therefore it is essential that birds are killed immediately poststun. Air pressures >120 psi resulted in the death of all the birds.

Further investigations, using broilers, chickens and turkeys, need to be carried out to determine the effects of air pressure, velocity and bolt-head design.

REFERENCES

AVMA Panel on Euthanasia (1986) *Journal of the American Veterinary Medical Association* 188, 252.

Gregory, N.G. and Wotton, S.B. (1990) Comparison of neck dislocation and percussion of the head on visual evoked responses in the chicken's brain. *Veterinary Record* 126, 570.

POSTER ABSTRACT

Effect of current frequency during water bath stunning on physical recovery and on the kinetic of bleed out in turkey

M. Mouchoniere[1], V. Sante[1], G. Le Pottier[1] and X. Fernandez[2]

[1]CIDEF, 11, rue Plaisance, 35310 Mordelles, France; [2]INRA - Meat Research Centre, Theix, F-63122 Saint-Genes Champanelle, France

Two experiments were carried out to evaluate the influence of the frequency of an AC constant current (150 mA) stunning (4 s) on the physical recovery of turkey hens and toms and on the rate and extent of blood loss.

Physical recovery of 70 hens and 78 toms was estimated after stunning at one of five different frequencies. The incidence of cardiac arrest after stunning at 50, 300, 480, 550 and 600 Hz was respectively 100, 60, 30, 30 and 0%, in hens and 53, 38, 0, 0 and 0%, in toms. In hens, time to return of corneal reflex and neck tension and the onset of wing flapping decreased as frequency increased from 300 to 600 Hz: from 19.0 to 6.7 s, 112.7 to 61.5 s and 10.2 s to 7.0 s, respectively. Contrary to hens, about half the toms stunned at 50 Hz did not show cardiac arrest. In these animals, recovery was significantly longer than at the four other frequencies.

A total of 50 hens and 53 toms were bled out by severing one carotid artery 10 s after stunning at one of four different frequencies (50, 300, 480 and 600 Hz). The rate and extent of blood loss within 3 min was evaluated. Within the first 20 s, the extent of blood loss, relative to liveweight, increased as stunning frequency increased: from 1.1 to 1.9% in hens and from 1.2 to 1.8% in toms. At 480 and 600 Hz, the maximum blood loss was obtained after 100 s in hens and 140 s in toms, whereas at 50 and 300 Hz, it increased up to 180 s. Large differences in the rate and extent of blood loss were observed within turkeys stunned at 50 or 300 Hz, according to the occurrence of cardiac arrest; cardiac activity was associated with significantly higher rate and extent of blood loss in both sexes.

Overall, the work suggests that the duration of unconsciousness decreases as stunning frequency increases. Additional neurophysiological experiments recording EEG and evoked potentials are currently being carried out to confirm these results.

POSTER ABSTRACT

Surface heating patterns after microwave decontamination of chicken carcasses

E. Göksoy and C. James

Food Refrigeration and Process Engineering Research Centre, University of Bristol, Langford, Bristol BS40 5DU, UK

Bacteria are predominantly found on the surface of a poultry carcass. Studies have shown that rapid surface heating has the potential to decontaminate without surface cooking. Three published studies have claimed that microwave heating can successfully reduce the bacterial load on chicken carcasses and pieces without cooking, but these studies did not address the problems of reproducibility and uneven heating ('hot and cold spots') reported by many other studies. Such uneven heating would make adequate decontamination without cooking difficult.

Experiments were carried out to measure the rate and pattern of heating of poultry carcasses in a microwave oven by infrared non-contact thermometry. Overwrapped, chilled ($5 \pm 1°C$) whole chicken carcasses, *ca.* 2 kg, were heated for 3 min at full power in a domestic microwave oven (Sharp Inverter 1000). After heating, thermal image photographs were taken from different positions using an Agema IR camera in order to determine the final surface temperature pattern over the whole of the carcass.

The results show large temperature differences between different areas of the surface of the carcass. The temperature of the surface of wings, the legs and the vent area reached 95°C after 3 min heating. However, the upper back area only reached 25°C and breast area 50–60°C.

Accepting that there is no athermal effect on bacteria, these results contest the claims of previous studies, since in order to avoid cooking any areas, other surfaces are prevented from attaining temperatures capable of destroying bacteria. Further unpublished experiments have shown no evidence of any athermal antimicrobial action of microwaves. Given these findings, microwaves are unlikely to be successfully used to decontaminate whole chicken carcasses.

POSTER ABSTRACT

The effect of short heating times at high temperatures on the surface appearance of chicken flesh and skin

E. Göksoy and C. James

Food Refrigeration and Process Engineering Research Centre, University of Bristol, Langford, Bristol BS40 5DU, UK

The main drawback to heat-based (hot water or steam) methods of poultry decontamination is that they can cause partial cooking, i.e. denaturation of the muscle proteins. However, since more heat is required to denature protein than to destroy bacterial cells, carefully controlled rapid heating and cooling has the potential to destroy bacteria without surface cooking. The design of such systems requires information on the rate of bacterial death and the rate of change of surface appearance with temperature. Although data are available on the death kinetics of pathogenic bacteria, there are few on the relationship between surface temperature and the appearance of poultry tissues.

A controlled series of experiments was carried out using instrumental colour measurements and photographic methods to investigate the relationship between meat surface temperature and appearance changes. Small samples of skin-on chicken breast were vacuum packed and dipped into a hot water bath at a range of temperatures (100, 90, 80, 70, 60 and $50 \pm 1°C$). After immersion for a set period of time, samples were immediately cooled in a water bath running at $5 \pm 1°C$. Final appearance was assessed visually, and instrumentally using a Minolta Chroma Meter.

Preliminary results show that poultry tissues can be immersed in water at temperatures of 100, 90, 80, 70, 60 and $50 \pm 1°C$ for 1, 2, 6, 9, 60 and 120 s, respectively, without causing irreversible appearance changes. Temperatures of 45 and 30°C caused no significant appearance changes, irrespective of how long the poultry tissues were treated.

Noticeable changes were found between the time/temperature relationship for skin and those for exposed muscle. At temperatures of 70°C and above, changes occurred to the skin before the muscle. At lower temperatures initial changes were apparent in both the muscle and skin.

Preliminary colour measurements show that instrumentally it is difficult to pick up the slight changes in appearance that cause samples to be deemed unacceptable through visual assessment. Changes in the lightness (L) values of muscle appear the most useful. However, since changes at temperatures greater than 70°C are more apparent in the skin and, due mainly to a change in visual texture, instrumental measurements are less useful in assessing appearance changes after treatment at temperatures of ≥70°C.

POSTER ABSTRACT
Organoleptic properties of irradiated chicken

I.F. Kiss
University of Horticulture and Food Science, Budapest, Hungary

Irradiation is a very effective technique for reducing the microbiological contamination of foods. Relatively low doses, 2–4 kGy, reduce the viable cell count of chicken at chill and/or freezing temperatures by 2–3 log cycles. The main spoilage and pathogenic microorganisms are very sensitive to irradiation. Therefore, the shelf-life of the product at chill temperatures increases two–threefold and the microbial safety of frozen product can also be improved.

Chemical changes of irradiated foods might cause some organoleptic changes. This effect depends on the irradiated dose, conditions, temperature, type of foods, chemical composition, moisture content, etc.

In our experiments, chicken carcasses were packed in polyethylene and Saran foils, respectively, and irradiated 2, 3, 4 or 5 kGy with cobalt-60 and stored at 4–8°C, or –18°C. For organoleptic tests scoring, ranking methods with 10 panellists were carried out with various prepared chicken dishes, i.e. soup, cooked and fried meat. Assessment was made over 1–58 weeks.

The results of sensory evaluations proved that irradiation up to 2 kGy in the fresh state and up to 4 kGy in the frozen state had no effect on the hedonic value of dishes made by different culinary methods. No significant differences were found in sensoric properties at the 95% probability level between dishes made of irradiated and untreated samples. Though some changes in the flavour of the soup and cooked meat made of poultry irradiated with 4 kGy was noted at the beginning, this difference disappeared during storage. The quality scores for samples packed in Saran foil were little higher, but this type of difference was neither characteristic nor statistically significant.

POSTER ABSTRACT

Natural antioxidants in feed: effects on quality and storage stability of poultry meats

C. Jensen, L. Skibsted and G. Bertelsen

Department of Dairy and Food, Royal Veterinary and Agricultural University, Frederiksberg C, Denmark

Oxidative changes are the major non-microbial cause of deterioration of meats, as products of autoxidation of unsaturated fatty acids affect wholesomeness and nutritive values. Heat-treated meat products are especially susceptible to lipid oxidation, resulting in a rapidly developing off-flavour denoted warmed-over flavour (WOF), caused by oxidation of the membrane phospholipids. Membrane lipids are protected against oxidation by a number of naturally occurring antioxidants. A strategy to improve the quality of precooked poultry meat products is to supplement antioxidants in the feed to increase the tissue level and increase the oxidative stability of poultry meat and meat products.

A number of chicken feeding experiments were conducted using different combinations of antioxidants. A number of products were made and stability measured during storage. These and several other studies have shown that elevated dietary α-tocopherol levels in feed increase tissue concentration, resulting in increased oxidative stability of poultry meats. The level of α-tocopherol in the tissue, however, also depends on the quality of the lipid fractions of the feed. A diet containing oxidized oil, compared to a diet containing fresh oil, results in a lower concentration of α-tocopherol in the tissue, as a result of oxidation of the natural content of α-tocopherol in the oil of the feed. Supplementation with ascorbic acid does not seem to have an effect on the oxidative stability of either raw poultry meat or cooked meat.

Supplementation with carotenoids has in some studies been found to increase the oxidative stability of meats. However, in our experiments a higher level of retinol, β-carotene or canthaxanthin in the feed did not affect the oxidative stability of the meats. The latter is expected to be a result of sufficient levels of α-tocopherol in the diets. Thus, supplementation with α-tocopherol is a simple approach to ensure optimum storage stability of poultry meats.

POSTER ABSTRACT

Sensory descriptive profiles of deboned poultry classified by shear values of two devices

B.G. Lyon and C.E. Lyon

USDA, Agricultural Research Service, Richard B. Russell Agricultural Research Centre, P.O. Box 5677, Athens, Georgia 30604-5677, USA

Innovative techniques, such as pulsed electric stimulation, wing restraints or tensioning, postchill flattening or extended holding of the deboned breasts and various combinations, have been devised to minimize post-mortem ageing. However, texture (tenderness) of the meat may be compromised. Processors need reliable, rapid and economical ways to measure texture to determine efficacy of new processing techniques. Instrumental devices, such as the Warner-Bratzler and the Allo-Kramer, measure force to shear of muscle fibres and these correlate statistically with sensory texture. However, correlations often oversimplify texture measurements. Instruments do not consider juiciness, other moisture-related characteristics or changes in meat as it is chewed.

Previous studies in our laboratory reported shear values from four devices that correlated with consumer sensory tenderness ('very tough' to 'very tender') for broiler breast meat. These shear value 'benchmarks' allowed commercial processors to attach a meaning of relative tenderness to instrumental shear values of cooked breast meat. The objective of this study was to determine the sensory descriptive texture profiles of cooked chicken breast fillets according to their deboning treatment (2, 6, and 24 h post-mortem) and consumer tenderness classification based on shear values from two commonly used devices (Warner-Bratzler and Allo-Kramer blades). Trained descriptive sensory panels identified and quantified specific texture attributes.

Sensory texture attributes were separated by variable cluster analysis into five groups representing mechanical, moisture and chewdown characteristics. Warner-Bratzler and Allo-Kramer shear values indicated differences due to deboning time and correlated highly ($r \geq 0.90$) with mechanical and chewdown sensory characteristics. However, texture profiles of samples in shear value ranges corresponding to consumer 'tender—tough' categories showed that texture remained differentiated by deboning times. Particle size, bolus and wetness characteristics interacted with minor attributes of saliva, ease of swallow and mouth coating to contribute to sensory perceptions and differentiation of texture.

Index

Note: page numbers in *italics* refer to figures and tables